Key Clinical Topics in

Paediatric Surgery

Max Pachl BSc MB ChB MRCS
Specialist Registrar in Paediatric Surgery
Birmingham Children's Hospital NHS Foundation Trust
Birmingham, UK

Michael N de la Hunt MS FRCS
Consultant Paediatric Surgeon
Royal Victoria Infirmary
Newcastle-upon-Tyne Hospitals NHS Trust
Newcastle-upon-Tyne, UK

Girish Jawaheer MBChB MD FRCS (Eng) FRCS (Paed)
Consultant Paediatric Surgeon
Birmingham Children's Hospital NHS Foundation Trust
Honorary Senior Lecturer, University of Birmingham
Specialty Tutor for Paediatric Surgery
Royal College of Surgeons of England
Paediatric Surgery Specialist Advisory Committee (SAC) Member
Intercollegiate Specialty Board Examiner for Paediatric Surgery
Birmingham, UK

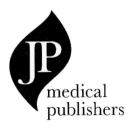

JP
medical
publishers

London • St Louis • Panama City • New Delhi

© 2014 JP Medical Ltd.
Published by JP Medical Ltd,
83 Victoria Street, London, SW1H 0HW, UK
Tel: +44 (0)20 3170 8910   Fax: +44 (0)20 3008 6180
Email: info@jpmedpub.com   Web: www.jpmedpub.com

ISBN: 978-1-907816-58-1

British Library Cataloguing in Publication Data
A catalogue record for this book is available from the British Library

Library of Congress Cataloging in Publication Data
A catalog record for this book is available from the Library of Congress

JP Medical Ltd is a subsidiary of Jaypee Brothers Medical Publishers (P) Ltd, New Delhi, India

Publisher: Richard Furn
Development Editor: Thomas Fletcher
Design: Designers Collective Ltd

Indexed, copy-edited, typeset, printed and bound in India.

Preface

This new book aims to fill a longstanding void. Its principal purpose is to provide senior trainees in the UK with a concise revision aid for the Intercollegiate Specialty Board Examination in Paediatric Surgery. In addition, its international authorship ensures that candidates attempting Paediatric Surgery Board Examinations in their respective countries will also derive benefit.

The topics have been set out in alphabetical order. The start of each topic provides the reader with clearly defined learning outcomes. The broad content then reflects the generality of paediatric surgery. It has been our aim to focus on the principles of management rather than minutiae and, as such, this book will also appeal to more junior surgeons. It is important to emphasise the beneficial effect of a multidisciplinary team approach upon clinical outcomes and this resonates throughout the text. Specific and general information about operative approaches has been incorporated where possible. The experienced paediatric surgeon requires a sound knowledge not only of paediatric surgery but also of closely allied topics such as anaesthesia, medicine, orthopaedics, ophthalmology, otorhinolaryngology, cardiac surgery, neurosurgery, and plastic surgery, all of which have been included.

Max Pachl
Michael N de la Hunt
Girish Jawaheer
August 2013

Contents

Contributors

Edgardo Abelardo MD MRCS DOHNS
Topic 101
Tracheal Fellow, Department of Cardiothoracic
Surgery, Great Ormond Street Hospital for
Children NHS Trust, London, UK

Aanand N Acharya FRCS (ORL-HNS)
Topic 76
Specialist Registrar, Department of ENT,
Birmingham Children's Hospital NHS
Foundation Trust, Birmingham, UK

Oluwasegun Akilapa MRCS PG Dip. (Sports
and Exercise Medicine)
Topic 75
Paediatric Orthopaedic Clinical Fellow,
Birmingham Children's Hospital NHS
Foundation Trust, Birmingham, UK

Jane Armstrong MBChB MRCPCH
Topic 14
Consultant Community Paediatrician,
Designated Doctor for Safeguarding,
Birmingham Community Healthcare NHS Trust,
Birmingham UK

G Suren Arul MD FRCS (Paeds)
Topics 12, 42 & 65
Chairman, UK Children's Cancer and
Leukaemia Group (CCLG) Surgeons Group;
Surgical Representative, National Paediatric
Germ Cell Working Group;
Consultant General Surgeon with Paediatric
Surgical Oncology, Birmingham Children's
Hospital NHS Foundation Trust,
Birmingham, UK

Navoda Atapattu MD MRCPCH
Topic 31
Senior Registrar in Paediatric Endocrinology,
Lady Ridgewell Hospital, Columbo, Sri Lanka

Christopher E Bache FRCS (Orth)
Topic 75
Consultant Orthopaedic Surgeon, Birmingham
Children's Hospital NHS Foundation Trust,
Birmingham UK

Sami Bansal MD
Topic 63
Clinical MIS Fellow, The Rocky Mountain
Hospital for Children, Denver, USA

David J Barron MD FRCP FRCS (CTh)
Topic 71
Consultant Paediatric Cardiac Surgeon,
Birmingham Children's Hospital NHS
Foundation Trust, Birmingham, UK

Alison Bedford-Russell BSc (Hons) MBBS
FRCPCH MD
Topic 85
Clinical Director, West Midlands Strategic
Clinical Network for Maternity and Children;
Neonatal Lead for Surgery liaison with
Birmingham Children's Hospital NHS
Foundation Trust;
Consultant Neonatologist, Birmingham
Women's NHS Foundation Trust,
Birmingham, UK

James Bennett MBBS FRCA
Topic 12
Consultant Anaesthetist, Birmingham
Children's Hospital NHS Foundation Trust,
Birmingham, UK

Hugh S Bishop MBChB MRCPCH
Topic 44
Consultant Paediatric Oncologist, Royal
Aberdeen Children's Hospital,
Aberdeen, UK

Peter Bromley MBBS FRCA
Topic 12
Consultant Paediatric Anaesthetist,
Birmingham Children's Hospital NHS
Foundation Trust, Birmingham, UK

Abraham Cherian MBBS MS DNB FRCS FRCS
(Paed Surg)
Topic 6
Consultant Paediatric Urologist, Great Ormond
Street Hospital for Children NHS Foundation
Trust, London, UK

Alexander Cho MBBS BSc (Hons) MRCS (Eng)
Topic 39
Specialist Registrar in Paediatric Surgery,
Norfolk and Norwich University Hospital,
Norwich, UK

Simon Clarke FRCS (Paed Surg)
Topic 58
Consultant Paediatric Surgeon, Chelsea and
Westminster NHS Foundation Trust; Honorary
Senior Lecturer, Imperial College London,
London, UK

Stewart Cleeve MBChB FRCS (Paed)
Topic 49
Locum Consultant Paediatric Surgeon, St
George's NHS Healthcare Trust, London, UK

Ed Copley MBBS FRCA
Topic 12
Specialist Registrar in Anaesthesia,
Birmingham Children's Hospital NHS
Foundation Trust, Birmingham, UK

Peter Cuckow MBBS FRCS FRCS (Paed Surg)
Topic 34
Consultant Paediatric Urology Surgeon,
University College Hospital NHS Foundation
Trust, Great Ormond Street Children's Hospital
NHS Foundation Trust, London, UK

Joe Curry MBBS FRCS (Eng) FRCS (Paed Surg)
Topics 40 & 55
Consultant Neonatal and Paediatric Surgeon,
University College Hospital NHS Foundation
Trust, Great Ormond Street Children's Hospital
NHS Foundation Trust, London, UK

Haitham Dagash MBBS MRCS (Ed)
Topic 87
Specialist Registrar in Paediatric Surgery,
Leicester Royal Infirmary, Leicester, UK

Dipankar R Dass MRCS (Eng) MBChB
Topic 7
Paediatric Surgical Registrar, Sheffield Children's
Hospital, Sheffield, UK

Mark Davenport ChM FRCS (Paeds)
Topics 9 & 15
Professor of Paediatric Surgery, Kings College
Hospital, London, UK

Carl Davis MB MCh FRCSI FRCS (Paeds)
Topic 20
Consultant Paediatric and Neonatal Surgeon,
Royal Hospital for Sick Children; Barclay
Lecturer, University of Glasgow,
Glasgow, UK

Michael N de la Hunt MS FRCS
Topics 10, 33 & 83
Consultant Paediatric Surgeon, Royal Victoria
Infirmary, Newcastle-upon-Tyne Hospitals NHS
Trust, Newcastle, UK

Chamaleeni de Silva MBChB BMedSc MRCPCH
Topic 100
Paediatric Specialty Registrar, Birmingham
Heartlands Hospital, Birmingham, UK

Ashish P Desai FRCS (Paed) FEBPS MCh (Paed
Surg) MS
Topic 70
Consultant Paediatric Surgeon, King's College
Hospital, London, UK

Renuka P Dias MBBS MRCPCH PhD
Topic 27
Academic Clinical Lecturer in Paediatric
Endocrinology and Diabetes, Centre for Rare
Diseases and Personalised Medicine, University
of Birmingham; Department of Endocrinology,
Birmingham Children's Hospital NHS
Foundation Trust, Birmingham, UK

Alistair Dick MD BCh BAO FRCS (Paed Surg)
Topics 1 & 84
Consultant Paediatric Surgeon, Belfast Hospital
and Social Care Trust, Belfast, UK

Belinda Hsi Dickie MDPhD
Topics 35, 48 & 56
Assistant Professor of Surgery, Cincinnati
Children's Hospital Medical Center,
Cincinnati, USA

Martin J Elliott MD FRCS
Topic 101
Professor of Cardiothoracic Surgery, University
College London; Director, National Service for
Severe Tracheal Disease in Children; Co-Medical
Director, The Great Ormond Street Hospital for
Children NHS Foundation Trust,
London, UK

Marianne D Elloy MBBS FRCS (ORL-HNS)
Topic 91
Paediatric ENT Consultant, University Hospitals
of Leicester NHS Trust, Leicester, UK

Bala Eradi FRCS (Paed)
Topics 1 & 98
Consultant Paediatric Surgeon, Leicester Royal
Infirmary, Leicester, UK

Ross Fisher MBChB MPhil MSc FRCS (Paed
Surg)
Topics 1 & 98
Consultant Paediatric Surgeon, Sheffield
Children's Hospital, Sheffield, UK

Oluwafikayo Fayeye MBChB BMedSc
(Neuroscience) MRCS (Eng)
Topic 46
Specialty Registrar in Neurosurgery,
Birmingham Children's Hospital NHS
Foundation Trust, Birmingham, UK

Prasad P Godbole MBBS FRCS FRCS(Paeds)
FEAPU
Topic 107
Consultant Paediatric Urologist, Sheffield
Children's NHS Foundation Trust, Honorary
Senior Lecturer, University of Sheffield,
Sheffield, UK

Philip J Hammond FRCSEd (Paed Surg)
Topic 37
Consultant Paediatric Surgeon, Royal Hospital
for Sick Children, Glasgow, UK

Fraser MJ Harban MBBS Dip IMC RCS(Ed) FRCA
Topic 69
Consultant Paediatric Anaesthetist,
Birmingham Children's Hospital NHS
Foundation Trust, Birmingham, UK

Benjamin EJ Hartley MBBS BSC FRCS
Topic 91
Consultant Paediatric Otolaryngologist,
Great Ormond Street Hospital for Children NHS
Foundation Trust, London, UK

Richard E Hill BSc (Hons) MBChB MRCS MSc
Topic 62
Specialist Registrar in Paediatric Surgery,
Queen's Medical Centre, Nottingham, UK

Rowena JI Hitchcock MB BCH MA MD FRCS
(Paed)
Topics 50, 51 & 105
Consultant Paediatric Urologist,
Oxford University Hospitals, Oxford, UK

Gareth P Hosie MB ChB FRCS (Paed)
Topic 81
Consultant Paediatric Surgeon, Royal Victoria
Infirmary, Newcastle-upon-Tyne, UK

Simon N Huddart MA MBBS FRCS FRCS (Paed)
Topics 19 & 86
Consultant Paediatric Surgeon, University
Hospital of Wales, Cardiff, UK

John M Hutson AO BSMD (Monash) MDDSc
(Melb) FRACS FAAP (Hon)
Topic 26
Chair of Paediatric Surgery, University of
Melbourne; Consultant Surgeon, Royal
Children's Hospital Melbourne; Honorary
Fellow, Surgical Research Group, Murdoch
Children's Research Institute,
Melbourne, Australia

Andrew M Ibrahim MD
Topic 52
General Surgery Resident, Case Western
Reserve University School of Medicine,
Cleveland, USA

Girish Jawaheer MBChB MD FRCS (Eng) FRCS
(Paed)
Topics 16 & 97
Consultant Paediatric Surgeon, Birmingham
Children's Hospital NHS Foundation Trust;
Honorary Senior Lecturer, University of
Birmingham; Specialty Tutor for Paediatric
Surgery, Royal College of Surgeons of England;
Paediatric Surgery Specialist Advisory
Committee (SAC) Member; Intercollegiate
Specialty Board Examiner for Paediatric Surgery,
Birmingham, UK

Andrea Jester FRCS MD
Topic 77
Consultant Plastic Surgeon Hand Surgeon,
Birmingham Children's Hospital NHS
Foundation Trust, Birmingham, UK

Ingo Jester FRCS (Eng)
Topics 92 & 102
Consultant Paediatric Surgeon, Birmingham
Children's Hospital NHS Foundation Trust,
Birmingham, UK

Timothy J Jones MD FRCS (CTh)
Topic 71
Consultant Paediatric Cardiac Surgeon,
Birmingham Children's Hospital NHS
Foundation Trust, Birmingham, UK

Arielle E Kanters BS BA
Topic 28
Case Western Reserve University, Cleveland,
USA

Larissa Kerecuk BSc MB BS (Lon) MRCPCH
FRCPCH
Topic 89
Consultant Paediatric Nephrologist,
Birmingham Children's Hospital NHS
Foundation Trust, Birmingham, UK

Charles Keys FRCS (Paed)
Topic 3
Consultant Paediatric Surgeon, Royal Hospital
for Sick Children, Edinburgh, UK

Jeremy Kirk MD FRCP FRCPCH
Topics 25, 27, 31, 43 & 100
Consultant Paediatric Endocrinologist (Honorary
Reader), Birmingham Children's Hospital NHS
Foundation Trust, Birmingham, UK

Victoria A Lane MBChB MRCS
Topics 18, 54 & 88
Paediatric Surgical Registrar, Leeds General
Infirmary, Leeds, UK

Nick Lansdale MB ChB MRCS (Eng)
Topic 32
Specialty Registrar in Paediatric Surgery, Royal
Manchester Children's Hospital,
Manchester, UK

Marc A Levitt MD
Topics 4, 5, 18, 35, 48 & 56
Director, Colorectal Center Cincinnati Children's
Hospital; Professor of Surgery, University of
Cincinnati, Cincinnati, USA

Richard M Lindley MBChB BMedSci MD FRCS (Paed Surg)
Topic 95
Consultant Paediatric Surgeon, Sheffield Children's NHS Trust, Sheffield, UK

Joana Lopes MB ChB MRCS
Topics 19 & 86
Specialty Trainee in Paediatric Surgery, University Hospital of Wales, Cardiff, UK

Georgina Malakounides MBBS MRCS (Eng)
Topic 66
Paediatric Surgery Specialist Registrar, The Great Ormond Street Hospital for Children NHS Foundation Trust, London, UK

Sean S Marven MB ChB FRCS (Paed)
Topics 7 & 41
Consultant Paediatric Surgeon, Sheffield Children's NHS Foundation Trust, Sheffield, UK

Majella Mc Cullagh MCh FRCS (Paeds)
Topic 72
Consultant Paediatric Surgeon, Royal Belfast Hospital for Sick Children, Belfast, UK

Janet McNally MBBCh FCS (SA) (Paed Surg)
Topic 21
Consultant Paediatric Surgeon, Bristol Royal Hospital for Children, Bristol, UK

Alastair JW Millar FRCS (Eng) FRACS (Paed Surg)
Topic 78
Charles F M Saint Professor of Paediatric Surgery, University of Cape Town and Red Cross War Memorial Children's Hospital, Cape Town, Republic of South Africa

Pankaj K Mishra MS MCh FRCS (Paed Surg)
Topic 61
Clinical Fellow, Department of Paediatric Surgery, Norfolk and Norwich University Hospital NHS Trust, Norwich, UK

Bruce Morland MBChB MRCP DM FRCPCH
Topic 47
Consultant and Honorary Reader in Paediatric Oncology, Birmingham Children's Hospital NHS Foundation Trust, Birmingham, UK

Rafeeq Muhammed MMBBS MD MRCPCH
Topic 92
Consultant Paediatric Gastroenterologist, Birmingham Children's Hospital NHS Foundation Trust, Birmingham, UK

Barry O'Donoghue MB BCh BAO DCH MRCPCH
Topic 25
Registrar in Paediatric Endocrinology, Birmingham Children's Hospital NHS Foundation Trust, Birmingham, UK

Channa Panagamuwa MMedED FRCS (Eng) ORL-H&N Surgery
Topic 76
Consultant Paediatric ENT Surgeon, Birmingham Children's Hospital NHS Foundation Trust, Birmingham, UK

Max Pachl BSc MB ChB MRCS
Topics 11, 17, 23, 36, 38, 60, 64, 68, 70, 79, 90, 94, 103, 104, 106, 108 & 109
Specialist Registrar in Paediatric Surgery, Birmingham Children's Hospital NHS Foundation Trust, Birmingham, UK

Manoj V Parulekar MS FRCS (Ophth)
Topic 74
Consultant Ophthalmologist, Birmingham Children's Hospital NHS Foundation Trust, Birmingham, UK

Yatin Patel MBBCh FRCS (Paed Surg)
Topic 13
Consultant Paediatric Surgeon, Royal Aberdeen Children's Hospital, Aberdeen, UK

Todd A Ponsky MD FACS
Topics 28 & 52
Associate Professor of Surgery and Pediatrics,
Akron Children's Hospital, Akron, USA

Mark Powis BSc (Hons) MBBS FRCS (Eng) FRCS
(Paed Surg)
Topics 57 & 112
Consultant Paediatric Surgeon, Leeds Teaching
Hospitals NHS Trust, Leeds, UK

Neil R Price BMedSc MBChB DCH FRACS
(Paed Surg)
Topics 29 & 111
Consultant Paediatric Surgeon and Urologist,
Starship Children's Health; Professional
Teaching Fellow, Faculty of Medical and Health
Sciences, University of Auckland, Auckland,
New Zealand

Clare M Rees MD MRCS MBChB
Topics 82 & 99
Specialty Registrar in Paediatric Surgery, Barts
Health NHS Trust; NHS Clinical Leadership
Fellow, NHS Leadership Academy,
London, UK

Giuseppe Retrosi MD
Topic 58
Clinical Fellow and Specialty Registrar in
Paediatric Surgery, Chelsea and Westminster
Hospital NHS Trust, London, UK

Andrew Robb MCh FRCSEd (Paeds) DipIMC
(RCSEd)
Topics 45 & 110
Paediatric Urology Fellow, Birmingham
Children's Hospital NHS Foundation Trust,
Birmingham, UK

Desiderio Rodrigues MBBS FRCS (SN)
Topics 46 & 73
Consultant Paediatric Neurosurgeon,
Birmingham Children's Hospital NHS
Foundation Trust, Birmingham, UK

Steven S Rothenberg MD FACS FAAP
Topic 63
Chief of Surgery, The Rocky Mountain Hospital
for Children, Denver; Clinical Professor of
Surgery, Columbia University College of
Physicians and Surgeons, New York, USA

Vrinda Saraff MBBS MRCPCH
Topic 43
Speciality Registrar in Paediatrics, Birmingham
Children's Hospital NHS Foundation Trust,
Birmingham, UK

Gregory J Shepherd BMBS BMedSci (Hon)
MRCS (Edin)
Topics 24 & 62
Specialty Registrar, Department of Paediatric
Surgery, Nottingham Children's Hospital,
Nottingham University Hospital NHS Trust,
Nottingham, UK

Michael Singh MBBS FRCS (Paed Surg)
Topics 30 & 53
Consultant Paediatric Surgeon, Birmingham
Children's Hospital NHS Foundation Trust,
Birmingham, UK

Giampiero Soccorso MBBS MRCS (Ed) MRCS
(Glasg)
Topic 41
Specialty Registrar in Paediatric Surgery,
Sheffield Children's NHS Foundation Trust,
Sheffield, UK

Henrik Steinbrecher BSc MBBS FRCS (Eng) MS
FRCS (Paeds)
Topics 59 & 80
Consultant Paediatric Urologist, University
Hospital Southampton NHS Trust,
Southampton, UK

Richard J Stewart MD FRCS FRCS (Paed)
Topics 24 & 62
Consultant Paediatric Surgeon, Queen's Medical
Centre, Nottingham University Hospitals NHS
Trust, Nottingham, UK

Ian D Sugarman MBChB FRCS (Paed)
Topics 18, 54 & 88
Consultant Paediatric Surgeon, Leeds Teaching
Hospital NHS Trust, Leeds, UK

Jonathan Sutcliffe MB ChB FRCS (Paed Surg) MD
Topics 4 & 5
Consultant Paediatric Surgeon, Leeds General
Infirmary, Leeds, UK

Thomas Tsang FRCS
Topics 39 & 61
Consultant Paediatric Surgeon, Norfolk and
Norwich University Hospital Trust,
Norwich, UK

Robert Wheeler MS FRCS LLB (Hons) LLM
Topics 22 & 96
Consultant Paediatric and Neonatal
Surgeon, Senior Lecturer in Clinical Law,
University Hospital Southampton NHS Trust,
Southampton, UK

David J Wilkinson MB ChB BMedSci (Hons)
MRCS (Eng)
Topic 93
Clinical Research Fellow and Specialty Registrar
in Paediatric Surgery, University of Liverpool,
Alder Hey Children's Hospital, Liverpool, UK

Ruth Wragg MBBS MRCS
Topic 21
Specialty Registrar, Department of Paediatric
Surgery, Bristol Royal Hospital for Children,
Bristol, UK

Iain E Yardley BM DPH FRCS (Paed Surg)
Topics 8 & 82
Specialist Registrar in Paediatric Surgery, Royal
Manchester Children's Hospital, Former Clinical
Advisor to WHO Patient Safety,
Birmingham, UK

Acknowledgements

Figure 2 was originally published in Tunstall R, Pocket Tutor Surface Anatomy, London: JP Medical, 2012. The photograph is reproduced courtesy of Sam Scott-Hunter.

Figure 22 is reproduced courtesy of Stephen Parker and was originally published in MRCS Applied Basic Science and Clinical Topics, London: JP Medical, 2012.

We are grateful to all the authors who kindly accepted the challenge of conveying to the reader the fundamentals of evidence-based medicine whilst remaining concise.

Thanks also go to our families, without whom this work would not have been possible, and to all the children, to whose care this book is dedicated.

We extend our gratitude to Richard Furn, Hannah Applin, Katrina Rimmer and Thomas Fletcher at JP Medical Publishers for all their help and support.

MP, MdlH, GJ

Abdominal trauma

Learning outcomes

- To appreciate the significant anatomical and physiological differences between children and adults
- To learn when to suspect and how to diagnose intra-abdominal injury
- To develop a pragmatic and tailored approach to imaging and treatment based on the above

Overview

Accidental injury is the leading cause of death among 10- to 19-year-olds and is a leading cause of disability. While prevention is the key, appropriate recognition and management of childhood injuries is also paramount.

Compared with adults, children have a compliant ribcage, which allows direct transmission of force to the thoracic and abdominal viscera. The diaphragm is relatively flat and the liver and spleen are comparatively large. In addition, the abdominal musculature is less developed and there is little fat or connective tissue to cushion the organs. The pelvis is shallow, such that the urinary bladder is an intra-abdominal organ in young children. The abdominal viscera are therefore poorly protected from blunt or penetrating trauma.

Children have good cardiac function, which is able to compensate well for hypovolaemia. While adults manifest hypotension after a 15% loss of blood volume, children can compensate for up to 40% blood loss. Hypotension in a child is an ominous sign.

Although children have a greater circulating blood volume per unit mass (70–80 mL/kg), the absolute volume is very small compared to an adult. Therefore, loss of a small amount of blood may be critically important. The body surface area to volume ratio is greater in children, allowing rapid heat loss and the onset of hypothermia.

Epidemiology and aetiology

More than 75% of trauma cases are caused by road traffic accidents, in which the child may be involved as a pedestrian or as a passenger. Risky sports also cause some of these injuries, especially in the older child or adolescent. The majority of injuries are blunt and in Europe, where use of firearms is controlled, penetrating injury during peacetime is rare. Males are involved two to three times more often than females. Thoracic and abdominal trauma occurs most often before the end of the first decade of life, when children have achieved a degree of autonomy.

Clinical features

Signs of abdominal injury are usually apparent on secondary survey, and these include abrasions and contusions on the abdominal wall, abdominal tenderness and distension. Especially in young children, distress leads to aerophagia and gastric distension. Placement of a nasogastric tube and aspiration of gastric content may assist clinical evaluation, especially if consciousness is impaired. The groin, external genitalia and perineum are carefully inspected. The anus is inspected at the time of assessment of the back by logrolling. There is insufficient published evidence to support the use of routine rectal examination in the assessment of paediatric trauma patients.

Splenic injury

The spleen is the most frequently injured abdominal organ in children. Injury to the spleen typically results from impact to the left upper abdomen or lower chest, and fractured lower ribs on the left side should raise strong suspicion. Left shoulder tip pain (Kehr's sign) as a result of diaphragmatic irritation by blood is often present.

Liver injury

The liver is the second most commonly injured abdominal organ. The right lobe is more frequently involved than the left lobe. Right shoulder tip pain (Kehr's sign) is a frequent accompaniment. Elevated transaminases are strongly suggestive of liver injury, as are fractured lower ribs on the right side.

Bowel injury

A frequent mechanism of intestinal injury is due to a lap belt or seat belt, usually because of inadequate fit between the child and the restraint. Patterned abrasions due to the restraint are often seen. Lumbar spine fractures, called Chance fractures, are detected in a number of children with lap belt injury. The children most at risk are those who are generally too big for a children's car seat but too small for adult belting systems.

In young children, absence of a plausible mechanism must raise suspicion of child abuse. These injuries often present late. A fall down stairs is not usually associated with bowel injury.

Pancreatic and duodenal injury

The classic mechanism causing this injury is the bicycle handlebar injury where the child is impaled in the epigastrium by the handlebar. This can lead to transection of the pancreas where it crosses over the lumbar spine or injury to the duodenum. Vehicular accidents and child abuse are other causes. A patterned abrasion in the epigastrium is common.

Renal injury

Microscopic haematuria following abdominal injury is very common and is of no consequence. Frank haematuria resulting from trivial injury may signify underlying renal anomaly, such as pelvi-ureteric junction obstruction or renal tumour.

Investigations

Blood is sent for full blood cell count, cross-matching, liver and renal function tests, amylase and lipase as a baseline and as indicators of liver, renal or pancreatic injury, though laboratory studies are seldom useful in the acute phase.

In the haemodynamically unstable child, abdominal ultrasound can be used to differentiate between intraperitoneal and extraperitoneal blood loss. It can also be used as an adjunct to serial abdominal examination when physical examination is not straightforward. Focused assessment with sonography in trauma (FAST) is used in some trauma centres, and its primary goal is to detect free fluid in Morrison's pouch, pelvis, perisplenic region and pericardium.

In the haemodynamically stable child, further abdominal imaging is not required if there is no suspicion of intra-abdominal injury based on the mode of injury and a reliable clinical examination or, even better, on serial abdominal examinations. In all other situations, intravenous contrast-enhanced computed tomography (CT) is the standard of care for the evaluation of the child with abdominal injury. It helps with the diagnosis and grading of solid organ and other associated injuries. CT detects 60–70% of pancreatic injuries. Fluid in the lesser sac is a useful marker. In addition, the radiologist may instil enteral contrast via the nasogastric tube. This may be useful to delineate duodenal injury. Frank haematuria should instigate prompt imaging by CT.

Treatment

Initial management follows the airway, breathing and circulation (ABC) of trauma resuscitation. Large-bore intravenous access is vital. Intraosseous infusion of fluid for resuscitation is life-saving when venous access proves difficult.

Splenic injury

Non-operative management without blood transfusion is now the standard of care. In one large series, > 95% of splenic injuries in children were managed in this way. Only 10–12% require blood transfusion, usually due to other injuries. Non-operative management requires significant expertise and is more successful in dedicated paediatric centres. Long-term results demonstrate that missed injuries are rare, as is delayed splenic rupture. Routine follow-up imaging studies are not required.

Operative management is indicated in the presence of haemodynamic instability and may merit splenectomy. Splenorrhaphy and partial splenectomy are spleen-conserving techniques.

The risk of overwhelming post splenectomy infection is the main reason for spleen conservation. Antibiotic prophylaxis with oral penicillin V and vaccination with polyvalent pneumococcal vaccine are essential in children who lose splenic function.

Liver injury

In children, 85–90% of liver injuries can be managed non-operatively, though a greater proportion will require blood transfusion. Other aspects of non-operative management are similar to the management of splenic injury. Bleeding into the biliary tree (haemobilia) and, very rarely, bile in the bloodstream (bilhaemia) are specific long-term complications.

In the presence of major haemorrhage, the vicious cycle of blood loss necessitating transfusion, leading to hypothermia and coagulopathy, is the real killer. Thus, operative management of liver injury is based on the 'damage control' philosophy. Tamponade of bleeding with abdominal packs, followed by a planned second look when hypothermia and coagulopathy have been corrected, is preferred over major hepatic resection.

Bowel injury

Operative management involves segmental resection with primary anastomosis. Mesenteric lacerations may lead to an ischaemic perforation or stricture. A stricture may present several weeks after the initial injury in the form of intestinal obstruction. Laparoscopy has diagnostic and therapeutic potential that must not be overlooked.

Pancreatic and duodenal injury

Pancreatic contusion is managed conservatively along the lines of pancreatitis. Spleen-preserving distal pancreatectomy in cases of ductal transection of the pancreatic body is associated with fewer complications than non-operative management. Treatment of major ductal injury involving the head of the pancreas is more controversial, though most authors support initial non-operative management, followed by drainage of resulting pseudocysts. Alternatively, some authors advocate transductal pancreatic stenting.

Formation of a pancreatic pseudocyst is the most common complication of non-operative management. Small pseudocysts may resolve with time while larger ones (> 5 cm) that persist for > 4–6 weeks require drainage. Internal drainage is standard, in the form of either cyst-gastrostomy or cyst-enterostomy into a Roux-en-Y limb.

Duodenal injury may be in the form of a haematoma or perforation. Haematomas may compromise the duodenal lumen. The majority can be managed non-operatively by nasogastric decompression and parenteral nutrition.

Duodenal perforations are often contained in the retroperitoneum and are difficult to diagnose even by CT. Operative management depends upon the degree of contamination and the extent of injury. Small fresh injuries can be dealt with by primary closure, omental patch and nasogastric drainage. Larger injuries in the presence of significant contamination may necessitate pyloric exclusion and gastrojejunostomy.

Renal injury

Renal injuries are managed non-operatively. The chance of renal salvage by urgent operation in cases of complete devascularisation is small as the warm ischaemia time of the kidney is very short.

Injury to the renal collecting system may result in formation of a urinoma. This is managed either by internal stenting (double-J ureteric stent) alone or in conjunction with percutaneous external drainage. Pelvi-ureteric junction obstruction is a long-term complication.

Extraperitoneal bleeding

Haemodynamic instability in the scenario of extraperitoneal bleeding, as can be seen secondary to pelvic fracture or renal pedicle injury, warrants the involvement of the interventional radiology team to diagnose the source of the blood loss and for potential embolisation.

Further reading

Gaines BA, Ford HR. Abdominal and pelvic trauma in children. Crit Care Med 2002; 30:S416–S423.

Hughes G. Children's injuries: a global problem. Emerg Med J 2009; 26:236.

Scaife ER, Rollins MD. Managing radiation risk in the evaluation of the pediatric trauma patient. Semin Pediatr Surg 2010; 19:252–256.

Thomas DFM, Duffy PG, Rickwood AMK. Essentials of paediatric urology. London: Informa Healthcare, 2008.

Related topics of interest

Achalasia

Learning outcomes

- To understand the pathophysiology of achalasia of the oesophagus
- To understand the clinical presentation and approaches to treatment of achalasia of the oesophagus in children

Overview

Achalasia of the oesophagus is classified as a functional disorder of the oesophagus leading to bolus obstruction in the distal oesophagus.

Epidemiology and pathology

The incidence in the population is 1 per 100,000, with only 2–5% occurring in the paediatric age group. The presence of coexisting structural anomalies is variable in children. Symptoms have been reported from as early as the 5th day of life to the teenage years. Various conditions have been associated with achalasia – Addison's disease, Alport's syndrome, alacrima/achalasia/adrenocorticotropic hormone deficiency syndrome, Binder's syndrome, hereditary dysautonomia of the nervous system, microcephaly and trisomy 21. Association with *Trypanosoma cruzi* (Chagas' disease) or other infective aetiologies has been reported.

Aetiology

Deficiencies in inhibitory neuropeptides have been frequently reported. Abnormal ganglion cell innervations and smooth muscle structure have been proposed but are not consistently observed in resected specimens. The proposed pathophysiology in achalasia is unopposed excitatory (cholinergic) neurotransmission due to the deficiencies of inhibitory neuropeptidases. This results in impaired peristalsis and a failure of relaxation of the distal portion of the oesophagus.

Clinical features

Most (90%) will have dysphagia, and vomiting or regurgitation (50%). Respiratory symptoms (20%), poor growth (20%) and retrosternal pain (20%) are also often found.

In younger children, the main symptoms are failure to thrive, regurgitation and repeated aspiration pneumonia. Ingestion of solid food will give rise to dysphagia and retrosternal pain in children who have attained competency in communicating their symptoms. Symptoms can be mistaken for gastro-oesophageal reflux.

Investigations

Upper gastrointestinal contrast study

This is the most universally used investigation in the diagnosis of oesophageal achalasia. The diagnostic features are dysmotility, aperistalsis or 'free fall' of the contrast in the oesophagus proximal to the diseased segment, the appearance of a 'rat tail' or 'beaking' and impaired oesophageal clearance. Other supportive features are a dilated oesophagus and epiphrenic diverticulae.

Upper gastrointestinal endoscopy

This is not diagnostic but may be of value in excluding luminal or intramural obstructions causing a pseudo-achalasia.

Manometry

This is diagnostic of achalasia if the lower oesophageal sphincter (LOS) zone pressure is high (>30 mmHg), there is an absence of propulsive waves, no relaxation in response to swallowing and incoordinated tertiary contractions. It may present with normal LOS pressures, but is rarely seen with low LOS pressures.

pH studies

These are not helpful in the diagnosis of achalasia.

Differential diagnosis

- Gastro-oesophageal reflux
- Diffuse oesophageal obstruction

- Intra- or extra-luminal obstruction (pseudo-achalasia)

Treatment

Calcium channel blockers and nitrates

These have been shown to reduce the LOS pressure, but the effect is transient and they are not recommended as a long-term treatment.

Oesophageal balloon dilatation

This is believed to be the most effective non-surgical procedure for adults and children. The limitation of this technique in children is an unsustained therapeutic response. Whilst initial response rates can approach 80–93%, 5- and 10-year relapses occur in 60–74% of patients. The majority of recurrences occur in the first 12 months after pneumatic dilation. Single and planned dilation programmes have been evaluated with similar outcomes. The majority of studies in children are small volume (10–50 cases), and long-term follow-up is frequently deficient.

Dilatation is generally carried out under general anaesthesia in children. Using endoscopic and image intensifier control, a guidewire is passed into the stomach. A 20–40 mm balloon dilator is passed over the guidewire and positioned to lie across the affected segment of oesophagus. A small amount of contrast in the balloon helps in identifying the correct position. The balloon is usually inflated to pressure of 100–775 mmHg (2–15 psi) for 60 seconds. The patient is observed for the next 5–6 hours and, if there are any concerns about oesophageal injury, a contrast study should be performed before discharge.

The perforation rate is 2% and the gastro-oesophageal reflux complication rate is 0–9%. The best predictors of post dilatation outcome are pressure in the LOS region of < 10 mmHg and age. This method appears to be less effective in younger patients.

Botulinum toxin A injection

This can be an effective treatment in the short term by inhibiting calcium-dependent release of acetylcholine from nerve terminals, thereby counterbalancing the effect of the selective loss of inhibitory neurotransmitters. It is injected into the oesophagus about 1 cm above the oesophageal sphincter using a sclerotherapy needle. Symptomatic relief develops over 1–3 days, but a significant number of patients have symptomatic recurrence 6–12 months after treatment. This can be repeated, but has been shown to cause fibrosis in the oesophageal wall, is less effective in subsequent doses and may lead to antibody formation. One third of patients may not show any sustained response, but it has been shown to be effective in recurrences following previous pneumatic dilatation and surgery.

Complications of transient chest pain and heartburn have been reported at 25% and 5%, respectively, but concern has been expressed that surgical myotomy is more difficult after injection. The possibility of scarring and the high recurrence rate has led to the procedure being reserved for patients with significant comorbidities where other strategies pose a more significant risk.

Heller's myotomy

Whether open, laparoscopic or thoracoscopic and used with or without an antireflux procedure, Heller's myotomy is still believed to give the most sustained response in the management of achalasia, certainly in younger patients. This involves dividing the serosa and muscularis propria of the distal oesophagus and extending this 1–2 cm onto the cardia of stomach (depending on age). The underlying mucosa should be left intact. A concomitant antireflux procedure may be performed to minimize the possibility of gastro-oesophageal reflux, which may occur in 11–22% of cases. A myotomy can produce a sustained remission in at least 83% of cases. The possibility of reduced postoperative pain and a quicker recovery from the operation has popularised the minimally invasive route.

Further reading

Pehlivanov N, Pasricha PJ. Medical and endoscopic management of achalasia. GI Motility Online 2006; 10:1038.

Sato TT. Esophageal achalasia. In: Stringer MD, Oldham KT, Mouriquand PDE (eds), Pediatric surgery and urology: long-term outcomes, 2nd edn. Cambridge: Cambridge University Press, 2006:232–241.

Spitz L. Achalasia. In: Spitz L, Coran AG (eds), Operative pediatric surgery, 6th edn. London: Hodder Education, 2007:321–330.

Related topics of interest

- Gastro-oesophageal reflux (p. 133)

Acute scrotum

Learning outcomes

- To be able to recognise the acute scrotum
- To outline the differential diagnosis of the acute scrotum with regard to age
- To describe the successful diagnosis and management of acute scrotal pathologies

Overview

The presentation of infants and boys with acute scrotal pain is relatively common. The most common pathologies in order of frequency are

- Torsion of testicular appendages
- Testicular torsion
- Idiopathic scrotal oedema
- Infections of the testicle or epididymis

Acute testicular torsion can cause infarction of the testicle within 6–8 hours making prompt evaluation, diagnosis and management of all boys with testicular pain important. The management of testicular torsion is urgent surgical exploration aiming to salvage the testicle. Most other pathologies can be managed conservatively. Other conditions presenting primarily with scrotal swelling and causing pain or discomfort are herniae, hydroceles and tumours.

Testicular torsion

This is axial rotation of the testicle and cord upon itself, cutting off the blood supply to the testicle and epididymis, resulting in venous engorgement, ischaemia and infarction.

Epidemiology and aetiology

Testicular torsion has an incidence of approximately 1 in 4000 males and a bimodal frequency. The first peak occurs perinatally, with a reported incidence of 6 per 100,000 births, followed by a second larger peak in adolescence. Approximately 90% of testicular torsions occur in teenage boys, with a median age of 14 years. The ratio of right to left torsion is 3:2.

Bilateral torsion has been described in the neonatal group, but is rare. However, it may influence the management in neonates. In neonates, the testicle and all of its coverings twist together within the scrotum – an extravaginal torsion. This occurs because the testicle and coverings in the newborn are loosely arranged and unfixed. It remains unclear whether it is due to lack of fixation between external spermatic fascia and dartos, or between tunica vaginalis and scrotum.

In older boys, the testicle twists on its cord within the covering of the tunica vaginalis – an intravaginal torsion. The testis sits within the covering of the tunica vaginalis that attaches to the posterior aspect of the testicle, epididymis and spermatic cord, keeping it relatively fixed. To twist within its coverings, there must be abnormal fixation resulting in an unusually mobile testicle. The most common anomaly is high attachment to the spermatic cord and no attachment to the posterior aspect of the testicle – the bell clapper anomaly. These testicles are freely mobile on a long mesorchium, tend to lie horizontally and are predisposed to torsion. Autopsy reports estimate the bell clapper anomaly to be present in 12% of males, and it has been shown to be bilateral in approximately 90%.

Not all boys with a bell clapper testicle develop a torsion; the initiating event may be minor trauma. Rotation of the testicle on the right is usually anticlockwise and on the left clockwise. It may twist from 90° to five complete turns. The consequences depend on the duration and the degree of the twist. The normal sequence is venous engorgement, followed by ischaemia and infarction. Histologically there is loss of architecture, haemorrhagic infiltration, extravasation and subsequent necrosis.

Clinical features

Perinatal torsion presents in two groups:

1. In the first group, testicular signs are obvious at birth and this torsion has

almost certainly occurred antenatally. The testis is almost invariably necrotic. This is the most common perinatal scenario
2. In the second group, there are no signs at birth, but they develop within the first 30 days presumably because the torsion occurs postnatally. The testicle may be salvageable

The hemiscrotum is discoloured black or red, and the testicle is swollen and hard. It is not usually tender as by birth the testicle is often necrotic. The scrotal skin may be oedematous. Rarely the condition may be bilateral.

In older boys, there is a short history of severe testicular pain. There may be a history of preceding trauma. The pain often radiates to the abdomen and may be associated with vomiting.

Examination reveals a red, swollen testicle in a high position due to shortening of the twisted cord. Cord shortening may abolish the cremasteric reflex. The entire testicle is usually exquisitely tender. Scrotal oedema develops over a period of hours. The other testicle may have a low or horizontal lie if it also has a bell clapper anomaly.

The less common scenario of intermittent torsion can occur in a boy with a bell clapper anomaly. This presents with self-limiting episodes of pain and a horizontally lying testicle on examination whilst standing upright. Bilateral orchidopexy is recommended.

Investigations

- A mid-stream specimen of urine (MSSU) is taken
- Doppler ultrasound is occasionally used in equivocal cases in younger boys with pain but minimal examination findings, to demonstrate testicular blood flow. This test has low sensitivity and is very operator dependent
- Other investigations include high-resolution ultrasound of the cord to detect the twist, contrast-enhanced ultrasound, computed tomography and near-infrared spectroscopy, but these are not performed routinely

Treatment

Emergent surgical scrotal exploration is the treatment for acute or suspected torsion. Fasting status should not delay surgery. Surgery involves the following steps:

- A horizontal incision in each hemiscrotum or a single vertical lower midline raphe incision is made allowing access to both sides
- The tunica vaginalis is opened and the testicle delivered
- The testicle is untwisted and assessed for viability. In doubtful cases, options include
  - Covering the testis in warm packs and waiting for 5–10 minutes
  - Opening the tunica albuginea to assess for intratesticular blood flow
- If viable, then it should be fixed; if non-viable, then it should be excised by ligating and dividing the cord
- Fixation methods include everting the tunica vaginalis, then either
  - Placing the testicle in a subdartos pouch and allowing scar tissue to fix it
  - Performing three-point suture fixation with a non-absorbable suture
- The contralateral testicle is then fixed in the same way

The treatment of neonatal torsion remains a subject of debate. As this condition is rare, there is no evidence base to guide practice. The majority of these testicles are already necrotic at presentation to the tertiary unit and practice varies between

- Emergent exploration and/or contralateral orchidopexy
- Excision of the torted testicle and contralateral orchidopexy
- Conservative management and counselling of the parents to present urgently in the presence of contralateral symptoms

The primary aim of the latter two is to avoid anorchia. The arguments for emergent surgical exploration include the small chance of saving the twisted testicle especially if signs developed postnatally.

The argument against emergent exploration includes the low chance of saving the affected testicle, the low rate of positive contralateral findings and the risk of iatrogenic damage. Reports of neonatal synchronous asymptomatic contralateral torsion make contralateral orchidopexy logical.

Surgical complications include bleeding or infection. If an ischaemic testicle is left in situ, there is a risk of severe infection in the dead testicular tissue, requiring repeat exploration and excision. The other adverse outcome is excision of a testicle in the mistaken belief that it is infarcted when it is only ischaemic. With fixation of the contralateral side, there is a small but measurable risk of damaging the testicle, especially in neonates.

Torsion of testicular appendages

Epidemiology

This condition is most common in boys aged between 5 and 10 years and there is no laterality difference.

Aetiology

The testicle may have appendages at several sites. The most common is the hydatid of Morgagni at the superior pole of the testicle, which is a vestigial remnant of the Müllerian duct. Less common sites are the epididymis and the lower end of the spermatic cord. Most are 2–15 mm long and mushroom-like in shape predisposing them to torsion.

Clinical features

The main difficulty is differentiating torsion of testicular appendages from a testicular torsion. In the former:

- Pain with or without scrotal swelling in a prepubertal boy
- Examination findings may be less severe than a torted testicle, but this is not always reliable
- Testicular position will commonly be normal with an intact cremasteric reflex although not all boys normally have a bilateral cremasteric reflex
- The testicle and cord will not be swollen, but this may be concealed by scrotal oedema
- Tenderness is usually limited to the upper pole of the testicle at the site of the appendage

- An infarcted appendage generally turns black and this is often seen through the skin as a blue dot; this is pathognomonic of a twisted appendage, and no further investigation is required.This appearance is not always present

Investigations

- A MSSU is taken
- If diagnostic doubt exists, a surgical exploration is the definitive investigation
- A Doppler ultrasound demonstrating blood flow supports the diagnosis in borderline cases but is of limited help in making a decision not to operate

Management

If the clinical diagnosis is certain, this can be conservative and the patient is reassured that the symptoms will settle in 2–5 days with simple analgesia and rest. Some children return with ongoing pain, and surgery is indicated for analgesia rather than diagnosis.

Surgery is performed as described above, and a torted appendage found at exploration is excised. Testicular fixation or contralateral exploration is not required.

Idiopathic scrotal oedema

This is a self-limiting swelling of unknown aetiology. It may be recurrent.

Most commonly, it occurs in children between 2 and 7 years of age, often presenting incidentally at bath time with a swollen red scrotum. Pain may be the presenting feature, but it is not as severe as conditions involving torsion.

The diagnosis is clinical and is based on a characteristic superficial pink swelling in the scrotal skin resembling an allergic wheal. The swelling can spread to the other hemiscrotum, penis, groin and perineum. The testicle is not swollen or tender although this is often difficult to appreciate. No investigations are necessary.

Treatment

- Reassurance that the symptoms will resolve spontaneously in 3–5 days
- Symptomatic relief with anti-histamines, simple analgesics and rest

Testicular infections

Infections of the testicle and epididymis are rare. These may be caused by a virus or bacteria.

Viral orchitis

Mumps is a viral disease primarily affecting the parotid glands and is self-limiting. Testicular symptoms occur in approximately 30% of postpubertal boys, is bilateral in approximately 30% of cases and may cause testicular atrophy in half of these. Testicular pain, swelling and oedema commence approximately 8 days into the illness and are usually self-limiting after 5–10 days. The diagnosis is usually apparent in the context of the systemic illness. There is no specific treatment.

Bacterial testicular infection

This is rare and usually caused by reflux of urine into the vas deferens due to an ectopic vas insertion, persistent Müllerian remnants, an ectopic ureter or by elimination disorders causing urinary stasis. The causative organisms are those commonly accounting for urinary tract infections with *Escherichia coli* the most common. In adolescent boys, it may be caused by sexually transmitted diseases.

Clinical features

Clinical features include acute unilateral testicular pain and swelling. Examination tends to reveal an intensely hot and tender testicle with surrounding scrotal oedema. This diagnosis is extremely difficult to differentiate from acute testicular torsion.

Investigations

- A MSSU is taken
- As clinical findings are often extremely similar to those of torsion, surgical exploration is often performed as an investigation. Often the only way to avoid this is a positive urine culture and a Doppler ultrasound demonstrating blood flow in the context of either recurrent episodes or a known predisposing renal tract anomaly
- The renal tract should be investigated with an ultrasound scan

Treatment

- Systemic antibiotics
- The functional outcome of a testicle that has been bacterially infected is unknown

Further reading

Rhodes H, et al. Neonatal testicular torsion. A survey of current practice amongst paediatric surgeons and urologists in the United Kingdom and Ireland. J Pediatr Surg 2011; 46:2157–2160.

Srinivasan A, Cinman N, Feber KM, et al. History and physical examination findings predictive of

testicular torsion: an attempt to promote clinical diagnosis by house staff. J Pediatr Urol 2011; 7:470–474.

Tekgül S, Riedmiller H, Gerharz E, et al. Guidelines on paediatric urology: the acute scrotum. European Society of Paediatric Urologists, 2008:13–18.

Related topics of interest

Anorectal malformation in females

Learning outcomes

- To know how to assess a female neonate with an anorectal malformation
- To be aware of when and how to form a colostomy
- To understand the principles of definitive surgery

Overview

Anorectal malformations in females should be recognised in the neonatal period and accurately characterised. Common abnormalities are the rectoperineal fistula, the rectovestibular fistula and the cloaca. The cloaca represents the severe end of the spectrum. Associated abnormalities are common.

Clinical assessment of the neonate will determine if a temporary stoma is required. If so, definitive surgery is then deferred, and performed during the first few months of life. The approach is through a posterior midline approach, the posterior sagittal anorectoplasty (PSARP). Long-term outcome can be optimised with careful management of functional sequelae.

Epidemiology and aetiology

The overall incidence is approximately 1 in 4000. The most common defects in a female are shown in **Figure 1**. The aetiology remains poorly understood but is the focus of ongoing work.

Clinical features

An absent or abnormal anus should be identified clinically at the neonatal assessment. However, some patients have a fistula opening onto the perineum or into the vestibule that allows meconium to be passed into the nappy. This has the potential to lead an unsuspecting examining clinician to miss the diagnosis, a situation that remains common.

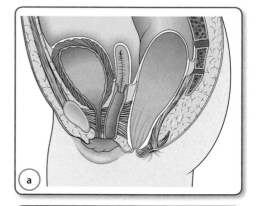

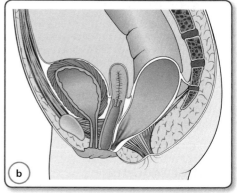

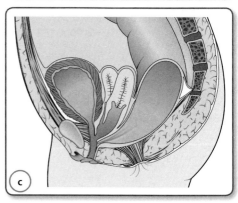

Figure 1 Rectoperineal (a), rectovestibular (b) and cloacal (c) defects. Reprinted from: Chapter 4 – Female defects. In: Peña A. Atlas of surgical management of anorectal malformations, Springer Verlag: New York, 1989. With kind permission of Springer Science+Business Media.

There is a spectrum of abnormalities; a perineal fistula is usually easily differentiated from a vestibular fistula, which is hidden in the posterior wall of the vestibule. A small single orifice in the perineum suggests a cloaca.

Associated abnormalities tend to become increasingly common with the severity of the anorectal abnormality. These defects may fall within the VACTERL association and include vertebral (often dysraphism or sacral abnormalities), anorectal, cardiac (septal defects), tracheo-oesophageal (OA-TOF), renal (e.g. vesicoureteric reflux or bladder dysfunction) and limb abnormalities (e.g. radial limb deformities). Gynaecological abnormalities have been found to be common in rectovestibular fistulae.

Investigations

Careful clinical assessment of the perineum is usually sufficient to characterise the anorectal malformation. General examination, spinal ultrasound scanning (USS) and X-ray, echocardiography and renal tract USS are required to exclude associated abnormalities and are increasingly important with more severe anorectal defects.

Anteroposterior and lateral sacral films allow the length of the sacrum in comparison to that of the pelvis to be calculated ('sacral ratio') (**Figure 2**). A poorly developed sacrum is usually associated with poor innervation,

poor musculature and therefore poor prognosis. If the ratio is < 0.4, continence is very unusual without careful management, often with washouts. Conversely, in patients with a low defect and good ratios, a favourable outcome may be predicted. Parents will benefit from having a realistic expectation of outcome from early on either way.

Differential diagnosis

The most common mistake is to fail to recognise the abnormality at all, usually because meconium is not adequately cleaned from the perineum in the neonatal period. Rectoperineal fistulae are incompletely surrounded by sphincteric muscle and usually lie anteriorly on the perineum. Rectovestibular fistulae open just inside the introitus, the vestibule. Cloacal abnormalities are defects in which the anorectum, genital and urinary tract all open into a single, common channel.

The term 'rectovaginal fistula' implies the opening lies above the hymen and is probably overused; many of these defects will have an unrecognised abnormal urethral opening and therefore actually be cloacae. This is more than semantics as potentially significant urogenital abnormalities may require correction.

Anal or rectal stenosis can exist with a normally placed anus. One important feature of this type of anorectal abnormality is its

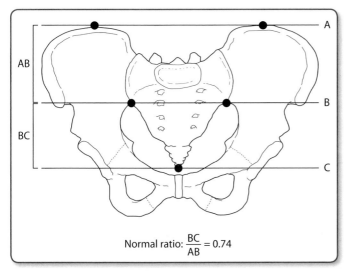

Figure 2 Landmarks used to determine the sacral ratio.

AB

BC

A

B

C

Normal ratio: $\dfrac{BC}{AB} = 0.74$

association with the presence of a presacral mass (potentially a teratoma) and an abnormal sacrum as part of the Currarino triad.

Treatment

In the neonatal period, a decision must be made about the need for a colostomy; the purpose of a colostomy is to divert the faecal stream if further investigations are required or there is some technical advantage to delay surgical correction. Cloacal defects require cover with a stoma, whilst the need is less fixed for a rectovestibular fistula; in some centres, definitive repair may be completed in the neonatal period without stoma coverage, but in others it may be felt that a staged approach is associated with better long-term outcomes. Both approaches are acceptable in experienced hands. Rectoperineal fistulae rarely require a stoma; if obstructed in the neonatal phase, definitive repair can be performed without a stoma. If asymptomatic, the need for surgical repair is contentious. Some patients become symptomatic with time, and for these girls, stoma cover is an option.

Formation of a colostomy for an anorectal malformation involves a left lower quadrant incision and identification of the most proximal loop of sigmoid colon. The bowel is frequently distended, limiting vision, so particular care is needed to make sure that the proximal end is identified and the distal limb thoroughly washed out. The colostomy is brought out at the lateral end of the wound and a mucous fistula at the medial end of the incision, just far enough away to allow placement of a stoma bag over the colostomy alone. This prevents spillover of effluent into the distal limb. The configuration of this type of stoma, a 'divided descending colostomy', allows the child to decompress, has a low chance of stomal prolapse (the proximal limb is fixed to the retroperitoneum), gives access to the distal limb for washouts and leaves sufficient downstream bowel for a future pullthrough.

The principle of definitive repair in girls is to mobilise the anorectum or fistula into the sphincteric muscle through a posterior sagittal (PSARP) incision, as first described by Pena. Since perineal innervation and musculature are paired, a midline approach minimises iatrogenic injury to these structures whilst providing excellent exposure. Parasagittal fibres can be seen running just under the perineal skin (probably representing external sphincter) and 'muscle complex' running in a perpendicular direction up to the levator. Accurate placement of the neoanus and rectum within these structures will give the best chance of a good functional outcome. Additional considerations in a rectovestibular fistula are the need for meticulous dissection of the anorectum or fistula from the back of the vagina (the plane is often so thin that it is considered as a common wall) and creation of an adequate perineal body.

Following repair, anal dilatation is performed on a daily basis to prevent cicatrisation of the neoanus. Once an adequate size is reached, the colostomy is closed and dilatations reduced before being stopped. Central to good long-term outcome is close follow-up and early management of sequelae, which may include constipation, incontinence and urogenital symptoms.

Further reading

Haider N, Fisher R. Mortality and morbidity associated with late diagnosis of anorectal malformations in children. Surgeon 2007; 5:327–330.

Levitt MA, et al. Rectovestibular fistula—rarely recognized associated gynecologic anomalies. J Pediatr Surg 2009; 44:1261–1267.

Pena A, Devries PA. Posterior sagittal anorectoplasty: important technical considerations and new applications. J Pediatr Surg 1982; 17:796–811.

Related topics of interest

Anorectal malformation in males

Learning outcomes

- To know how to assess a male neonate with an anorectal malformation
- To know when and how to form a colostomy
- To understand the principles of definitive surgery

Overview

Anorectal malformations in males fall into a spectrum of abnormalities. Severe abnormalities ('high abnormalities') are usually associated with a congenital fistula between the hindgut and the urinary tract. Determining the location of this fistula will reduce the chance of urological injury during exploration to find the rectum. Placement of a colostomy in the neonatal period will allow investigations to be completed before definitive treatment. High abnormalities have an increased frequency of associated anomalies, typically within the vertebral, anorectal, cardiac, tracheo-oesophageal, renal and limb (VACTERL) association.

At the milder end of the spectrum ('low abnormalities'), the hindgut opens onto the perineum. For many of the patients in this group, exploration and repair of the defect can be performed in the neonatal phase with the knowledge that the risk of urological injury is low. Colostomy can be avoided.

The approach for both groups is usually through a midline approach, the posterior sagittal anorectoplasty (PSARP), as described by Pena. For high abnormalities, access into the peritoneal cavity may be required. Laparoscopy may be a useful adjunct. Long-term outcomes can be optimised with careful management of functional sequelae.

Epidemiology and pathology

The overall incidence is approximately 1 in 4000. The most common defects in a male are shown in **Figure 3**.

Aetiology

The aetiology remains poorly understood but is the focus of ongoing work.

Clinical features

An absent or misplaced anus should be identified on the neonatal examination although this is occasionally missed. The primary objectives of the neonatal assessment are

- To establish if a colostomy is required or not (i.e. is it a low or high defect?)
- To look for evidence of associated abnormalities

A low abnormality usually does not need a colostomy and is characterised by the presence of a fistula between the hindgut and the perineal skin. This is typically anterior to the normal position of the anus and is small in calibre. The presence of meconium on the perineal skin indicates a low defect. One exception is a 'bucket-handle defect'; although meconium may not actually be seen in the neonatal phase, the hindgut is very close to perineal skin and this abnormality can be treated as a low defect. The appearance of a raised bridge of skin over a well-formed, but non-patent, anal dimple is pathognomonic to an experienced clinician. Typically, low abnormalities are associated with near-normal-sized gluteal musculature and good 'sphincter' contraction on stimulation of the anal dimple.

Conversely, high abnormalities are usually connected to the urinary tract (at the bulbar urethra, prostatic urethra or even the bladder neck) by a fistula. Presence of meconium in the urine is therefore pathognomonic of a high defect (although this will often take 24 hours or so to appear). An exception to this rule is 'imperforate anus without fistula' in which no connection exists to the urinary tract and which is most commonly seen in Down's syndrome. A rare variant is rectal atresia, whereby the anal canal is normal but the very distal rectum is stenotic or atretic.

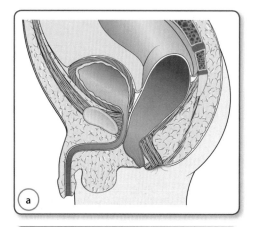

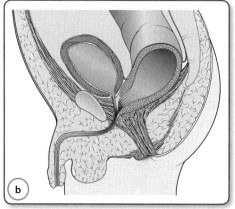

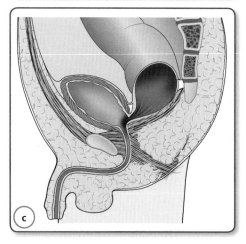

Figure 3 Rectoperineal (a), rectobulbar urethral (b) and rectobladder neck (c) fistulae. Reprinted from: Chapter 3 – Male defects. In: Peña A. Atlas of surgical management of anorectal malformations, Springer Verlag: New York, 1989, 50, 61. With kind permission of Springer Science+Business Media.

Typically, high abnormalities are associated with poorly formed gluteal musculature (a flat bottom) and little in the way of 'sphincter' contraction on stimulation.

Given that the repair of high abnormalities requires dissection close to the urethra, formation of a colostomy in the neonatal period allows detailed imaging of the hindgut to be performed (see below). Occasionally, even children with low abnormalities require a stoma, particularly if their diagnosis is delayed and distension severe.

The technique of stoma formation for anorectal malformations and an outline of associated defects encountered are covered in 'Anorectal malformation in females' (p. 12).

Investigations

Whilst differentiation of low from high abnormalities is usually possible on clinical grounds, occasionally imaging is required. A cross-table shoot-through radiograph with a radio-opaque marker on the anal dimple can indicate the distance of the terminal portion of the hindgut. Ultrasound can also be used but requires an experienced sonographer.

General examination, spinal ultrasound scanning (USS) and X-ray, echocardiography and renal tract USS are required to exclude associated abnormalities and become increasingly important with the severity of the anorectal defect.

After 4–6 weeks, a distal loopogram is performed to identify the point of insertion of the fistula into the urinary tract, allowing the surgeon to plan the approach. For the highest abnormalities, it is not possible to reach the fistula through a perineal incision alone and exploration from above is necessitated. The investigation comprises the instillation of water-soluble contrast into the mucous fistula under some pressure. This ensures that the contrast overcomes any resistance from the musculature of pelvic floor and enters any fistula.

Treatment

The principle of definitive repair is to separate the hindgut from the urinary tract and mobilise the anorectum or fistula into the sphincteric muscle through a posterior sagittal (PSARP) incision. Since perineal innervation and musculature is paired, a midline approach minimises iatrogenic injury to these structures whilst providing excellent exposure. Dissection of the fistula from the urinary tract is delicate and requires careful separation of these structures, joined by a common wall.

As indicated above, some high fistulae must be approached via the abdominal cavity. The question of this being open or laparoscopic should not affect the procedure undertaken, and the division of the fistula should be sufficiently close to the urinary tract to prevent formation of a posterior urethral diverticulum. Once the hindgut has been safely divided from the urinary tract, a posterior sagittal approach will allow the segment to be pulled through (see p. 000).

Following a period of time in which anal dilators are used, the stoma is closed, and dilatations tailed off. Central to good long-term outcome is close follow-up and early management of sequelae. This may include constipation (particularly for low defects) and incontinence (particularly for high defects).

Further reading

Bischoff A, Levitt MA, Pena A. Laparoscopy and its use in the repair of anorectal malformations. J Pediatr Surg 2011; 46:1609–1617.

Pena A, Devries PA. Posterior sagittal anorectoplasty: important technical considerations and new applications. J Pediatr Surg 1982; 17:796–811.

Wijers CHW, de Blaauw I, Marcelis CL, et al. Research perspectives in the etiology of congenital anorectal malformations using data of the International Consortium on Anorectal Malformations: evidence for risk factors across different populations. Pediatr Surg Int 2010; 26:1093–1099.

Related topics of interest

Antenatal hydronephrosis

Learning outcomes

- To discuss the differential diagnosis and outcomes of antenatal hydronephrosis
- To illustrate appropriate postnatal management pathways
- To briefly discuss the most common aetiology that requires intervention

Overview

Hydronephrosis is dilatation of the pelvis of the kidney and is the most common urological anomaly detected on prenatal scanning. This does not equate to obstruction, as >60% spontaneously resolve. Obtaining detailed information regarding prenatal ultrasound findings at all prenatal appointments is vital in the elucidation of a possible diagnosis, to offer appropriate antenatal counselling and to initiate the correct postnatal investigative pathway and management.

Epidemiology and aetiology

Most prenatal studies have reported significant dilatation as >1 cm renal pelvic diameter, and using this parameter the incidence is between 0.4% and 0.6%. Several European centres have reported incidences between 1 in 150 and 1 in 1200 and may only reflect differences in methodology and interpersonal variability.

Causes of antenatal hydronephrosis (most can cause unilateral or bilateral hydronephrosis) are:

- Transient or physiological hydronephrosis   63%
- Pelvi-ureteric junction obstruction (PUJO)   11%
- Vesicoureteric reflux (VUR)   9%
- Megaureter [obstructed (VUJO) or non-obstructed]   4%
- Multicystic dysplastic kidney   2%
- Ureterocoele   2%
- Renal cysts   2%
- Posterior urethral valves (PUV)   1%

Transient or physiological renal pelvic dilatation is not fully understood and may be due to immaturity of the pelvi-ureteric junction (PUJ) or vesicoureteric junction (VUJ), increased fetal urinary output in the third trimester, a prominent extrarenal pelvis or VUR.

Clinical features

By and large this population is an asymptomatic group and has raised a variety of controversial aspects in the definition of obstruction and the indications for intervention. Clinical presentation with a palpable mass is extremely rare with the advent of prenatal scanning. The most important parameter is the anteroposterior diameter (APD) of the renal pelvis in transverse section at the level of the renal hilum on ultrasound scan (US). This parameter should always be accompanied by taking note of the presence of calyceal dilatation, which suggests a significant pathology. A unilateral or bilateral abnormality, a dilated ureter (hydroureter or megaureter) or distended bladder, and the amount of liquor on US are other observations that are vital in the decision-making process.

Investigations

The postnatal management pathways are illustrated in the algorithm in **Figure 4**. Postnatal imaging includes:

- **US:** Within the first 72 hours of life, it may falsely reassure improvement in dilatation due to physiological dehydration and is ideally performed within the first week. In addition to APD, the presence of a dilated ureter, pre- and post-micturition upper tract status if possible, bladder outline and thickness should be noted. Other observations should include whether it is a simplex or duplex system and lesions within the bladder (e.g. ureterocoele). An abnormal bladder or upper tracts in the absence of an obvious cause should proceed to an ultrasound spine to look for any form of spinal dysraphism to support a neuropathic bladder
- **MAG3 renogram (Mercapto-acetyl triglycine tagged with technetium-99m) study:** This produces radioisotope uptake and drainage curves. Differential function of each kidney contributing to

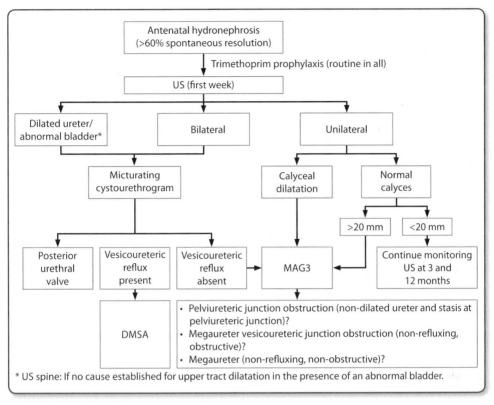

Figure 4 Postnatal management of antenatal hydronephrosis. DMSA, dimercaptosuccinic acid; MAG3, mercapto-acetyl triglycine; US, ultrasound scan. From Burge D, et al. Paediatric Surgery 2nd edition. London: Hodder Education, 2005;438, Figure 50.1. Reproduced by permission of Hodder Education.

total renal function is calculated during the early uptake phase. Most studies would incorporate a post-frusemide drainage curve to challenge or reinforce an abnormality in drainage. Drainage curves are unreliable to confirm the presence of obstruction, more so in the presence of severe hydronephrosis, and depend on hydration of the child, renal function and bladder emptying. The study is recommended ideally at around 3 months of age but can be done as early as 4 weeks in select cases (e.g. severe hydronephrosis and severe calyceal involvement)

- **DMSA kidney scan (Dimercaptosuccinic acid tagged with technetium-99m):** This usually follows the finding of VUR on cystogram. This is to establish areas of scarring, if any. It is also performed in unilateral poorly functioning kidneys when the choice is between a nephrectomy and renal preservation

because MAG3 scans can be less accurate in these settings to assess function

- **Micturating cystourethrogram (MCUG):** This is to demonstrate vesicoureteric reflux or bladder outflow pathology, if any. It is indicated when one or more of dilated ureter or ureters, distended or thick walled bladder, bilateral hydronephrosis, solitary or duplex hydronephrotic kidney and echogenic kidneys are noted on either pre- or post-natal ultrasound imaging. It is unnecessary in the case of a simplex system with unilateral isolated hydronephrosis
- **Blood tests:** Bilateral involvement should necessitate overall renal function assessment in the form of serum creatinine

Specific issues that require attention or understanding:

- Disproportionate dilatation between pelvis of the kidney and ureter should question the existence of dual pathology, e.g. VUR and PUJO

- Reflux can coexist with PUJO (10%) or VUJO (VUJ obstruction) as in a refluxing obstructive megaureter
- PUJO can coexist with a VUJO (<5%). A VUJO can be masked by a PUJO and may come to light only after pyeloplasty
- Early and prompt postnatal admission and investigations should be initiated in those with pre- or postnatal findings of an abnormal bladder, echogenic kidneys, oligo- or anhydramnios, hydronephrosis in a solitary kidney or severe bilateral hydronephrosis (>20 mm) because they may have significant renal impairment or be predisposed to life-threatening urosepsis (e.g. PUV)
- Prenatal intervention in the form of vesico-amniotic shunting has been performed in select male patients with bladder outflow obstruction in specialised centres. Selection criteria and outcomes of this intervention are still unclear

PUJO

Obstruction is rarely complete in which case the kidney would not function. Less than 5% cases of antenatally detected hydronephrosis have a PUJO that need pyeloplasty. Surgery is indicated if the differential function is <40%, there is progressive increase in APD, APD is >30 mm (APD >30 mm and dilated calyces – 90% chance of needing surgery), and the patient is symptomatic (urinary tract infection or pain). Exceptions to this guidance and a lower threshold for intervention should be considered in intrarenal type of hydronephrosis, gross calyceal involvement, solitary kidney and bilateral PUJO.

Treatment – PUJO

Anderson-Hynes dismembered pyeloplasty is the most common surgical intervention and is the gold standard. Most series report a >95% success rate. In infancy, an extraperitoneal, muscle-splitting approach is used to access the PUJ and excise it along with some of the hydronephrotic pelvis. The normal healthy ureter is then spatulated and anastomosed to the residual pelvis, with or without a transanastomotic stent. A variety of stent, perinephric drain and bladder catheter combinations exist among surgeons. The benefits of conventional laparoscopic (transperitoneal), retroperitoneoscopic and robot-assisted pyeloplasty seem to be more obvious in older children.

Other forms of treatment include endopyelotomy, using a variety of balloon devices employed in an antegrade or retrograde fashion, and vascular hitch procedure in pure extrinsic PUJO due to lower pole vessels.

Follow-up

Following surgery an US is performed at around 3 months and a MAG3 scan at around 6–9 months. Parameters to be monitored would be the APD on pre- and post-micturition US, and differential function with drainage on MAG3 scanning. In most, improving parameters need to be monitored over 3–5 years following surgery.

Further reading

Dhillon HK. Antenatal diagnosis of urinary tract anomalies. Paediatric surgery, 2nd edn. Hodder Arnold Publishers Ltd, 2005.

Thomas DFM. Prenatal diagnosis: what do we know of long-term outcomes? J Pediatr Urol 2010; 6:204–211.

Woodward M, Frank D. Postnatal management of antenatal hydronephrosis. BJU Int 2002; 89:149–156.

Related topics of interest

Appendicitis

Learning outcomes

- To be able to recognise and grade appendicitis
- To be aware of the treatment options
- To be aware of the complications of intervention

Overview

Acute appendicitis is inflammation of the vermiform appendix, which usually results in abdominal pain. Around 6% of the UK population will develop appendicitis at some point in life. Unfortunately, its presenting features overlap with many other conditions, and diagnostic delay does increase morbidity. On analysis of appendicitis patients, 56% of preschool children have perforated appendicitis at presentation, and in older children, 67% have acute appendicitis at presentation. Surgery is still the definitive management of this condition although low-quality studies of antibiotic therapy alone in simple appendicitis show that it may be a viable treatment option in the future.

Epidemiology and aetiology

Appendicitis forms 25–40% of the diagnosis of children admitted with acute abdominal pain. In acute appendicitis, the appendix is congested and oedematous and has submucosal or transmural infiltration by neutrophils. This may be secondary to intraluminal obstruction by lymphoid hyperplasia, faecal matter or parasites. Once obstructed, distension with mucus and bacterial proliferation result in venous congestion, arterial flow obstruction and gangrenous appendicitis. The lumen may be pus-filled and peritoneal fluid is increased. There is loss of normal tissue architecture on histology. Ischaemia can then result in necrosis and perforation.

In perforated appendicitis, the perforation may be micro- or macroscopic and is normally located on the antimesenteric border. Peritonitis may be local or generalised. Rarely portal pyaemia and hepatic abscess occur due to infective emboli.

Appendix masses are made up of an inflammatory mass and/or abscess. The mass is usually appendix, small bowel and omentum.

Clinical features

Appendicitis may be inferred by a pattern of typical features in the history and examination in around half of all cases. Recognition of this pattern can be used to make a decision to admit, investigate and operate. A full, detailed pain history should be taken.

Typical features

1. History

- Central colicky abdominal pain that migrates to the right iliac fossa and becomes constant and peritonitic in nature (highest predictive value)
- Anorexia
- Nausea and vomiting
- Fever and malaise

2. Examination

- Features of sepsis – fever, tachycardia and flushing
- Signs of peritonism
  - Pain exacerbated by movement
- Simple palpation
  - Coughing
  - Percussion tenderness
  - Rovsing's sign
  - Shuffling gait
  - Pain on hopping
- Signs of muscle spasm
  - Loss of abdominal wall excursion with breathing
  - Involuntary guarding in the right iliac fossa
  - Scoliosis concave to the right
  - Flexed right hip

In many cases, patients with appendicitis have an atypical pattern.

Atypical features

1. History

- Pain on micturition or dysuria
- Diarrhoea

- Non-specific, diffuse abdominal pain
- Pyrexia and malaise

2. Examination
- Abdominal distension in children younger than 8 years
- Palpable mass in the right iliac fossa

Alarm signals
- Painful gastroenteritis
- Repeated presentation
- More than two doctors seen
- History > 3 days
- History of recent antibiotic use
- Preschool children (< 5 years) with abdominal pain. These are more likely to present with perforation. This is due to the failure of the protective greater omentum to relocate to the right iliac fossa and localise the appendicitis. They are also unable to vocalise and difficult to assess thus making diagnosis troublesome
- Parental suspicion
- Overweight children
- Teenage females
- Children with learning difficulties or neurological impairment

Routine examination should also include assessment of external genitals, hernial orifices and chest. Rectal examination is rarely helpful in diagnosing acute appendicitis in children and should be avoided unless there are strong specific indications. Assessment for rebound tenderness should also be avoided if there are already signs of peritonism.

Investigations

The decision to operate can be made by clinical assessment alone; however, it is increasingly common to use other investigations, often to rule out other pertinent causes of such abdominal symptoms:
- Blood tests – leucocyte count and C-reactive protein – are non-specific but may help to exclude active infection. Liver function tests and serum amylase may also be helpful in selected patients
- Urinalysis, including pregnancy test for postmenarchal females, is recommended

- Ultrasound scanning is becoming widely accepted as a first-line investigation tool in the diagnostic process and can also evaluate the pelvis for other causes of abdominal pain
- Computed tomography scanning in the UK is usually reserved for the most complicated presentations of appendicitis

Differential diagnosis

In many children with abdominal pain, no specific diagnosis will be made. The following should be considered:
- Acute non-specific abdominal pain
- Urinary tract infection
- Gynaecological causes – ovarian torsion, ovarian cyst, pelvic inflammatory disease and endometriosis
- Acute testicular pain
- Hernia
- Constipation
- Mesenteric adenitis

Management

Simple decisions that need to be made:
- Admit or discharge
- Observe or investigate
- Observe or operate

In general, antibiotics should not be given until a diagnosis is made or a decision has been made to operate.

Early appendicitis

Surgical removal of the appendix is curative. Depending on the availability of equipment and surgical expertise, appendicectomy may be performed laparoscopically or by open incision. There is growing evidence to suggest that simple appendicitis may be managed non-operatively using intravenous antibiotics.
- Open
  - Muscle splitting right lower quadrant incision centred on McBurney's point
  - Excision of appendix following ligation and coagulation of meso-appendix
  - Peritoneal lavage
- Laparoscopic
  - Umbilical 10 mm port (Hasson), 5 mm left lower and right lower quadrant ports

- Meso-appendix coagulation
- Appendix ligation – double or triple endoloop
- Removal of appendix via the 10 mm port (with or without endocatch bag)
- Peritoneal lavage

Advanced appendicitis

Appendicitis is considered to be advanced when the body has made attempts to seclude the infection and is associated with greater morbidity. Often palpable as a mass, the omentum migrates to the infected area and local inflammation of bowel results in fluid-filled loops of bowel, with thickened walls called 'phlegmon'. Open approach to surgery is generally favoured, though with increasing competence appendicectomy can still be achieved laparoscopically. Dissection through these inflamed tissues has increased complication risks. As a result many centres will treat these children, if the infection is well localised, with antibiotics, and an interval appendicectomy may or may not be performed at a later date.

Prognosis and follow-up

Complications following removal of simple appendicitis include:
- Formation of intra-abdominal abscess
- Adhesive bowel obstruction
- Fistula
- Wound infection
- Delayed return to feeding (ileus)

Further reading

Hall NJ, et al. Is interval appendicectomy justified after successful nonoperative treatment of an appendix mass in children? A systematic review. J Pediatr Surg 2011; 46:767–771.
Masoomi H, Mills S, Dolich MO, et al. Comparison of outcomes of laparoscopic versus open appendectomy in children: data from the Nationwide Inpatient Sample (NIS), 2006–2008. World J Surg 2012; 36:573–578.
Svensson JF, et al. A review of conservative treatment of acute appendicitis. Eur J Pediatr Surg 2012; 22:185–194.

Related topics of interest

Balanitis xerotica obliterans

Learning outcomes

- To recognise balanitis xerotica obliterans
- To know the underlying aetiology
- To be aware of the management options and potential complications

Overview

Balanitis xerotica obliterans (BXO) is lichen sclerosus of the male prepuce, which creates a progressive, scarring, inflammatory dermatosis.

Epidemiology and aetiology

There are several theories relating to its cause:

- **Autoimmune:** BXO is associated with several autoimmune conditions, including type 1 diabetes, thyroid disease and vitiligo. Patients with lichen sclerosus have also been found to have a variety of serum auto-antibodies
- **Hormonal:** There is an association between BXO in adulthood and reduced serum levels of both testosterone and dihydrotestosterone
- **Infection:** Human papilloma virus has been detected, coexisting with BXO

None of these associations are consistent and the cause of BXO remains unknown. What is striking is that BXO is almost unheard of in boys who have been circumcised as infants, giving strength to the theories of an infective or chronic irritant aetiology. There are also marked racial differences, with black and Hispanic men being more than twice as likely to develop BXO as white men, in turn giving weight to the suggestion of a genetic cause. It seems most likely that the origins of BXO are multifactorial and lie in an underlying susceptibility that is triggered by an as yet unidentified environmental factor.

Clinical features

BXO in childhood most commonly presents between the ages of 8 and 13 years. Although it has been reported in boys younger than 3 years, it is very unusual to find BXO in the preschool age range. The incidence has been estimated at 3 cases in 1000 boys younger than 15 years.

Early in its course, BXO may produce non-specific symptoms of itching or burning sensations in the penis, with or without dysuria. The majority of boys with BXO present with a phimosis, often in a previously retractile foreskin. This can in turn lead to difficulty or pain on passing urine. In very severe cases, the phimosis can cause an outflow obstruction and upper tract dilatation. Older boys may report painful erections.

Typical findings on examination are a non- or partly retractile foreskin, often with a very tight phimosis, preventing glans visualisation. The presence of pearly white sclerotic plaques is pathognomic and clearly differentiates BXO from a normal developmental phimosis.

Investigations

A definitive diagnosis requires histological confirmation, but BXO can usually be diagnosed on clinical examination alone, meaning biopsy is rarely indicated. Where biopsy is performed or tissue obtained as part of a therapeutic procedure, the histological findings are of hyperkeratosis, with degeneration of the basal layer, marked dermal oedema and blood vessel dilatation. There is often a lymphocytic infiltrate.

Differential diagnosis

- Developmental ('physiological') phimosis
- Acquired phimosis following recurrent balanitis

Treatment

- **Topical steroid preparations, e.g. betamethasone:** This may be sufficient in early cases to control the disease and allow the foreskin to become retractile and is often used as an adjunct to more invasive measures. Because the condition is chronic, long-term topical steroids may be necessary following treatment, preserving the foreskin or for BXO extending onto the glans

- **Intralesional steroid injections, e.g. triamcinolone:** This is used in more advanced cases and is often combined with preputioplasty or stretching to retract the foreskin
- **Preputioplasty:** The foreskin is incised longitudinally in several places, and closed transversely to widen the aperture and allow the foreskin to be retracted. A recent study has reported good outcomes following preputioplasty combined with intralesional steroid. The incidence of meatal stenosis was lower when compared to circumcision, and the overall reoperation rate was similar
- **Circumcision:** This is the preferred treatment of many surgeons because circumcision has the potential to be curative, even when the BXO can be seen to involve the glans at operation. There are a myriad of ways of performing a circumcision – given below are the operative steps in two commonly used methods. It should be remembered that the oedema and sclerosis associated with BXO can make circumcision considerably more difficult than when done for other reasons:
  - Forceps technique
    - The phimosis is dilated using an artery clip to allow foreskin retraction
    - Preputial adhesions are divided and the glans cleaned with antiseptic
    - The foreskin is elevated with artery clips
    - A clamp or forceps is passed across the foreskin at the level of the coronal sulcus
    - This clamp is elevated clear of the glans and, taking care to avoid damaging the glans, the foreskin is divided with a scalpel or bipolar electrocautery
    - The mucosa is trimmed, leaving approximately 3 mm around the coronal sulcus
    - Careful haemostasis is carried out
    - The shaft skin and mucosal cuff are approximated using interrupted absorbable suture
  - Sleeve technique
    - This removes the surface layer of skin, avoiding blood vessels and connective tissue layers
    - The foreskin is slid back along the shaft, and a freehand incision is made around the shaft as far back as the scar line is to be placed
    - The foreskin is returned to cover the glans, and another incision is made around the shaft at the same position along its length as the first
    - A longitudinal incision is made between the two circumferential ones and the skin is removed
    - The edges are pulled together and sutured
    - The frenulum can be included in the main incision or divided separately
    - Results depend on the skill of the surgeon, but can be as tight or loose as desired with the scar line anywhere that is wanted
    - Since no blood vessels have been divided, bleeding is minimal – no dressing is needed, and healing is rapid
    - The skin can be marked prior to resection to aid dissection

Complications

- **Meatal stenosis:** This can form part of the initial presentation or occur later following treatment for BXO, affecting the prepuce. Treatment with dilatation or meatoplasty needs to be followed by topical steroids to prevent recurrence
- **Urethral stricture:** This is a rare sequel to childhood BXO and is difficult to treat, often requiring excision and grafting, for example a buccal mucosal graft, followed by urethroplasty
- **Obstructive uropathy:** This is an unusual complication that occurs in late-presenting BXO. Failure of hydronephrosis to resolve following successful treatment of preputial and meatal disease should prompt investigation for a urethral stricture

Further reading

Jayakumar S, Antao B, Bevington O, et al. Balanitis xerotica obliterans in children and its incidence under the age of 5 years. J Pediatr Urol 2012; 8:272–275.

Wilkinson DJ, Lansdale NK, Everitt LH, et al. Foreskin preputioplasty and intralesional triamcinolone a valid alternative to circumcision for balanitis xerotica obliterans. J Pediatr Surg 2012; 47:756–759.

Yardley IE, Cosgrove C, Lambert AW. Paediatric preputial pathology: are we circumcising enough? Ann R Coll Surg Engl 2007; 89:62–65.

Related topics of interest

- Meatal stenosis (p. 200)

Biliary atresia

Learning outcomes

- To be aware of possible causes of surgical jaundice arising in infancy
- To be familiar with the methods of investigation
- To understand the management options
- To be aware of the surgical outcome and results

Overview

Biliary atresia (BA) is characterised by conjugated jaundice, pale stools and dark urine, arising in an otherwise well infant of only a few weeks old.

Epidemiology and aetiology

There is an incidence of 1 in 17,000 in the UK. There is a higher incidence in Asia, specifically in Japan, China and Taiwan.

Three types of BA are recognized, based on where the most proximal level of obstruction is: type 1 (obstructed common bile duct), type 2 (obstructed common hepatic duct) and type 3 (solid proximal portal plate) (**Figure 5**).

Although for most patients the aetiology is not known, there is a proportion in whom the onset is clearly congenital and results from failure of bile duct development. Examples include the biliary atresia splenic malformation (BASM) syndrome and cystic biliary atresia. Both these variants have a female predominance. Otherwise BA is usually an isolated anomaly, and some (10%) may be associated with perinatal viral infection, the most well-defined being those with cytomegalovirus (CMV) immunoglobulin M (IgM) antibodies at presentation.

Experimental BA can be created in certain species of mice by perinatal intraperitoneal injection of certain viruses (e.g. rhesus rotavirus). An inflammatory process can then be identified that targets biliary cholangioles and ductules.

Clinical features

The infant may present with one or more of the following features:

- Conjugated jaundice
- Pale stools (lack of bile in gastrointestinal tract)
- Dark urine (passage of water-soluble conjugated bilirubin into renal tubules)
- Vitamin K deficiency and coagulopathy
- Antenatally detected subhepatic cyst
- Cirrhosis (ascites and hepatosplenomegaly), rarely younger than 3 months

Investigations

A split bilirubin test (including conjugated and unconjugated fractions) distinguishes most surgical causes of jaundice from non-surgical causes. All surgical causes will be associated with elevated γ-glutamyl transpeptidase and aspartate transaminases levels. Medical causes, such as α_1-antitrypsin deficiency, Alagille's syndrome, cystic fibrosis and neonatal hepatitis, should be excluded.

Biliary ultrasound should identify the presence of bile duct dilatation (not seen in BA, but characteristic of other surgical causes) and whether the gallbladder is atrophic, dilated or abnormal. The 'triangular cord sign' may be identified and represents the solid proximal bile ducts within the porta hepatis between right and left portal veins. The appearance of the liver is usually homogeneous, becoming irregular with the onset of cirrhosis.

Percutaneous liver biopsy will identify histological features of 'large duct obstruction', including biliary ductule proliferation and bile plugs. Radioisotope hepatobiliary scan is a useful diagnostic procedure. The presence of radioisotope in the intestine excludes the diagnosis of BA.

Differential diagnosis

- Obstructed choledochal malformation (invariably cystic at this age)

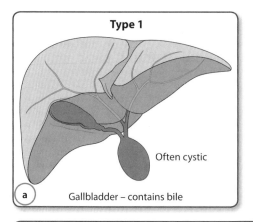

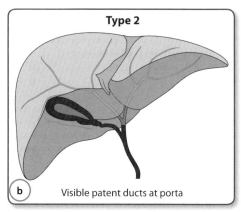

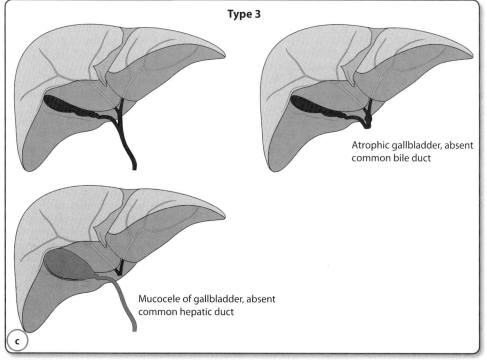

Figure 5 Classification of biliary atresia: (a) type 1, which is found in ~5% of patients; (b) type 2, which is found in ~2% of patients; and (c) type 3, which is found in > 90% of patients.

- Inspissated bile syndrome (usually preterm, may have had surgery and parenteral nutrition)
- Spontaneous perforation of bile duct (from 2 to 8 weeks of life)
- Tumours (**Table 1**)

Treatment

- Kasai portoenterostomy (> 90%)

- Liver transplantation (up to 10% depending on availability) – indicated in older infants (older than 100 days), with features of irretrievable cirrhosis

Operative details: Kasai portoenterostomy

- Confirmation of BA by visualisation ± cholangiogram

Table 1 Surgical jaundice in infancy

Cause	Antenatal features	Postnatal features	Investigations	Interventions
Biliary atresia	5% will have detectable cyst present	↑Jaundice	US: non-dilated ducts, atrophic gallbladder Liver biopsy: biliary ductule proliferation and bile plugs	Kasai portoenterostomy (>90%) Liver transplant
Choledochal malformation	Most common cause of 'subhepatic or hepatic cyst'	↑Jaundice	US and MRI scan: dilated intrahepatic ducts, obvious cyst	Laparotomy: excision and hepaticojejunostomy
Inspissated bile syndrome or gallstones	Nil	Intermittent jaundice; often preterm, history of sepsis or haemolysis	US and MRI scan: dilated CBD, bile sludge, even stones, visible	Ursodeoxycholic acid if CBD <3 mm diameter Consider percutaneous transhepatic cholangiogram if CBD >3 mm
Spontaneous perforation of bile duct	Nil	Delay in onset of jaundice; abdominal distension, vomiting with pigmented umbilicus or hydroceles	US: subhepatic collection, usually non-dilated ducts Radioisotope: shows leakage into abdominal cavity	Laparotomy: T tube, primary repair or hepaticojejunostomy
Tumours (rare), e.g. haemangiomas	Liver lesion(s)	Hepatomegaly, cardiac failure, ↓ platelet count	US and CT scan: mass lesion within liver or head of pancreas	Depends on tumour type

CBD, common bile duct; MRI, magnetic resonance imaging; US, ultrasound scan.

- Looking for other elements of BASM syndrome (situs inversus, preduodenal portal vein and absence of vena cava)
- Mobilisation of liver (division of left triangular and falciform ligaments) and extraction of at least left lobe from abdominal cavity
- Dissection of gallbladder from bed and mobilisation of (usually) obliterated biliary tract from vascular elements of portal triad; division of common bile duct and separation of remnants to the level of proximal porta hepatis – requires visualisation of right and left portal veins
- Complete resection of all biliary remnants from porta
- Creation of 40 cm long Roux loop
- Wide portoenterostomy using absorbable monofilament sutures (6/0)

Postoperative care

Antibiotics, such as tazocin and gentamicin, and high-dose steroids (prednisolone) are administered. Fat-soluble vitamin deficiencies are corrected. High-calorie formula infant feeds (supplemented with medium chain triglycerides) are provided.

Complications

- Cirrhosis and liver failure
- Ascites
- Portal hypertension, leading to splenomegaly, hypersplenism and oesophagogastric varices
- Pulmonary arteriovenous shunting

Outcome

- Those with cystic BA and non-cirrhotic livers at presentation have a better prognosis. BASM and CMV IgM-positive-associated BA have a poor prognosis
- More than 50% of patients will clear their jaundice to normal levels, which is the best guide to medium- and long-term outcome
- The 5- and 10-year native liver survival in the UK is about 45–50%, with overall survival being >90%

Further reading

Caponcelli E, Knisely AS, Davenport M. Cystic biliary atresia: an etiologic and prognostic subgroup. J Pediatr Surg 2008; 43:1619–1624.

Davenport M, Ong E, Sharif K, et al. Biliary atresia in England and Wales: results of centralization and new benchmark. J Pediatr Surg 2011; 46:1689–1694.

Mack CL. The pathogenesis of biliary atresia: evidence for a virus-induced autoimmune disease. Semin Liver Dis 2007; 27:233–242.

Related topics of interest

Bladder dysfunction

Learning outcomes

- To understand the fundamental principles of bladder innervation and function
- To understand the principles of assessment and treatment of children with bladder problems
- To learn the clinical features suggestive of high-risk bladder dysfunction

Overview

Bladder dysfunction includes a very wide spectrum of clinical abnormalities that can damage kidney function as well as cause lower urinary tract symptoms (LUTS) and social difficulties. Bladder dysfunction usually presents with LUTS or urinary tract infections (UTIs). For some, neuropathic bladder can be predicted from congenital or acquired neurological problems and needs proactive management from the outset. Detailed clinical assessment and investigation is needed to enable formulation of an individualised treatment plan, usually delivered in a multidisciplinary setting. This should be directed towards preserving renal function, preventing progressive bladder damage and reducing the frequency and impact of UTIs as well as optimising continence and social integration.

Epidemiology and pathology

To work effectively, the bladder needs be able to store an adequate volume of urine at a safe pressure and empty voluntarily and completely. Most children become dry during the day by the age of 3 years, and 90–95% become dry at night by 7 years.

The cerebral cortex exerts conscious and unconscious control over the pontine micturition centre and spinal micturition centres to control normal bladder function. This is mediated through:

- **Pelvic parasympathetic nerves (S2–S4):** these stimulate the detrusor and bladder muscle
- **Sympathetic nerves (T10–L2) from the hypogastric plexus:** these contract the trigone and urethral muscle and also relax the detrusor muscle
- **Somatic nerves (S2–S4) from the sacral plexus:** these provide bladder sensation and motor innervation to the voluntary external urethral sphincter and pelvic floor

Bladder dysfunction can be classified simply in relation to its normal function:

- Failure to store urine:
  - **Detrusor:** poor compliance, involuntary contractions, small capacity bladder and sensory abnormalities
  - **Bladder outflow tract inadequate resistance:** physiological, anatomical or psychological
- Failure to empty voluntarily and completely:
  - **Detrusor weakness:** neurogenic, myogenic, psychological and idiopathic
  - **High outlet resistance:** neurogenic, anatomical, physiological (e.g. sphincter dyssynergia) and psychological

Many patients with neuropathic bladders will have complex associated problems (e.g. paraplegia), but others may have only bladder problems and some may even have no other demonstrable neurological abnormality.

Functional voiding disorders are those not associated with any neurological abnormality. They include a wide spectrum, from benign but troublesome conditions to those that place the kidneys at risk (e.g. Hinman syndrome). Many are also associated with constipation and/or faecal soiling.

Aetiology

Bladder dysfunction has many causes:

- **Congenital:** spinal dysraphism, syringomyelia, diastematomyelia, sacral anomalies and caudal regression
- **Traumatic:** direct spinal cord injury or ischaemia and extensive pelvic surgery
- **Inflammatory:** infection and transverse myelitis
- **Neoplastic:** sacrococcygeal teratoma, neuroblastoma and bladder and prostate rhabdomyosarcoma

- **Vascular:** spinal cord ischaemia and thrombosis
- **Functional:** disturbed voiding patterns and toilet phobia or refusal
- Idiopathic

Clinical features

Many patients with neuropathic bladders will present at birth (e.g. spina bifida and those with prenatally diagnosed or suspected spinal abnormalities), but many are diagnosed later, usually presenting with continence problems and/or urine infection. Some may present acutely with severe urosepsis and renal failure.

Features suggestive of more serious conditions are recurrent UTI and secondary day or night wetting (having been dry for a period of at least 6 months) and features of renal compromise, including hypertension, proteinuria and dilatation.

A full history is needed, taking note of the pattern and severity of wetting, voiding habit (including strength and quality of the urine stream), whether it is primary or secondary, urine infection and bowel function. A full social and developmental history is also needed. Clinical examination should include the abdomen, blood pressure, the spine for stigmata of spinal disease, perineum and genitalia, assessment of perineal sensation, lower limb reflexes and gait, and also urine microscopy and dipstick testing. Initial assessment should also include an assessment of overall development, behaviour and family dynamics.

Investigations

Investigations are guided by a very detailed clinical history and clinical examination:
- Urine culture and biochemical renal function assessment are useful
- Non-invasive urodynamic assessment enables a diagnosis to be made in almost all children and can be done in the outpatient setting. This includes a detailed bladder diary (including voided volume, frequency and time and severity of wetting), urine flowmetry and post void residual volume

- Ultrasonography can identify upper urinary tract dilatation, gross scarring, bladder muscle hypertrophy, bladder emptying and can also be used to assess the spinal cord in infants younger than 4 months
- Other imaging investigations may be needed, depending on the initial clinical presentation, such as urine infection or obstruction (micturating cystourethrogram, DMSA kidney scan, MAG3 excretion urogram or MAG3 indirect cystogram)
- A videocystometrogram may be needed to help make a diagnosis or provide reassurance but is usually used to assess the degree of risk (safe capacity of the bladder) and for planning surgical reconstruction. It also enables assessment of the shape and wall of the bladder, and the presence of vesicoureteric reflux and diverticulae. The normal bladder holds urine at low pressure until micturition is initiated. Storage pressures > 30 cm H_2O indicate a major risk to the upper tracts and need urgent attention
- Investigation of underlying cause and associated anomalies (e.g. spinal MRI) is required

Differential diagnosis

Other causes of urine infection or urinary tract dilatation need to be considered:
- Anatomical causes of incontinence – epispadias, fistula, ectopic ureter in girls, cloaca

Treatment

Treatment needs to be tailored to the individual and considered from the physiological, pharmacological, psychosocial and surgical perspectives. For functional disorders, the first steps are to make a diagnosis, identify potential risk to renal function and then to optimise the voiding pattern and treat any coexisting constipation. A strong programme of education and support is essential. The following additional measures may be helpful:
- To increase urine storage:

- Gentle stretching of the bladder by increasing fluid intake and improving bladder habit
- Anticholinergics (e.g. oxybutynin) to relax the detrusor – caution is needed if bladder emptying is incomplete
- Sympathomimetics (e.g. ephedrine) to increase outflow resistance but only if bladder pressures are not high and emptying is adequate
- To improve emptying:
  - Double micturition and timed regular voiding
  - Alpha-blocking agents to reduce outflow resistance, as in dysfunctional voiding or sphincter dyssynergia
  - Clean intermittent catheterisation (CIC) may need to be considered if emptying remains poor and the above measures fail

Urine infection should be treated with short courses of antibiotics or low-dose prophylaxis if indicated.

Injection of botulinum toxin (see below) has been used in children with functional voiding disorders but does carry the risk of needing bladder catheterisation acutely or exacerbating incontinence. More specific forms of functional problems need a different approach.

- Nocturnal enuresis is an underrated problem causing a lot of distress, sleep disturbance, reduced school performance and social disruption. It occurs largely as a failure to wake to pass urine and may be exacerbated by poor nocturnal concentration of urine, small bladder capacity and bladder overactivity. Most children are dry at night by 7 years, but for 1%, particularly those who have never had a single dry night, this can persist into adulthood. Desmopressin (particularly for those with poor nocturnal urine concentration) and nocturnal enuresis alarms help in about 70% of cases and are usually started from the age of 7 years
- Mild stress incontinence may respond to pelvic floor exercises
- The extreme daytime frequency syndrome occurs sporadically in children, usually aged 3–8 years, and is associated with extreme frequency during the day but without wetting and without any disturbance at night. It is a self-resolving condition of unknown cause and strong reassurance is the principal focus of management. Anticholinergics have been used but usually make little difference to the natural history of this condition, which tends to remit after weeks or even several months
- Giggle incontinence is associated with complete and uncontrollable bladder emptying, associated with giggling or being tickled. It is triggered by a central reflex and is not caused by primary bladder dysfunction. Many respond well to methylphenidate
- Post void dribbling in girls occurs as a result of vaginal pooling during micturition and can be improved or cured by modifying posture during micturition
- Management of functional voiding disorders at the more severe end of the spectrum (e.g. Ochoa syndrome, Hinman syndrome or 'non-neuropathic neuropathic bladder') requires treatment along the same lines as neuropathic bladder

Children with neuropathic bladders require close surveillance and a proactive approach to protect the kidneys throughout childhood and adult life. The principles of treatment are similar. Most will need CIC supported with anticholinergic agents to improve capacity and dry interval. Ephedrine can also be used to increase sphincter tone but only if the bladder has a good capacity at safe pressures (<20–30 cm H_2O). If conservative measures fail, surgery needs to be considered.

There are many surgical approaches and all require thorough assessment of the bladder, child and family before going ahead, and include:

- **Suprapubic catheter or button:** This is generally a short-term emergency measure
- **Vesicostomy:** This is a good temporising measure in children of nappy age who have an unsafe bladder
- **Botulinum toxin:** This is gaining in popularity. It can be injected into the bladder to increase compliance or into the

sphincters to reduce outflow resistance It does need to be repeated at 6-month intervals, and the long-term effects are still unknown

- **Catheterising conduits:** Appendicovesicostomy (Mitrofanoff procedure) is performed for those unable to catheterise urethrally for anatomical reasons or urethral sensitivity
- **Bladder augmentation:** This increases capacity using a segment of ileum, colon or stomach
- **Bladder neck repair and urethral sling procedures:** This is usually used in conjunction with augmentation if there is little or no outlet resistance. Many techniques are in use, including the Young–Dees, Kropp and Pippe-Salle procedures, complete bladder neck closure, bladder neck suspension, urethral sling procedures or artificial urethral sphincters
- **Urinary diversion:** Ileal conduit or continent complete bladder replacement procedures are used with a pouch of bowel. These are now less popular because of long-term problems with dilatation and sepsis and are usually carried out as salvage procedures

Further reading

Abrams P, Cardozo L, Fall M, et al. The standardisation of terminology in lower urinary tract function. Report from the Standardisation Sub-committee of the International Continence Society. Urology 2003; 61:37–49.

Related topics of interest

Branchial remnants

Learning outcomes

- To know the relevant embryology
- To understand the pathology of branchial arch remnants
- To know the operative steps

Overview

There are four pairs of branchial arches interposed by clefts which develop between 4 and 8 weeks after fertilisation. There are also two pairs of rudimentary arches. The fifth arch is normally absent in humans.

Branchial remnants occur due to either the failure of these embryonic structures to fully mature or their persistence in an aberrant fashion. Being congenital they are present at birth, but may not be noticed until they are symptomatic. Elective excision of a non-inflamed remnant is the treatment of choice.

Epidemiology and aetiology

The head and neck structures are derived from these arches and clefts.

- **First arch:** This forms the mandible with a contribution to the maxillary process of the upper jaw and auditory ossicles
- **First cleft:** This contributes to the tympanic cavity, eustachian tube and external auditory meatus
- **Second arch:** This forms part of the hyoid bone and the tonsillar fossa cleft
- **Second cleft:** This forms the tonsils and adenoids
- **Third arch:** This produces the remainder of the hyoid bone
- **Third cleft:** This forms the inferior parathyroids and the thymus
- **Fourth and sixth arches:** These form the laryngeal cartilage, including thyroid and cricoid cartilages
- **Fourth cleft:** The dorsal portion forms the superior parathyroids, and the ventral portion contributes to the ultimobranchial body, which in turn contributes to

thyrocalcitonin, producing parafollicular cells in the thyroid gland

First branchial anomalies (~8% of all branchial remnants) are rare, and cysts may occur around the ear or inferior to the earlobe. External openings can be found in a suprahyoid position inferior to the mandible. The tract may be associated with or course through the parotid and may be deep to the facial nerve; 30% open into the external auditory canal.

Second branchial anomalies (~92%) occasionally form cysts, and if they have an external opening it is along the anterior border of sternocleidomastoid muscle at the junction of the middle and lower thirds. The tract passes through platysma and cervical fascia. It ascends along the carotid sheath, then through the carotid bifurcation and behind the posterior belly of digastric, anterior to the XII nerve, and ends in the tonsillar fossa. The internal opening is generally found here, but can be anywhere in the naso- or oropharynx; 10% are bilateral.

Third branchial cleft anomalies are unusual, but are in the same area as second anomalies. However, they ascend behind the carotid artery rather than through the bifurcation, and the fistula passes through the thyrohyoid membrane and into the piriform sinus.

Fourth cleft remnants are exceedingly rare and can be difficult to differentiate from the other anomalies. The tract originates at the piriform sinus and travels inferiorly in the tracheoesophageal groove, posterior to the thyroid gland, and into the thorax, looping below the aorta on the left and subclavian artery on the right. The descending part of this tract before the first loop is the most common location of clinical infection. The tract then courses superiorly, posterior to the common carotid artery, and ascending in the neck to reach the hypoglossal nerve. It then makes a second loop around the hypoglossal nerve and finishes its course at the medial border of the sternocleidomastoid muscle. They occasionally form cysts which must be differentiated from laryngoceles. Malignant degeneration has been reported in branchial cleft remnants which have persisted to adulthood.

Clinical features

Sinuses, fistulae and cartilaginous remnants are typically noted in infancy, whereas cysts are more commonly noted in childhood or early adulthood.

Signs and symptoms include the following:

- Mucoid drainage from a small opening along the border of sternocleidomastoid indicates a sinus or fistula. The tract should be palpated and discharge observed to confirm the diagnosis
- Cysts lie deep to the skin along the anterior border of sternocleidomastoid
- Infected cysts and tracts can be the first symptom of a branchial remnant

Investigations

- Ultrasound scan to identify the cystic nature of the mass if not clinically obvious

Differential diagnosis

- Cystic hygroma, other lymphatic and vascular malformations
- Dermoids
- Parotid lesions
- Primary or metastatic neoplasm
- Torticollic mass
- Skin lesions

Treatment

If infected at presentation, antibiotic therapy and warm soaks should be used to encourage the spontaneous drainage of mucoid plugs, but incision and drainage is sometimes required. Definitive surgery should be undertaken when no inflammation is present to decrease the risk of recurrence.

Surgical procedure

- Under general anaesthesia
- Supine position with neck hyperextended
- In the case of cysts, a transverse incision over the cyst should be made with dissection deepened to enucleate the entire cyst. If a fistula or sinus is present dissection should proceed as below:
- A small, elliptical incision is made around the external opening and deepened beneath the cervical fascia
- Initial dissection along the lower border of the incision, so the tract is uninjured
- Dissection superiorly staying on the tract until visualising the upper portion becomes difficult. At this point a 'step ladder' second transverse incision can be made to give better exposure
- The tract is pulled through the second incision and dissection continued to the point of insertion into the pharynx. The tract should be ligated with a non-absorbable suture
- The tract can be filled with a methylene blue stain to facilitate dissection in more difficult cases, for instance in those with multiple previous infections
- The entire tract should be excised to prevent recurrence up to the
  - external auditory meatus in first cleft anomalies
  - tonsillar fossa in second cleft anomalies
  - piriform fossa in third cleft anomalies
- Care must be taken to avoid injury to associated structures
  - Facial nerve branches in first cleft anomalies
  - Hypoglossal, glossopharyngeal, spinal accessory and vagus nerves in second cleft anomalies

The recurrence rate is reported as < 7% in most series.

Further reading

Bajaj Y, Ifeacho S, Tweedie D, et al. Branchial anomalies in children. Int J Pediatr Otorhinolaryng 2011; 75:1020–1023. Epub 15 June 2011.

Nicoucar K, Giger R, Pope HG Jr, et al. Management of congenital fourth branchial arch anomalies: a review and analysis of published cases. J Pediatr Surg 2009l; 44:1432–1439.

Related topics of interest

Central venous access techniques

Learning outcomes

- To understand the indications for central venous access
- To be familiar with the different types of central lines
- To be aware of the range of line insertion techniques and to recognise common complications

Overview

Central venous access is essential to modern paediatric practice and is gained by either surgical cut-down or percutaneous cannulation, using anatomical landmarks or real-time ultrasound guidance. The latter improves safety and success. The techniques can be difficult and risky, and many institutions provide a vascular access service to coordinate the scheduling and insertion of devices with appropriate radiological and theatre support.

Indications and devices

Indications include:
- Parenteral nutrition
- Chemotherapy
- Haemodialysis or plasmapheresis
- Drug delivery – inotropes, irritant drugs
- Difficult peripheral access
- Sampling and measurement

Long-term central venous access devices (peripherally inserted central catheters and neonatal long lines)

Long-term central venous access devices are small-bore catheters inserted via peripheral veins. The tip should lie in a central vein or the right atrium. Peripherally inserted central catheter (PICC) lines have the advantage of relatively easy placement but malposition is common.

Tunnelled catheters (Hickman and Broviac)

These devices are intended for long-term use and are made of silicone to ensure biocompatibility. They are available in a range of diameters, chosen according to the size of the child, and may have up to three lumina depending on the proposed therapy. Subcutaneous tunnelling reduces microbial entrance, and an internal dacron cuff near the exit site anchors the line by fibrous adhesion. The catheters are cut to length at the time of insertion, leaving them open ended distally.

Tunnelled lines with valved endings (Groshong) are similar to Hickman lines, but have a blind distal end with a slit-like opening which acts as a valve to prevent inflow of blood and clot formation within the catheter.

Tunnelled dialysis catheters (Haemocath) are of large internal diameter to maximise blood flow. Additionally, the tips of each lumen are staggered or separated and sited within the right atrium to minimise recirculation of afferent and efferent blood. The internal jugular vein is preferred to avoid thrombosis of the subclavian vein or impaired run-off from potential sites for arteriovenous fistulae.

Totally implantable ports (e.g. vascuport and portacath) consist of a catheter connected to an internal chamber, which is secured with sutures and which does not require a cuff. Access to the line is gained with a needle inserted through the skin and the port membrane. The need to pierce the skin may make it unacceptable to some children. The absence of any permanent external part reduces infection risk.

Investigations

A clotting screen and platelet count are requested because haemorrhage is a common complication and is potentially life-threatening. Indicators of sepsis such as white cell count, C-reactive protein and blood cultures may be helpful, as localised or systemic sepsis is a relative contraindication.

Previous difficult central access or multiple large superficial collateral veins suggest possible thrombosis of the great vessels. The operator may choose to investigate venous patency preoperatively with Doppler ultrasound, venography, computed tomographic angiography or magnetic resonance venography, or to proceed directly with line placement, with on-table ultrasound and venography.

Insertion techniques

PICC and neonatal long lines

A peripheral intravenous cannula, of an appropriate diameter to allow passage of the central line, is placed by locating a peripheral vein, either visually or with ultrasound guidance. Before placement, the required length of the catheter should be estimated by measuring from the point of insertion, along the path of the veins to the required location of the catheter tip. Following insertion, the redundant catheter is coiled on the skin and the line is secured with dressings.

Tunnelled lines

Tunnelled lines are inserted using either an open cut-down or a percutaneous technique. The patient is placed on a radiolucent operating table, and the skin is prepared with 2% chlorhexidine gluconate and draped.

In both techniques, a subcutaneous tunnel is created by the passage of an introducer, drawing the catheter towards the point of entry in the vein from a relatively distant skin incision, chosen as the exit site; this should be in a comfortable position and away from stoma sites. The dacron cuff is placed under the skin close to the exit site.

The open technique involves skin incision followed by location and mobilisation of a suitable vein. Once secured, the vessel is incised longitudinally, and the catheter is advanced from the tunnel, cut to the correct length and inserted into the vein. Haemostasis is achieved with sutures.

The percutaneous method involves needle cannulation of the vein, with or without ultrasound guidance, introduction of a Seldinger wire towards the heart and advancement of a splittable introducer sheath over the wire with fluoroscopic guidance – the relatively large rigid sheath has the potential to damage internal structures, with occasional disastrous consequences. The portion of the line to be placed within the vein is drawn out of the tunnel and introduced via the peel-away sheath into the vein. Haemostasis is achieved with gentle digital pressure and the skin is closed.

Common to both techniques is the need to ensure good flow in the catheter and suitable line tip position with fluoroscopy. The line should then be flushed, usually with a heparinised solution and secured with sutures and sterile dressings.

The relative benefits of the two techniques, the use of ultrasound guidance and line tip position, are matters of considerable debate. Very narrow-bore lines such as neonatal long lines and 2.7 Fr Broviac lines should be radiographed with contrast if tip position cannot be visualised without contrast. The literature suggests that specialist teams reduce complication rates.

Complications

Complications can be divided into early and late.

Early complications include:
- Malposition
- Haemorrhage
- Damage to adjacent structures
- Haemo- or pneumothorax
- Air embolism and thromboembolism
- Internal displacement
- Accidental removal

Late complications include:
- Infection (local or systemic)
- Catheter damage, including complete separation and potential embolisation
- Blockage from an external fibrin sheath or intra luminal thrombus

Future developments are likely to include refinements in ultrasound imaging and improved catheter materials to reduce infection and fibrin sheath formation. Obligatory registration and follow-up of implantable devices would allow more accurate estimation of complication rates and improve comparison between devices and insertion techniques.

Further reading

Arul GS, et al. Ultrasound-guided percutaneous insertion of Hickman lines in children. Prospective study of 500 consecutive procedures. J Pediatr Surg 2009; 44:1371–1376.

Arul GS, et al. Ultrasound-guided percutaneous insertion of 2.7Fr tunnelled Broviac lines in neonates and small infants. Paediatr Surg Int 2010; 26:815–818.

Hatfield A, Bodenham A. Portable ultrasound for difficult central venous access. Br J Anaesth 1999; 82:822–826.

National Institute for Clinical Excellence. Guidance on the use of ultrasound locating devices for placing central venous catheters. London: NICE, 2002.

Chest wall deformities

Learning outcomes

- To be able to recognise and assess common chest wall abnormalities
- To know indications and timing of interventions
- To be aware of the surgical options available

Overview

Pectus excavatum (PE) and carinatum (PC) are the result of an overgrowth in ribs and cartilage. Sternal defects (including ectopia cordis and pentalogy of Cantrell), Poland syndrome, Jeune and Jarcho–Levin syndromes result from agenesis, atresia or dysplasia of various chest wall structures. Many of these, fortunately very rare, conditions are incompatible with life. The complex multidisciplinary management of the remainder is beyond the scope of this topic.

Epidemiology and aetiology

Chest deformities occur in 1 per 1000 children. Ninety per cent are PE, most of the remainder being isolated PC or mixed pectus deformities. The other defects between them comprise < 1% of all chest wall abnormalities.

Up to 80% of pectus deformities occur in males and one-third of patients report a positive family history. However, no firm genetic link has yet been established.

The exact pathophysiology of pectus defects is unknown; the theory is that abnormal cartilage growth causes the sternum to be displaced. In PE there is a dipping of the sternum, and in PC there is a protrusion of the sternum. Both defects can be symmetrical or asymmetrical and have varying torsion of the sternum. Up to 30% are associated with scoliosis or connective tissue disorders, such as Marfan and Ehlers–Danlos syndromes. Acquired deformities can occur after repair of large congenital diaphragmatic herniae.

Clinical features

PE can be present at birth but most, along with PC, become evident during the pubertal growth spurt. Most patients present with psychosocial and body image issues which affect their willingness to expose themselves for participation in sporting activities. However, easy fatigue, breathlessness, wheeze and palpitations are frequently reported during exercise. Upper respiratory tract infections as well as chest and back pain are also frequently reported. Pectus patients have a typical hunched forward posture, trying to hide the defect. This enhances the cosmetic appearance of PE.

Investigations

- A detailed physical examination recording features of the defect and signs of associated conditions
- Plain chest radiograph
- Clinical photographs
- CT scan with Haller index (internal transverse diameter/anteroposterior diameter at the level of defect) in PE
- Static and exercise pulmonary function testing
- Echocardiogram in PE
- Nickel allergy testing for Nuss procedure

Treatment

Patient selection is paramount to the appropriate management of pectus deformities. The following elements should be considered:

- Haller index > 3.2
- Cardiac or pulmonary compression or cardiac displacement
- Progressive defect
- Mitral valve prolapse, cardiac conduction abnormalities
- Restrictive or obstructive lung disease
- Significant body image issues

Operative intervention should be delayed until mid to late adolescence when the patient has gone through their growth spurt and can make independent informed decisions. Only significantly symptomatic younger children require earlier intervention. Asymptomatic mild-to-moderate defects are managed conservatively with breathing and postural physiotherapy.

The non-operative treatment of PC has advanced over the last 10 years with bracing techniques. The dynamic compression system uses curved aluminium segments to form a rigid belt attached to a unique cushioned compression plate that applies a constant preset pressure over the protrusion (**Figure 6**). Patients are advised to wear the device at night and during as much of the day as possible except for sporting activities and bathing. Good to excellent results have been reported in 88.4% of patients who used the device for a mean of 7.2 hours per day for 7 months (range 3–20). These exciting results suggest that it should be the first option in the management of PC; moreover, patients with lesser defects could be treated and at a younger age.

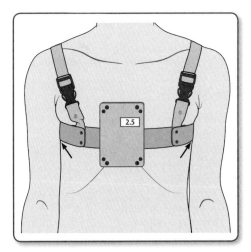

Figure 6 Illustration of the dynamic compression system. The docking device, which sets the treatment pressure at consultation, is attached. Arrows indicate space for thoracic expansion during inspiration.

- Nuss procedure – minimally invasive correction of PE. Not suitable for asymmetric and mixed defects
  - The bar is custom bent at the table except for nickel allergy when a custom built titanium bar is ordered
  - Lateral transverse incisions are made in line with the midpoint of the depression
  - A subcutaneous tunnel is created from the lateral chest to the top of the pectus ridge on each side
  - A 1 cm wide curved metal introducer is passed through the tunnel and into the thoracic cavity at the right pectus ridge. Careful dissection between the underside of the sternum and the pericardium is conducted under thoracoscopic guidance
  - The introducer is brought out through the left pectus ridge and opposite tunnel
  - Repeated simultaneous elevation of the sternum with the introducer and downward pressure applied to the lower costal margin corrects the sternal depression
  - The introducer is withdrawn after attaching a guide tape
  - The inverted bar is then placed by attaching the tape and following the dissected tunnel
  - The bar is turned to correct the sternal depression
  - The bar is stabilised on both sides using the supplied stabilisers with strong non-absorbable sutures
  - Bar in situ for 2–4 years. Consider two bars for longer or deeper defects
- Complications:
  - Pain (premedication, epidural or patient-controlled analgesia, pain-modifying drugs)
  - Pneumothorax, haemothorax, pleural effusion or cardiac tamponade
  - Damage to the internal mammary artery
  - Wound or bar infection, pericarditis, consider nickel allergy
  - Bar displacement
  - Overcorrection

- Ravitch operation
  - Midline sternal or transverse inframammary incision, skin flaps elevated
  - Pectoralis major and rectus abdominis muscles reflected off sternum
  - Longitudinal perichondrial incision, remove entire deformed cartilage
  - Anterior sternal osteotomy at angle of Louis:
    - In PE, the posterior table is fractured, sternum elevated and osteotomy closed with non-absorbable sutures
    - In PC, the osteotomy is wedged open with some of the resected costal cartilages to place the sternum in a neutral position
    - In both, some ingenuity is required to correct any sternal torsion
  - A metal sternal bar may be placed and secured to adjacent ribs to stop the sternum being flail or sinking
  - Perichondrial 'sleeves' are resutured, drains left in situ and the muscles resutured
- Excellent results but it is a major procedure
- Complications:
  - Bleeding (significant but rarely requiring transfusion)
  - Post–operative pain, shorter reported duration and severity than with Nuss procedure
  - Cartilage protrusion
  - Hypertrophic scars
  - Acquired asphyxiating chondrodystrophy

Further reading

Lopushshinsky SR, Fecteau AH. Pectus deformities: review of open surgery in the modern era. Semin Pediatr Surg 2008; 17:201–208.

Martinez-Ferro M, Fraire C, Bernard S. Dynamic compression system for the correction of pectus carinatum. Semin Pediatr Surg 2008; 17:194–200.

Nuss D. Chest wall deformities. Pediatric surgery and urology long-term outcomes, 2nd edn. Cambridge University Press, 2006:135–148.

Related topics of interest

- Congenital diaphragmatic hernia (p. 65)

Child protection

Learning outcomes

- To understand that safeguarding children is everyone's business
- To recognise the main types of child abuse
- To know what features of history and examination may be of concern
- To be aware of how to seek advice and make a child protection referral

Overview

Safeguarding children is everyone's business. The Children Act applies to all children younger than 18 years, including older teenagers presenting to adult services. Child protection refers to activities that protect children who are suffering, or are likely to suffer, significant harm. Harm may be physical (including fabricated or induced illness), emotional, sexual or neglect.

Epidemiology

Department of Education (UK) figures from 31 March 2011 show that there were 42,300 children who were the subjects of a child protection plan in England.

Aetiology

According to 2010 data, the proportions of different types of abuse were:

- Neglect – 44%
- Emotional – 28%
- Physical – 13%
- Sexual abuse – 6%

Clinical features

Physical abuse

Features of the history which may raise concerns about the possibility of abuse include:

- Injury is unexplained
- History is implausible, e.g. multiple fractures and brain haemorrhage following a low fall
- History is inconsistent and keeps changing
- Delayed presentation
- Injury out of keeping with child's development, e.g. long bone fracture in a non-mobile infant
- Direct disclosure by the child

Types of injuries that may be seen include:

- Bruises
- Burns and scalds
- Fractures
- Abdominal injury
- Oral or dental injury
- Fabricated or induced illness

Injuries such as bruises become more common because children become more mobile. Any unexplained injury in a non-mobile infant requires referral to safeguarding colleagues and thorough investigation to look for hidden injuries and exclude medical causes.

Clinicians may be asked by the social care provider or the police to age bruises to help their investigation. Clinicians should not attempt to estimate the age of a bruise by its colour because there is a lack of evidence to support this. Many factors influence the colour, including the degree of force used and whether the bruise is on a bony prominence or soft tissue. Factors which may help determine whether an injury is more likely to be due to accidental or non-accidental cause are shown in **Table 2**.

Morbidity and mortality rates in abdominal injuries are higher for abusive rather than accidental causes. Bowel and solid organ injuries both occur. It is extremely rare for children under 5 years to present with accidental small bowel injuries, and if there is inadequate explanation, child abuse must be excluded. Bruising may be absent in abused children and there needs to be a low index of suspicion in children with non-specific abdominal symptoms and other abusive injuries.

Neglect

Neglect is the persistent failure to meet a child's physical and psychological needs and may manifest as:

- Failure to thrive, which resolves when the child is admitted to hospital

Table 2 Patterns of injury in accidental versus non-accidental injuries		
Injury type	More common (but not exclusive) in accidental injury	Suspicious for non-accidental injury
Bruise	Front of body Bony prominences Sites – shins, knees, forehead, mouth, chin, nose	Back of body Soft tissues Pattern of an implement (belt, shoe) Sites – eyes, ears, buttocks, abdomen, neck, cheeks Petechiae are a strong predictor of abusive injury
Burn	Poorly demarcated	Well demarcated Imprint of an object (cigarette, iron)
Scald	Asymmetrical Splash marks, often upper body (pulling hot drink over self) Varied burn depth	Symmetrical Glove and stocking (immersion of limbs in hot water) Consistent burn depth
Fracture	Children with greater mobility Single	Infants under 18 months, especially if non-mobile Multiple Metaphyseal Ribs, vertebrae, sternum, pelvis
Skull fracture	Single, linear, parietal	Single, linear, parietal (difficult to distinguish) Multiple, complex, wide fractures raise suspicion but evidence is conflicting

- Recurrent, persistent infestations (head lice and scabies)
- Very poor hygiene
- Inadequate clothing
- Severe dental caries
- Carers failing to bring a child for appointments
- Non-compliance with treatment plans
- Lack of supervision, which may result in accidental injuries

Emotional abuse

Emotional issues are found in all forms of abuse, but may particularly present with behavioural problems, including
- Secondary enuresis
- Encopresis
- Eating disorders
- Self-harm
- Risk-taking

Sexual abuse

Sexual abuse may be of two types: contact (genital touching or penetration) or non-contact (grooming online). It may be perpetrated by either gender. The examination may be normal or non-specific even following penetrative abuse. If a child makes a disclosure or if there is clinical suspicion about the possibility of sexual abuse, specialist advice should be sought.

Common symptoms include vaginal discharge, anogenital bleeding, recurrent urinary tract infections and secondary enuresis. Because these symptoms are common in non-abused children, sexual abuse should be considered when symptoms do not respond to usual treatments or when there are concerning behaviours such as inappropriate sexualised behaviour or self-harm.

Disabled children

Disabled children are particularly vulnerable because they may be unable to make a disclosure, have different bruising patterns (no bruising on shins) and in cases of inadequate nutrition, it may be difficult to determine whether the cause is organic disease or neglect.

Investigations

All child protection issues should be discussed with senior paediatric colleagues. Investigations may be arranged to identify hidden injuries, particularly in children younger than 2 years, or to exclude other differential diagnoses. Children in whom sexual abuse is suspected may require sexually transmitted infection screening, serology for blood-borne viruses or pregnancy testing.

Differential diagnosis

Physical abuse

- Bruises:
  - Coagulation defects
  - Mongolian blue spots
- Burns and scalds:
  - Impetigo mimicking cigarette burns
  - Staphylococcal scalded skin syndrome
- Fractures:
  - Osteogenesis imperfecta
  - Osteopenia

Neglect

- Organic failure to thrive such as coeliac disease

Emotional abuse

- Constipation with overflow soiling

- Attention deficit hyperactivity disorder
- Other mental health problems

Sexual abuse

- Straddle injuries
- Urethral prolapse
- Vulvovaginitis
- Constipation causing fissures

Treatment

If the clinician is concerned that a child may be at risk of or has suffered significant harm, then he or she should make a referral to social services or the police as per local policy. Trusts have safeguarding teams who can provide advice and support regarding making referrals (**Figure 7**). All aspects of child protection work should be documented fully, including conversations.

Information sharing is an important part of safeguarding children from abuse and neglect. If it is safe to do so, parents or carers should be informed that information is being shared, including referrals to children's social

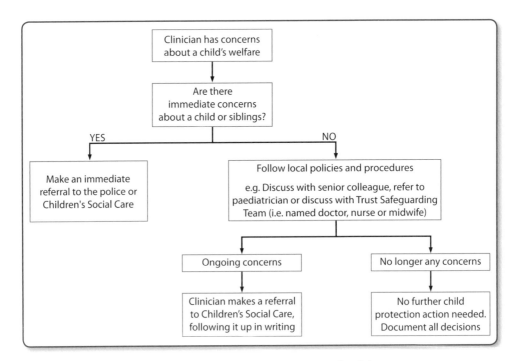

Figure 7 Actions to take if you are worried a child may be at risk or has suffered abuse.

care. The sharing of information should be appropriate, timely and proportionate. Physicians have a duty to share information if a child or young person is at risk of abuse, if sharing information would prevent or assist in the prosecution of a criminal offence or if a child or young person's actions are putting themselves or others at risk.

Further reading

Department of Health. What to do if you're worried a child is being abused. London: Department of Health, 2003.

Maguire S. Which injuries may indicate child abuse? Arch Dis Child Educ Pract Ed 2010; 95:170–177.

Working Together to Safeguard Children. A guide to inter-agency working to safeguard and promote the welfare of children. London: Department for Children, Schools and Families, 2013.

Related topics of interest

- Abdominal trauma (p. 1)
- Consent in paediatric surgery (p. 72)
- Faecal incontinence and idiopathic constipation (p. 115)

Choledochal malformation

Learning outcomes

- To be aware of variations in choledochal malformation
- To be familiar with methods of investigation
- To understand the nature of surgical approach

Overview

Choledochal malformation is a generic term to include different patterns of bile duct dilatation not associated with obstruction primarily. Most are probably of congenital origin.

Epidemiology and aetiology

There is a higher incidence in Asia, specifically in Japan, China and Taiwan. **Figure 8** illustrates King's College Hospital classification of choledochal malformation. The three most common variants are type 1c (choledochal cyst), type 1f (fusiform malformation) and type 4 (both intra- and extra hepatic dilatation).

Caroli's disease is distinct from most malformations because it has a clear genetic aetiology, liver fibrosis occurs irrespective of high biliary pressures and renal involvement is almost invariable.

The aetiology is not known. There are two broad theories of origin: distal bile duct stenosis and proximal dilatation versus reflux of pancreatic juice into the bile duct through the so-called common channel, allowing damage to bile duct lining and dilatation (Babbitt hypothesis). A common pancreatobiliary channel is a congenital anomaly found in >95% of primary choledochal malformations.

Recent studies have suggested that most dilatation arises as a result of sustained intrabiliary pressure due to a distal stenotic segment and that there is an inverse relationship between bile amylase (as a marker of pancreatic reflux) and pressure. Furthermore, epithelial damage and change is associated with elevated pressures, not elevated bile amylase levels.

Clinical features

The child may present with one or more of the following features:

- Conjugated jaundice (~50%)
- Acute pancreatitis (~25%)
- Antenatally detected hepatic or subhepatic cysts (15%)
- Palpable right upper quadrant mass (<5%)
- Cholangitis (<5%)
- Cirrhosis (<5%)
- Malignancy – needs time to develop and very rare in children

Investigations

Liver biochemistry may show elevated conjugated bilirubin, γ-glutamyl transpeptidase and aspartate transaminase levels. Elevated plasma amylase and lipase levels suggest ongoing pancreatic inflammation.

Biliary ultrasound should identify the degree of bile duct dilatation (cystic > fusiform) and any evidence of intrahepatic bile duct dilatation. Magnetic resonance cholangiopancreatography (MRCP) is a key investigation in determining the anatomy of the dilatation and the relationship with the pancreatic duct and hence choledochal variant.

In those with minor degrees of biliary dilatation or where choledocholithiasis may be possible, endoscopic retrograde cholangiopancreatography (ERCP) may be needed to enable correct diagnosis or initiate duct clearance.

Differential diagnosis

- Intrahepatic cyst of parenchyma (non-bile containing)
- Obstructed bile duct (with stones)
- Obstructed bile duct due to stenosis or stricture (uncommon) – will not have the common channel

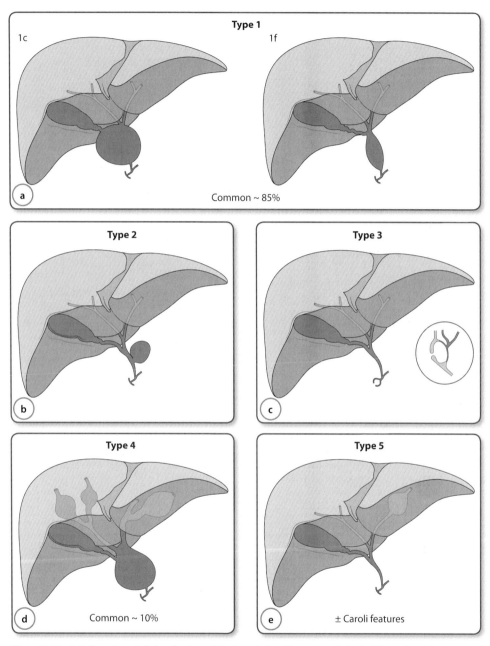

Figure 8 King's College Hospital classification of choledochal malformation. Note that 'forme fruste' choledochal malformation used to describe common channel and minimal biliary dilatation. Reproduced with permission from Makin E, Davenport M. Understanding choledochal malformation (review). Arch Dis Child 2012; 97:69–72.

Treatment

- Excision of choledochal malformation

Operative approach: choledochal malformation (open or laparoscopic)

- Antibiotics (e.g. tazocin and gentamicin), continued postoperatively
- Confirmation of diagnosis and anatomy by early cholangiogram
- Look for other anomalies of intrahepatic drainage
- Look for obstruction or dilatation of the common channel
- Dissection of gallbladder from bed and mobilisation of dilated extrahepatic biliary tract
- Division at the level of common hepatic duct – try to achieve single orifice
- Mobilisation within head of pancreas and identification of junction
- Consider endoscopy of the intrahepatic ducts and the common channel
- Consider transduodenal sphincteroplasty if ampullary stenosis or common channel dilatation and debris
- Roux loop (~40–50 cm) and hepaticojejunostomy using 5/0 or 6/0 polydioxanone (PDS) sutures

Complications

- Cirrhosis (< 5% at presentation)
- Cholangitis (uncommon if bile flow good)
- Intrahepatic stone formation (in dilated intrahepatic ducts)
- Recurrent pancreatitis (suspect common channel stenosis or obstruction – ERCP)

Outcome

- Should achieve close to 100% asymptomatic long-term survival with native liver
- Malignancy is a possible complication in the longer term but its current true prevalence is not known following change of surgical practice from simply internally draining cysts to actual resection and bile duct reconstruction

Further reading

Redkar R, Davenport M, Howard ER. Antenatal diagnosis of congenital anomalies of the biliary tract. J Pediatr Surg 1998; 33:700–704.

Stringer M, Dhawan A, Davenport M, et al. Choledochal cysts: lessons from a 20-year experience. Arch Dis Child 1995; 73:528–531.

Turowski C, Knisely AS, Davenport M. Role of pressure and pancreatic reflux in the aetiology of choledochal malformation. Brit J Surg 2011; 98: 1319–1326.

Related topics of interest

Cholelithiasis

Learning outcomes

- To understand the mechanism of formation of gallstones
- To be aware of the different modes of clinical presentation
- To be able to appropriately investigate children with cholelithiasis
- To develop the ability to formulate an appropriate management plan

Overview

Cholelithiasis is much more common in adults than in children. Management modalities have therefore been developed in adults and have been transposed to children. The applicability of adult-based investigations and treatment modalities to children has not been subjected to scrutiny, and therefore the evidence base is lacking.

Epidemiology and aetiology

The prevalence of gallstones in children is 0.13–1.9%. In England, the hospital admission rate for children in the age range 0–14 years was 1.1 per 100,000 in 1999–2000.

In an Italian population-based study, the median age at diagnosis was 7.3 (range 0–18) years with equal sex ratio, but gallstones were more common in girls in the adolescent age group (12–18 years). Adolescents share the same racial and genetic predisposition to cholelithiasis as adults.

Mechanism of stone formation

The process of gallstone formation is as follows:

- Supersaturation of bile is caused by either cholesterol or bile pigment
- Precipitation and crystal formation are accelerated. Haemolytic disorders cause formation of bilirubin at a rate which exceeds the conjugation capacity of the liver, thereby increasing the concentration of insoluble unconjugated bilirubin in bile. Similarly, infection leads to deconjugation of bilirubin glucuronide, causing a rise in the concentration of unconjugated bilirubin which is insoluble in bile and precipitates forming calcium bilirubinate crystals
- Gallbladder stasis enables cholesterol or calcium bilirubinate crystals to aggregate, resulting in stone formation
- Other predisposing factors are the immaturity of the bilirubin conjugation system in infants. Other risk factors in infants were noted to be systemic illness, parenteral nutrition (PN), congenital anomalies and necrotising enterocolitis
- Congenital duct stenosis also predisposes to choledocholithiasis

Stone composition

The distribution of gallstone type in children is different from that in adults, where cholesterol stones are most common. The constituents of paediatric gallstones are:

- Black pigment stones (50%)
- Calcium carbonate stones (35%)
- Cholesterol stones (10%)
- Brown pigment stones (5%) – composed of calcium bilirubinate and calcium salts of fatty acids (stearic acid, lecithin and palmitic acid). They form in the presence of stasis and bacterial infection (e.g. *Clonorchis sinensis*, *Ascaris lumbricoides*, *Escherichia coli*, and *Staphylococcus*, *Citrobacter*, *Enterobacter* and *Salmonella* species)

Haemolytic anaemias

The two most common haemolytic anaemias in children presenting with cholelithiasis in the UK are hereditary spherocytosis and sickle cell anaemia, in which the abnormal erythrocytes are prone to an increased rate of haemolysis, resulting in an increased rate of bilirubin formation. Supersaturation of bile with calcium bilirubinate, the calcium salt of unconjugated bilirubin, leads to black pigment stone formation. The latter is usually radio-opaque, and the higher the concentration of calcium bilirubinate within the stones, the more radio-opaque and the darker the stones. Other haemolytic disorders predisposing to stone formation are thalassaemia, haemoglobin C disorder and glucose-6-phosphate dehydrogenase deficiency.

Obesity and hyperlipidaemias

Supersaturation of bile with cholesterol leads to cholesterol stones. These may be composed of pure cholesterol or may be mixed with glycoproteins, bilirubin and calcium carbonate.

Miscellaneous causes

Other risk factors are prolonged PN, prolonged fasting, ileal disease, chronic hepatobiliary disease and cystic fibrosis. Major ileal resection interferes with the enterohepatic circulation of bile acids. Bile acid secretion in bile is reduced and cholesterol secretion is increased, causing cholesterol supersaturation of bile and stone formation.

Clinical features

Up to 67% of gallstones in children are symptomatic compared with 20% in adults. Modes of clinical presentation are as follows.

Biliary colic

A typical history comprises a sharp, colicky, right upper quadrant pain, which may radiate to the scapular area. An important feature to elicit in the history is fat intolerance, whereby the pain is triggered by fatty foods. Accompanying symptoms may be nausea and vomiting. Murphy's sign may be positive.

Acute cholecystitis

Migration of a stone into the cystic duct (CD) causes obstruction, acute dilatation of the gallbladder, oedema and stasis of bile with superimposed infection with *E. coli*, *Enterococcus* or *Klebsiella*. Inflammation ensues and common clinical features are right upper quadrant pain, which is severe and long-lasting, anorexia, nausea, vomiting and low-grade pyrexia. Murphy's sign is positive.

Acute pancreatitis

Stone migration may cause obstruction of the pancreatic duct, and clinical features are of an acutely unwell child with epigastric and back pain, vomiting, pyrexia, jaundice in some children, abdominal tenderness and elevated amylase and lipase levels. The acute episode may be followed by formation of a pancreatic pseudocyst.

Obstructive jaundice

Impaction of a stone in the common bile duct (CBD) causes obstructive jaundice. Typical clinical features are jaundice, pale stools, dark urine, and elevated conjugated serum bilirubin, alkaline phosphatase and gamma-glutamyl transpeptidase (GGT).

Asymptomatic stones

About 33% of stones in children are asymptomatic. They are either never diagnosed or noted as incidental findings during abdominal ultrasound. Gallbladder perforation, Mirizzi syndrome (obstruction of the CBD or common hepatic duct by a stone impacted in the CD or gallbladder neck causing obstructive jaundice) and gallbladder-enteric fistulae leading to gallstone ileus are rare in children.

Investigations
Blood

- Full blood count
- C-reactive protein
- Split serum bilirubin, GGT, alkaline phosphatase, transaminases
- Serum amylase and lipase
- Lipid profile
- Haemoglobinopathy screen

Radiology

- Ultrasonography is the study of choice, and no other radiological study is indicated for uncomplicated cholelithiasis
- Plain abdominal radiograph is not useful because gallstones, with the exception of calcium carbonate stones, are radiolucent
- Intraoperative cholangiography is performed selectively by some surgeons and routinely by others
- Magnetic resonance cholangiopancreatography (MRCP), endoscopic retrograde cholangiopancreatography (ERCP) or endoscopic ultrasound may have a role

to play in the small number of patients with CBD stones or complications of stone disease

Differential diagnosis

- Dyspepsia
- Peptic ulcers
- Non-specific abdominal pain
- Cholestasis
- Acalculous cholecystitis
- Non-functioning gallbladder
- Biliary dyskinesia
- Pancreatitis

Treatment

Asymptomatic stones are simply monitored with clinical assessment and regular ultrasound surveillance. The only exception is asymptomatic gallstones in children having splenectomy.

Children with cholecystitis are treated with analgesia and antibiotics, followed by cholecystectomy. Patients with sickle cell disease are kept well hydrated to prevent sickle cell crises.

Stone dissolution with ursodeoxycholic acid (25 mg/kg/day for median of 13 months) has been attempted with disappointing results. Although 65% of the patients became asymptomatic, stone dissolution was observed in only 7%. Of these, stones recurred in 38% after treatment cessation.

Operative technique for laparoscopic cholecystectomy

- Laparoscopic cholecystectomy (LC) is the treatment of choice for symptomatic gallstones
- No pre- or intraoperative antibiotics are given for uncomplicated cholelithiasis
- The patient is placed supine, in reverse Trendelenburg and rotated towards the left
- The procedure is performed using three to four ports (a single-port technique has been reported)
- The fundus of the gallbladder is retracted cephalad towards the diaphragm and to the right, to display open Calot's triangle
- Dissection starts in Calot's triangle close to the body of the gallbladder away from the CBD. The peritoneum is incised, staying

close to the gallbladder. The peritoneal incision is made in a U shape on either side of the gallbladder and across Hartman's pouch, staying away from the CBD
- A fundamental step is to develop a window in Calot's triangle at the level where the CD joins the gallbladder infundibulum, through which the liver can be visualised. No structure should be clipped or divided until this step has been completed. Adherence to this principle minimises the risk of CBD injury
- The cystic vessels are clipped with 5 mm endoclips and divided, taking care not to use diathermy between metal clips
- Any stones that may be present in the CD are milked towards the gallbladder. A 5 mm clip is then placed on the CD at its junction with the gallbladder neck
- The author's practice is to perform a routine intraoperative cholangiogram (IOC) at this point as there is population-based data which demonstrates that IOC reduces the risk of CBD injury and allows laparoscopic exploration and retrieval of CBD stones, if present
- Dissection of the CD to its junction with the common hepatic duct is not necessary and should not be performed. Diathermy should be used sparingly close to the CBD
- Two further 5 mm clips are placed on the CD between the previous clip and the CBD. The CD is divided, leaving two clips on the stump
- The gallbladder is dissected free from the liver bed, placed in a retrieval bag and extracted through the umbilical port

Common bile duct stones

About 8% of children with LC have CBD stones. There are two treatment options:

1. LC, on-table cholangiogram and laparoscopic bile duct exploration through a transcystic route or choledochotomy
2. A combination of ERCP and LC

Randomised controlled trials comparing these two treatment modalities in adults demonstrated the laparoscopic approach to be superior on the basis of a significantly shorter hospital stay, and both techniques were effective in clearing bile duct stones.

Outcomes

Complications

Complications are rare following LC. In a population-based study of 28,243 LCs, 0.4% incurred a bile duct injury.

Day case rate

Emphasis on adequate pain management and avoidance of postoperative nausea and vomiting results in a day case rate as high as 92% in children.

Further reading

Della Corte C, Falchetti D, Nebbia G, et al. Management of cholelithiasis in Italian children: a national multicenter study. World J Gastroenterol. 2008; 14:1383–1388.

Jawaheer G, Evans K, Marcus R. Day-case laparoscopic cholecystectomy in childhood: outcomes from a clinical care pathway. Eur J Pediatr Surg 2013; 23:57–62.

Stringer MD, Taylor DR, Soloway RD. Gallstone composition: are children different? J Pediatr 2003; 142:435–440.

Related topics of interest

- Biliary atresia (p. 27)
- Choledochal malformation (p. 48)
- Pancreatitis (p. 267)
- Spleen disorders (p. 329)

Chronic abdominal pain

Learning outcomes

- To be able to form a differential diagnosis for chronic or recurrent abdominal pain
- To understand the principles of managing chronic or recurrent abdominal pain

Overview

Chronic or recurrent abdominal pain is abdominal pain of any duration with two or more attacks over a 3-month period between the ages of 4 and 16 years. The majority have functional pain, but alarm symptoms indicate a requirement for further investigations. These include involuntary weight loss, deceleration of linear growth, gastrointestinal bleeding, significant vomiting (e.g. bilious, protracted or cyclical), chronic severe diarrhoea, persistent lateralisation, right upper or right lower quadrant pain, unexplained fever, family history of inflammatory bowel disease.

Epidemiology and aetiology

Chronic pain affects 15% of children, and 20% of these have bouts severe enough to significantly affect their activity and schooling. The prevalence of functional dyspepsia varies between 3.5% and 27%; that of irritable bowel syndrome (IBS) is reported as 0.2% of children with a mean age of 52 months. Abdominal migraine, cyclical vomiting syndrome and migraine-associated headache are a spectrum of a single disorder with affected patients progressing from one entity to another. It affects 1–4% of children and is more common in girls (3:2) with a mean age at onset of 7 years and a peak at 10–12 years.

Functional pain may be the result of disordered brain–gut communication involving the efferent and afferent pathways between the enteric and central nervous systems. The tendency of children to outgrow functional pain suggests self-limiting developmental factors.

The pain is thought to be secondary to alterations in motility and visceral hypersensitivity. Various motor and sensory phenomena occur and appear to be linked to the autonomic nervous system, but no motor abnormalities have been identified that are severe enough to account for these patients' symptoms. Children with functional bowel disorders, rather than having a motility disturbance, may have abnormal bowel reactivity to physiologic stimuli (e.g. meal, bowel distension and hormonal changes), noxious stressful stimuli (e.g. inflammatory processes) or psychological stressful stimuli (e.g. parental separation and anxiety). Evidence suggests that these disorders are associated with visceral hyperalgesia (a decreased threshold for pain in response to changes in intraluminal pressure). Mucosal inflammatory processes attributable to infections, allergies or primary inflammatory diseases may cause sensitisation of afferent nerves and have been associated with the onset of visceral hyperalgesia.

Functional abdominal pain is in group H2 of the categories of functional gastrointestinal disorders (FGIDs) defined by the Rome III criteria (2006). Functional disorders: children and adolescents:

- H1. Vomiting and aerophagia
  - H1a. Adolescent rumination syndrome
  - H1b. Cyclic vomiting syndrome
  - H1c. Aerophagia
- H2. Abdominal pain-related FGIDs
  - H2a. Functional dyspepsia
  - H2b. IBS
  - H2c. Abdominal migraine
  - H2d. Childhood functional abdominal pain
    - H2d1. Childhood functional abdominal pain syndrome
- H3. Constipation and incontinence
  - H3a. Functional constipation
  - H3b. Non-retentive faecal incontinence

Clinical features

In all cases, the criteria must be fulfilled at least once per week for at least 2 months before diagnosis (to eliminate the likelihood of acute disease and establish chronicity) and there should be no evidence of an inflammatory, anatomic, metabolic or neoplastic process that explains the symptoms.

H2a (functional dyspepsia) may occur following a viral illness, and diagnostic criteria must include all of

- Persistent or recurrent pain or discomfort centred in the upper abdomen (above the umbilicus)
- Not relieved by defaecation or associated with the onset of a change in stool frequency or form (i.e. not IBS)

Diagnostic criteria for IBS in H2b must include

- Abdominal discomfort (an uncomfortable sensation not described as pain) or pain associated with two or more of the following at least 25% of the time:
  - Improved with defaecation
  - Onset associated with a change in stool frequency
  - Onset associated with a change in stool form (appearance)

Symptoms cumulatively supporting IBS are abnormal stool frequency and form, abnormal stool passage, passage of mucus and bloating or abdominal distension. Anxiety, depression and multiple other psychological complaints are reported with IBS. It is important to explore potential triggers and psychosocial factors.

For the diagnosis H2c (abdominal migraine), all the following must be fulfilled:

- Paroxysmal episodes of intense, acute periumbilical pain lasting for 1 hour or more
- Intervening periods of good health lasting weeks to months
- Pain interferes with normal activities
- Pain is associated with two or more of the following:
  - anorexia, nausea, vomiting, headache and photophobia

When appropriate, urological or gastrointestinal obstruction, biliary tract disease, pancreatitis, familial Mediterranean fever and metabolic disorders should be considered, given the paroxysmal nature of the symptoms. They are not known to display any psychological features.

In group H2d, diagnostic criteria must include

- Episodic or continuous abdominal pain
- Insufficient criteria for other FGIDs

In group H2d1, there must be childhood functional abdominal pain at least 25% of the time and one or more of the following:

- Some loss of daily functioning
- Additional somatic symptoms, such as headache, limb pain or difficulty sleeping

H2d1 group is a subgroup in whom loss of daily functioning and/or accompanying somatic symptoms form an important part of their symptom complex. It includes some of the most challenging patients because pain is a subjective experience and these children often have pain in association with psychological events. Headache, limb pain and lower pain thresholds require further study.

Investigations

In H2a group, an upper gastrointestinal endoscopy assesses for *Helicobacter pylori*-associated disease. In all other groups, investigations are at the clinician's discretion to exclude an organic cause. These include full blood cell count, erythrocyte sedimentation rate, urinalysis, urine culture, liver and kidney biochemistry, stool analysis and breath hydrogen testing for sugar malabsorption.

Differential diagnosis

- Recurrent acute pain
- Twelfth rib syndrome

Treatment

Management of H2a disease includes avoidance of non-steroidal anti-inflammatory agents and aggravating foods. Antisecretory agents and prokinetics can be used along with antimicrobial management of *H. pylori* disease.

The goals of IBS management include modifying severity and developing strategies for dealing with symptoms. Peppermint oil may be therapeutic; serotonin and other antidepressants are efficacious in adults, but only anecdotal reports exist in children.

Potential triggers should be avoided in abdominal migraine. Medication includes pizotifen, propranolol, cyproheptadine or sumatriptan.

Functional abdominal pain syndrome requires a biopsychosocial approach.

Because pain is the specific target, it is vital to assess the contribution of psychosocial factors. Reassurance and explanation should be given, and there are reports of success with behavioural treatment with or without tricyclic antidepressants.

Further reading

Milla PJ. Irritable bowel syndrome in childhood. Gastroenterology 2001; 120:287–290.

Rasquin A, Di Lorenzo C, Forbes D, et al. Childhood functional gastrointestinal disorders: child/adolescent. Gastroenterology 2006; 130:1527–1537.

Subcommittee on Chronic Abdominal Pain. Chronic abdominal pain in children. Pediatrics 2005; 115:812–815.

Related topics of interest

- Appendicitis (p. 21)
- Faecal incontinence and idiopathic constipation (p. 115)
- Intussusception (p. 181)
- Meckel's diverticulum (p. 202)

Cloaca

Learning outcomes

- To be aware of epidemiology and pathology
- To gain an appreciation of the associated defects seen in infants with a persistent cloaca
- To gain an understanding of the initial management
- To have an overview of corrective surgical techniques

Overview

A cloaca is defined as a congenital defect in females where the rectum, vagina and urinary tract meet and fuse, creating a single common channel, rather than three discrete openings.

Epidemiology and aetiology

This congenital defect occurs in females. A persistent cloaca is the third most common defect in female patients after vestibular and perineal fistulae. The aetiology is unknown.

Clinical features

The diagnosis of persistent cloaca is a clinical one. This defect should be suspected in a female born with an imperforate anus and small-looking genitalia. Careful separation of the labia reveals a single perineal orifice.

Careful inspection of the perineum can help to predict the internal anatomy and the final functional prognosis. A well-formed midline groove and prominent anal dimple indicates the potential of a good anal sphincter mechanism, whereas a 'flat bottom' with no anal dimple carries a poor prognosis in terms of functional result.

Approximately 30% of patients will have a grossly distended vagina filled with fluid, with or without mucus called a hydrocolpos. Many of the patients with a hydrocolpos will also have a duplication of the Müllerian system, i.e. two hemiuteri and two hemivaginas. The hydrocolpos can be problematic. First, it can cause compression of the urinary tract at the trigone leading to megaureters and hydronephrosis. Second, if the hydrocolpos is left undrained, it can become infected and perforate.

Approximately 40% of patients have a double Müllerian system consisting of two hemivaginas and two hemiuteri. This duplication can be symmetrical or asymmetrical, partial or total. The asymmetrical type is often associated with an atresia of the Müllerian structure. If this is not recognised, it may lead to the accumulation of menstrual blood at the time of puberty together with retrograde menstruation.

Investigations

- VACTERL (vertebral anomalies, anal atresia, cardiovascular anomalies, tracheoesophageal fistula, renal or radial anomalies and limb defects) screening:
  - Abdominal or chest X-ray to assess spine and sacrum.
  - Spinal ultrasound for assessment of tethered cord
  - Echocardiogram
  - Passage of a nasogastric tube to rule out an oesophageal atresia
  - Ultrasound scanning of abdomen and urinary tract to assess the kidneys, degree of hydronephrosis and megaureters and to assess the hydrocolpos
  - Sacral X-ray to identify a hemisacrum and calculate the sacral ratio, a good predictor of functional outcomes
- Cystoscopy and vaginoscopy to assess the length of the common channel:
  - The longer the common channel, the worse the prognosis
  - More straightforward repairs have a common channel < 3 cm
  - This endoscopy is best done under a separate anaesthetic outside the newborn period
  - Contrast studies (tubes are left in situ when examined under anaesthesia) (**Figure 9**) – to delineate distal rectal, vaginal and urological anatomy. These images can be viewed in three dimensions

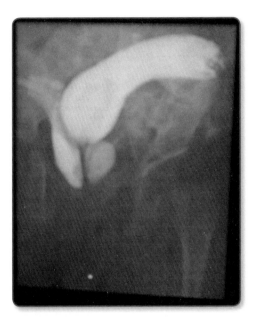

Figure 9 Contrast study via the common channel revealing a long common channel, two hemivaginas and the rectum entering between the hemivagina. Marker at the site of cloacal opening.

Differential diagnosis

- Urogenital sinus
- Rectovaginal fistula (cloaca often misdiagnosed as this)
- Ambiguous genitalia

Treatment

Neonatal period

In the first 24 hours after birth, the infant needs to be assessed for associated features that may pose a threat to a life, and these must be managed accordingly. Infants with a cloaca require a colostomy in the neonatal period. A distal transverse or descending colostomy and mucus fistula is recommended. Drainage of a hydrocolpos (vaginostomy) is required.

Definitive reconstruction (Figure 10)

- Vaginoscopy and cystoscopy outside the neonatal period to establish key features and aid decision-making:

  - The length of the common channel
  - Does the abdomen need to be opened for definitive repair?
  - Predict functional prognosis
  - Determine whether bowel preparation is necessary
  - Will a vaginal replacement be required?

Subtypes of cloacal malformation are as follows:

- Cloaca with a common channel < 1 cm
  - Posterior sagittal anorectal vaginoplasty - usually urethra can be left untouched
- Cloaca with a 1–3 cm common channel:
  - Posterior sagittal approach with total urogenital mobilisation (TUM, without laparotomy)
  - The incision is made in the posterior sagittal midline from the midsacral level to perineal orifice.
  - Incise through the sphincter mechanism to find the rectum which is then opened in the midline
  - Incision is extended through posterior wall of the common channel
  - Rectum is separated from the vagina which shares a common wall
  - TUM: vagina and urethra are brought to the perineum as a single unit
  - The previous common channel is used to create labia, the perineal body is reconstructed and the rectum is placed within the sphincter complex
  - These patients generally have a good prognosis
  - Less than 20% of patients require intermittent self-catheterisation
- Cloaca with a 3–5 cm common channel:
  - Extended TUM (requires laparotomy)
  - With or without vaginal replacement (using small bowel, colon or rectum)
  - With or without vaginal switch (suitable for patients with hydrocolpos and two hemivaginas)
  - Preoperative bowel preparation
  - The whole of the lower body should be prepared for theatre
  - As above, the rectum is separated from the vagina through a posterior midline incision
  - Laparotomy: bladder may need to be opened and catheters passed through

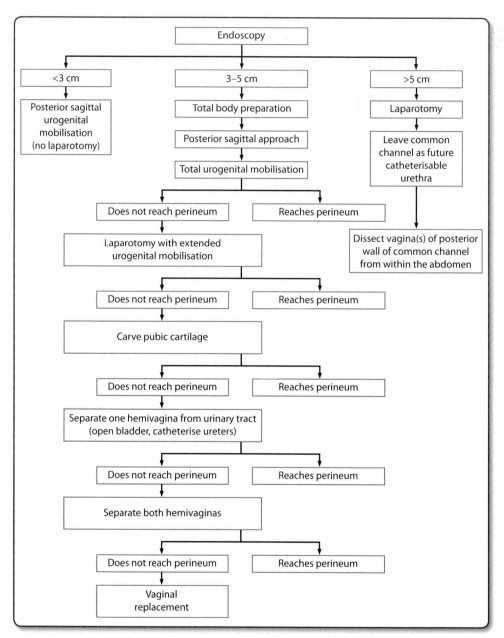

Figure 10 Algorithm for the surgical reconstruction of a cloaca. Reprinted from: Levitt MA, Pena A. Cloacal malformations: lessons learned from 490 cases. Semin Pediatr Surg 2010; 19:128–138, with permission from Elsevier.

the ureters (for identification) which pass through the common wall of vagina and bladder

- If TUM does not reach the perineum, the vaginas are dissected off and separated from the bladder neck, taking

great care to identify and protect the ureters

- Assess patency of Müllerian structures intraoperatively
- Assess the vagina and determine whether additional procedures are

required to enlarge the vagina or vaginal replacement is needed
- If there are a hydrocolpos and two hemivaginas, the patient may be suitable for the vaginal switch manoeuvre (see 'Further reading')

- Cloaca with a > 5 cm common channel:
  - Laparotomy first as should be able to separate structures intra-abdominally
  - Use the common channel as neourethra
  - There are various techniques for vaginal and anorectal reconstruction

Further reading

Bischoff A, et al. Hydrocolpos in cloacal malformations. J Pediatr Surg 2010; 45:1241–1245.

Levitt MA, Bischoff A, Pena A. Pitfalls and challenges of cloaca repair: how to reduce the need for reoperations. J Pediatr Surg 2011; 46:1250–1255.

Levitt MA, Pena A. Cloacal malformations: lessons learned from 490 cases. Semin Pediatr Surg 2010; 19:128–138.

Related topics of interest

Colonic atresia

Learning outcomes

- To learn the classification and aetiology of colonic atresia
- To be aware of the need to rule out Hirschsprung's disease in cases of colonic atresia
- To recognise the urgency of surgical correction of colonic atresia and the increase in mortality with delay in treatment

Overview

Colonic atresia is the second rarest cause of neonatal obstruction. However, it should not be overlooked as a delay in its recognition and treatment leads to a significant increase in morbidity and mortality.

- 1673 – Binninger recorded the first case of colonic atresia in the literature
- 1922 – Gaub reported the first surviving newborn with sigmoid atresia treated with colostomy
- 1947 – Potts reported the first surviving baby with transverse colonic atresia treated with primary anastomosis

Colonic atresia is classified in the same way as other bowel atresias:

- Type I – mucosal atresia with intact bowel and no mesenteric defect
- Type II – blind ends joined by a fibrous band without mesenteric defect
- Type IIIa – disconnected blind ends with mesenteric defect
- Type IIIb – apple-peel atresia
- Type IV – multiple atresias

Type III is the most common type found in colonic atresias overall (60%). It is also the most common atresia found in the ascending and transverse colon. Types I and II occur more commonly distal to the splenic flexure. Multiple colonic atresias are rare.

Epidemiology and aetiology

Colonic atresia is a rare cause of intestinal obstruction accounting for 1.8–15.0% of all gastrointestinal atresias. Its incidence is 1 in 20,000 live births. In common with jejunoileal atresia, its aetiology includes intrauterine mesenteric vascular impairment or intrauterine volvulus. It is less common than jejunoileal atresia as the colon is better protected from segmental ischaemia by its the vascular arcade.

Another aetiologic link has been recognised with congenital varicella syndrome. It is thought that intrauterine infections with varicella zoster virus within the first 20 weeks of gestation can result in injury to the enteric plexus that may lead to poor vessel development and ischaemic injury, resulting in atresia.

Colonic atresia can also occur in gastroschisis, with most cases resulting from bowel compression within the narrowing abdominal defect. A 'two-point constriction' may lead to a wide spectrum of bowel pathologies, and the morphology may depend on the viability of the intestinal segment between the atretic jejunum or ileum and the colon. It also seems that type II and IIIa atresias of the right colon may share a similar pathogenesis of temporary constriction within a closing umbilical ring.

Clinical features

Colonic atresia can be diagnosed antenatally by recognition of distended bowel indicating an obstruction. Postnatally it presents with the classic signs of large bowel obstruction – abdominal distention, bilious vomiting and failure to pass meconium.

The rate of associated anomalies with colonic atresia is much smaller than with other gastrointestinal atresias. However, up to one third of colonic atresias might have associated congenital anomalies. Colonic atresia occurs in 2.5–36.0% of neonates with gastroschisis.

It may also be associated with

- Hirschsprung's disease
- Malrotation
- Multiple small intestinal atresias – colonic atresia occurs in 5% of affected patients

- Cloacal exstrophy
- Vesicointestinal fistula
- Complex urological abnormalities
- Choledochal cyst
- Skeletal abnormalities

Differential diagnosis

Other causes of low bowel obstruction in neonates are
- Anorectal malformation
- Hirschsprung's disease
- Meconium ileus
- Meconium plug syndrome
- Ileal atresia
- Small left colon syndrome
- Megacystis microcolon syndrome

Investigations

Abdominal X-ray will show
- Air fluid levels
- Dilated loops of bowel
- Ground glass appearance of meconium mixed with air in a massively dilated, sometimes spherical, loop of bowel

Contrast enema is diagnostic and shows a small diameter distal colon that comes to an abrupt halt. Care is needed when performing the contrast enema as there is a risk of perforation of the distal colon if high intraluminal pressures are applied.

Management

Urgent surgery is mandatory because the risk of perforation is higher than with small bowel obstruction. This is due to the existence of a closed loop if there is a competent ileocaecal valve.

At surgery it is important to exclude other atresias, and frozen section rectal biopsy should be performed. The rate of association with Hirschsprung's disease is low with < 20 cases reported in the literature, but the consequences of not recognising it can be devastating with anastomotic leak, functional obstruction and enterocolitis. The surgical approach depends of the level of obstruction and presence or absence of associated atresias.

The disparity between the bowel ends is often large, with a 3 or 4:1 ratio not uncommon. The bowel does not tend to reduce in size over time, and studies show that a temporising stoma does not reduce the discrepancy in the calibre of the atretic ends in proximal colonic atresia, and that a right hemicolectomy and ileocolic anastomosis should be considered at the initial surgery.

Some centres in the UK perform primary resection and anastomosis, with or without tapering and with or without a temporary protective proximal stoma, in the standard fashion via a supraumbilical transverse incision.

The risk of anastomotic leak and poorer prognosis with primary anastomosis makes some centres prefer a staged procedure with primary colostomy and mucous fistula, followed by anastomosis at a later date. Resection of the bulbous proximal colon and a portion of the microcolon has been suggested by those who believe that both the proximal and distal ends adjacent to the atresia are abnormal in innervation and vascularity.

Due to the rarity of the disease, large prospective studies comparing different approaches and identifying the best surgical treatment are not yet available. In the absence of associations, the prognosis is excellent. The risk of short gut syndrome associated with other bowel atresias should not exist in isolated colonic atresia.

If there is no delay in the diagnosis, surgery is usually straightforward and uncomplicated. Mortality should be < 10%. A delay in diagnosis beyond 72 hours may result in > 60% mortality owing to more severe dehydration, electrolyte imbalance, acidosis, aspiration pneumonia, sepsis and closed loop obstruction (between the ileocaecal valve and the atresia) leading to perforation.

Further reading

England RJ, Scammell S, Murthi GV. Proximal colonic atresia: is right hemicolectomy inevitable? Pediatr Surg Int 2011; 27:1059–1062.

Etensel B, Temirb G, Karkiner A, et al. Atresia of the colon. J Pediatr Surg 2005; 40:1258–1268.

Seo T, Ando H, Watanabe Y, et al. Colonic atresia and Hirschsprung's disease: importance of histologic examination of the distal bowel. J Pediatr Surg 2002; 37:E19.

Related topics of interest

- Prenatal diagnosis and counselling (p. 287)
- Hirschsprung's disease (p. 161)
- Meconium ileus (p. 204)
- Small bowel atresia (p. 320)

Congenital diaphragmatic hernia

Learning outcomes

- To understand the antenatal assessment and counselling of congenital diaphragmatic hernia (CDH)
- To understand the principles of postnatal management and the role of extracorporeal life support (ECLS)
- To understand why CDH survivors require long-term multidisciplinary follow-up

Overview

CDH remains a challenging neonatal condition. Antenatal detection and evaluation aids counselling and delivery with stabilisation, using strategies of gentle ventilation and pulmonary hypertension (PHT) management. Surgical repair is delayed until PHT is controlled. ECLS should be considered if conventional management fails. Defect size should be graded at the time of surgery to evaluate outcome according to severity. Long-term multidisciplinary follow-up is essential.

The combination of pulmonary hypoplasia and PHT is the main determinant of postnatal survival. This has improved with antenatal diagnosis and advances in neonatal care. The International CDH Database reports an overall 70% survival, up from 63% in the mid-nineties, with an increased rate of repair in babies on ECLS from 23 to > 50% over the same period. The Extracorporeal Life Support Organization consistently report a 50% survival to discharge for babies with CDH who receive ECLS and CDH now accounts for 25% of all neonatal ECLS.

Epidemiology and aetiology

CDH has an incidence of 1 in 2000–5000 live births.

- Sporadic, though genetic factors are increasingly being recognised as playing a role
- Significant associated anomalies occur in about 20%

Clinical features

The diaphragmatic defect (80% left sided) is of varying size. Abdominal viscera can herniate into the chest from around the 10th week of gestation. Lung growth and development are impaired through limitation of space, reduced fetal breathing movements and loss of fetal lung liquid, leading to variable degrees of pulmonary hypoplasia.

Antenatal diagnosis

Antenatal diagnosis is more common in the UK since the introduction of universal fetal anomaly scans at 18–20 weeks. If a CDH is suspected, referral should be made to a specialist fetal medicine service for confirmation and investigations to assess the severity of the anomaly and search for associated malformations (especially cardiac defects) and chromosomal anomalies that will impact survival.

Postnatal diagnosis

- Seen on chest X-ray (CXR) soon after birth when investigating respiratory distress
- Can present later as an incidental finding

Investigations

- Antenatal – fetal ultrasound scanning (USS), with or without magnetic resonance imaging (MRI), with or without amniocentesis
- Postnatal – CXR, echocardiography

Differential diagnosis

- Congenital lung abnormality

Treatment

Antenatal management

Defect severity is most commonly measured using the lung-to-head ratio (LHR) on USS. Using the observed to expected (O/E) LHR and the position of the liver, the risk of death can be classified as low, moderate or severe.

MRI measurement of total fetal lung volume (TFLV) benefits in assessing both lungs. O/E TFLV is predictive of survival.

The mother should be offered multidisciplinary counselling, based on these findings. Some women will choose to terminate the pregnancy. Results of investigations and counselling should assist in this decision-making process. Fetal tracheal occlusion is a consideration for those with an isolated severe defect.

Delivery and early postnatal management

- Delivery should be planned and an experienced neonatal team should resuscitate the baby
- The main principles are
  - intubate early
  - avoid bag and mask ventilation (gas in the intrathoracic gut will compromise ventilation and cardiac output)
  - limit peak ventilation pressure
  - stabilise the newborn before transfer
  - there is no evidence to support the use of exogenous surfactant or caesarean section

Postnatal management should be undertaken following an evidence based protocol.

- Gentle ventilation strategy (peak inspiratory pressure ≤25 cm H_2O)
- Support systemic blood pressure with inotropes
- Assess for cardiac anomalies
- Assess and treat PHT, with inhaled nitric oxide (iNO), normally 20 ppm
- Relatively low PaO_2 and high $PaCO_2$ should be tolerated as long as measures of adequacy of perfusion and O_2 delivery are acceptable – pH ≥7.20, adequate BP, adequate urine output and blood lactate <2.0 mmol/L
- If there is evidence of compromised left ventricular function from a distended right ventricle, Prostin may be necessary to keep the duct open and offload the right-sided heart. This requires regular clinical and echocardiographic assessment
- If conventional mechanical ventilation (CMV) is failing, high frequency ventilation (HFV) should be considered.

Many units offer HFV from the start because they consider it a more gentle form of ventilation. If used, a low volume strategy should be applied

Should these fail to deliver adequate oxygenation and tissue perfusion, and based on antenatal markers of severity (if available) and the baby's behaviour postnatally, there should be early consideration of ECLS. In the UK, this involves discussion with an ECLS centre and often a potentially difficult transfer. The sooner this discussion is instigated, the greater the chance of a successful transfer because these infants are extremely unstable. If on HFV, most will not tolerate conversion to CMV for any length of time. Options then include transfer on HFV or cannulation at the referring site and transfer on ECLS, neither of which can be guaranteed at present.

Surgical repair

A baby with CDH should be delivered in a unit with a paediatric surgery service, thus avoiding a postnatal transfer, unless for ECLS. Ideally, high-risk cases should be born in a unit with full support.

CDH repair should be delayed until PHT is controlled and resolving. The aim is for FiO_2 ≤0.5 and reducing ventilation parameters, giving leeway to increase ventilation postoperatively, if required. If stable on HFV, surgery can be undertaken in the neonatal intensive care unit, without converting to CMV or transfer to the operating room. If the baby needs ECLS, the defect should be repaired early in the run unless there is evidence that the baby is likely to come off ECLS before repair. Modern ECLS circuits with centrifugal pumps and low-resistance hollow-fibre oxygenators allow low or no heparinisation strategies to be employed following repair, reducing bleeding risk.

At repair, the defect size should be graded as A, B, C or D (**Figure 11**) according to International CDH Study Group criteria. This relates to survival and may be used in staging CDH to compare outcomes between centres.

- Repair steps are as follows: Open subcostal route

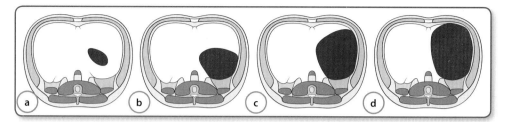

Figure 11 Grading of diaphragmatic hernia defect size at time of surgery: (a) defect A, (b) defect B, (c) defect C and (d) defect D.

- Thoracoscopic repair is presently associated with a high incidence of early recurrence and should only be considered for the most stable babies by very experienced surgical teams, as the potential for a high $PaCO_2$ could aggravate PHT
- Large defects (C and D) will always require a patch. At present polytetrafluoroethylene (GoreTex™) is the most reliable
- Unless repaired on ECLS, there is no indication for a chest drain
- Associated abdominal pathologies such as Meckel's diverticulum should be noted only. Non-rotation is expected and there is no benefit in undertaking a Ladd's procedure unless the base of the mesentery is obviously at risk of volvulus

Postoperative management

Postoperative management continues the same principles of ventilation and PHT control as preoperatively. If there is continuing evidence of PHT, oral sildenafil can be added because iNO is weaned off, increasing to a maximum dose of 2 mg/kg 4 hourly. Following extubation, ongoing supplemental O_2 is often required.

Long-term follow-up

Infants who have had CDH repair are likely to have long-term problems requiring systematic follow-up in a dedicated multidisciplinary clinic.

- There is a high incidence of readmission in the first year of life, even for infants with low grade defects
- In addition to the obvious need for respiratory and surgical follow-up, they have a number of other well-recognised needs:
  - Weight gain is problematic and regular dietetic input is necessary. Some require gastrostomy and a number of them need an antireflux procedure
  - Regular CXR will detect asymptomatic recurrence, especially in cases with large patches
  - Regular audiology review for late-onset hearing loss is essential
  - Neurodevelopmental follow-up should be undertaken (including Bayley score at 2 or 3 years)
  - Those with PHT during admission should be assessed to ensure it resolves. The sildenafil dose can be tapered and then stopped once PHT has resolved
  - Late cardiovascular and respiratory function testing should be part of the follow-up

Further reading

Jani JC, Benachi A, Nicolaides KH, et al. Prenatal prediction of neonatal morbidity in survivors with congenital diaphragmatic hernia: a multicenter study. Ultrasound Obstet Gynecol 2009; 33:64–69.

Lally KP, Lally PA, Lasky RE, et al. Defect size determines survival in infants with congenital diaphragmatic hernia. Pediatrics 2007; 120:e651–657.

The Congenital Diaphragmatic Hernia Study Group. Treatment evolution in high risk congenital diaphragmatic hernia: ten years experience. Ann Surg 2006; 244:505–513.

Related topics of interest

Congenital pulmonary adenomatous malformations

Learning outcomes

- To understand the spectrum of congenital lung malformations
- To understand the different ways in which these lesions may present
- To appreciate the arguments for and against surgical intervention

Overview

Congenital pulmonary adenomatoid malformations (CPAMs) and pulmonary sequestrations (PSs) are rare congenital lung lesions, which have traditionally been considered separately. However, in the context of growing evidence that up to 25% are hybrid lesions, they are increasingly being thought of as within the same spectrum.

Epidemiology and aetiology

The estimated incidence of CPAM has been reported to be 1 in 8000 to 1 in 35,000. CPAMs are hamartomatous cystic lesions found within the lung parenchyma which communicate with the tracheobronchial tree. There have been a number of different classifications of CPAMs described, of which Stocker's classification is probably the most well-known; however, these have limited clinical application. A more recent classification divides lesions into a microcystic (cysts < 5 mm) and a macrocystic (cysts > 5 mm) lesion and can be useful in guiding possible antenatal interventions. CPAMs occur with equal frequency in the right and left lungs. They occur more frequently in the lower lobes and, although single lobe involvement is more usual, they can affect more than one lobe.

PSs are segments of non-functioning lung tissue without a connection to the tracheobronchial tree, and they can be either intralobar sequestrations (ILSs) (75%) or extralobar sequestrations (ELSs) (25%). ILS may become aerated via the pores of Kohn. The majority of ILSs are found within the lower lobes, most commonly on the left. ELSs are invested in their own visceral pleura, are also more common on the left and are most often found in the posteromedial thoracic cavity. They can rarely be found within or below the diaphragm with 10% occurring in the abdomen.

PSs classically have a systemic blood supply, often originating from the aorta. Hybrid lesions have histological features of both CPAM and PS.

The embryogenesis of CPAM is not fully understood. There may be a hamartomatous overproliferation of the terminal bronchioles or alternatively a failure of apoptosis in the developing lung. PSs are thought to develop from an abnormal accessory lung bud. If this forms in early gestation, an ILS results. Conversely, if this forms in later gestation, the result is an ELS.

Clinical features

With the increased use of antenatal scanning in obstetrics, most CPAM and PS in the developed world are detected during routine anomaly scanning. The natural history of these antenatally detected lesions is variable with up to 40% resolving spontaneously. In those that do resolve antenatally, the pathogenesis may be that of transient bronchial obstruction.

Antenatal features

- Hyperechogenic lung lesions
- Pleural effusion
- Polyhydramnios
- Colour Doppler evidence of systemic arterial supply
- Pulmonary hypoplasia
- Mediastinal shift
- Hydrops

The only useful predictor of poor outcome is hydrops. Intrauterine death is rare (3.5%) and usually associated with hydrops.

Postnatal features

CPAM and PS are associated with a good prognosis. Most are asymptomatic at birth. Approximately 20% of newborns will exhibit some degree of respiratory distress, but most will settle spontaneously. Only a small number will require urgent surgical excision. Symptoms, however, may develop at any age. The true incidence of symptoms developing in these lesions is impossible to quantify without prospective long-term follow-up data, although a meta-analysis from 2009 suggested that 3.2% of children with an antenatal diagnosis would become symptomatic between 1 month and 16 years at a median age of 10 months.

Symptoms and signs may arise due to the following:

- Cyst enlargement and air trapping causing respiratory distress
- Infection causing recurrent pneumonia or lung abscesses
- Cyst rupture with resultant pneumothorax
- Haemoptysis or haemothorax
- Infarction secondary to torsion of an ELS
- Cardiac failure secondary to high volume flow through the systemic artery in PS

Although there is thought to be a risk of malignancy in these anomalies, the risk has not clearly been quantified:

- There are > 40 case reports in the literature of bronchioalveolar carcinoma and pleuropulmonary blastoma (PPB) associated with CPAM
- Pulmonary tumours associated with CPAM account for 4–9% of pulmonary neoplasms in childhood
- There are reports in the literature of carcinomas, mesotheliomas and PPB developing within sequestrations, but these are much less common than with CPAM

Associated anomalies in liveborn infants are rare.

Investigations

- **Chest X-ray (CXR):** An apparently normal postnatal CXR does not exclude the presence of a congenital lung lesion
- **Computed tomogram of the chest:** This investigation with intravenous contrast is the gold standard and should be performed even if there has been apparent antenatal regression or resolution on the antenatal scans and/or a normal postnatal CXR
- **MRI:** This may demonstrate a solid lesion and systemic blood supply

Differential diagnosis

- CPAM and PS cannot always be accurately radiologically categorised especially because some may be hybrid lesions
- PPB (especially the cystic subtypes) may appear identical to CPAM on imaging
- Neuroblastoma and PS may have similar appearances especially in a subdiaphragmatic lesion
- Bronchogenic cysts
- Gastrointestinal duplication cysts
- Teratomas
- Congenital diaphragmatic hernia can have a similar appearance to a CPAM on CXR.
- Congenital lobar emphysema

Treatment

Antenatal intervention for CPAM and PS should only be considered in those with a significant risk of intrauterine death, usually those with significant hydrops or significant mediastinal shift. The options for fetal intervention include fetal surgery (in limited centres worldwide), thoracoamniotic shunting, thoracocentesis and ultrasound-guided laser coagulation of feeding vessels.

Postnatally, surgical resection is the treatment of choice for all symptomatic cases. There is, however, considerable controversy regarding the treatment of asymptomatic CPAM and PS. True long-term follow-up data for conservatively treated malformations are currently not available. It is therefore unclear whether the risk of surgical resection is outweighed by the risk of conservative management. The advantages of both approaches are detailed in **Table 3**.

The standard surgical approach for CPAM and ILS is lobectomy of the affected lobe either via a posterolateral thoracotomy or using thoracoscopy, although some advocate a segmental resection. There is a far higher

Table 3 Advantages of operative and non-operative management of asymptomatic congenital pulmonary malformations	
Advantages of operative management	**Advantages of non-operative management**
Histology is the only way to reliably confirm the diagnosis	Risks of surgery are avoided
Prevention of complications, including infection, respiratory distress and malignancy	May never require surgery
Risk of surgery is low if performed electively (5% develop complications), and the risk of mortality is < 1%	
Risk of complications is approximately 2x higher in emergency surgery compared with elective surgery.	
Compensatory lung growth occurs following lobectomy in infants (with a return to near-normal pulmonary function) and to a certain degree in older children	

risk of residual disease (15% vs 0%) in those undergoing a segmental resection, presumably due to the difficulty in identifying the lesion's margins macroscopically. However, in cases where more than one lobe is involved, segmental resection may be a useful technique to attempt to preserve lung tissue. ELS can be simply excised after division of the systemic vessels.

Thoracoscopic techniques are becoming more popular, with reported advantages of shorter length of stay, lower risk of chest deformity and reduction in postoperative pain, although prospective randomised trials are needed to properly evaluate the results of muscle, sparing thoracotomy versus thoracoscopy. There remains a high conversion rate with thoracoscopy, especially in symptomatic patients.

Complications of surgery include infection, bleeding (potentially significant or life-threatening), bronchopleural fistula, residual disease, damage to remaining lung structures and chest deformity.

Further reading

Cavoretto P, et al. Prenatal diagnosis and outcome of echogenic fetal lung lesions. Ultrasound Obstet Gynaecol 2008; 32:769–783.

Laberge JM, Puligandla P, Flageole H. Asymptomatic congenital lung malformations. Semin Pediatr Surg 2005; 14:16–33.

Stanton M, et al. Systematic review and meta-analysis of the postnatal management of congenital cystic lung lesions. J Pediatr Surg 2009; 44:1027–1033.

Related topics of interest

Consent in paediatric surgery

Learning outcomes

- To differentiate between situations where capacity to consent can be presumed and when it must be established
- To identify adults with parental responsibility who are able to provide consent for a child
- To describe the information that must be disclosed when seeking consent
- To understand that confidentiality is grounded in consent

Overview

The legal rule governing consent for children and young people (adulthood commencing on the 18th birthday) is presented. It must be borne in mind that it describes the law in England and Wales; some Scottish variations are described but all jurisdictions have their local rules, which must be considered. Nevertheless, the common themes pervade all legal systems, namely competence, the role of the parent and what should be disclosed to achieve valid consent.

Age of capacity

Children may be divided into three groups when considering their capacity for consent. Young people of 16 and 17 years are presumed to be competent to provide their consent to treatment, independent of their parents. In reality, many young people defer to their parents, particularly for emergency procedures, and represent an unusual legal group, possessing the statutory capacity to consent yet being supported by an adult who can also provide consent.

Children of 15 years and below in England and Wales are presumed to be incompetent to provide consent but may establish their capacity by proving that they are 'Gillick competent'. To do so, they must demonstrate that they understand:

- That a choice exists
- The nature and purpose of the procedure
- Its risks and side effects
- The alternatives to the procedure

They need to be able to retain the information, weigh it up and arrive at a decision and to be free from undue pressure. It will be observed that it is a high threshold, arguably impassable by many adults, but nevertheless serves the public interest by protecting children, whilst empowering them to consent in the appropriate circumstances. It should be noted that in England and Wales neither the 16- and 17-year-old group nor the Gillick competent group has acquired the right to refuse life-saving treatment. There is no doubt that on the basis of pragmatism such children and young people successfully refuse treatment every day in this jurisdiction, but neither Parliament nor the judiciary will extend that veto to life itself. In Scotland, young people who are 16 years and over, if competent, can refuse all treatments.

On the basis of Gillick (or a statutory test on competence in Scotland), children unable to pass the test rely on the consent provided by an adult who has parental responsibility for them, or by the courts, in cases of disagreement.

Parental responsibility

The Children Act 1989 sets out the meaning and scope of parental responsibility, which amongst other things confers upon the holder the right and duty to provide consent for the child's medical treatment. The mother who delivers the child acquires parental responsibility automatically, as does the father if he is married to her at the time, or when and if he later marries the mother. Unmarried fathers whose children were registered after 1 December 2003 also acquire parental responsibility automatically, if they are named on the birth certificate. Otherwise, fathers can acquire parental responsibility by agreement with the mother, or by application to the court. Other family members or local authorities can acquire parental responsibility under certain circumstances. Parental responsibility is transferred by adoption, and extinguished as the child becomes an adult.

Anomalies can occur. One may encounter mothers who have yet to reach 16 years of age and the question arises whether she can consent for her baby's surgery. In general, if she is Gillick competent to consent for the proposed intervention, the young mother may consent for her child. In reality, it is likely that a grandparent will have been asked to share parental responsibility, which may allay any residual concerns over the mother's capacity.

What should be disclosed in obtaining consent?

It must always be remembered that the child or parent is unlikely to have a detailed grasp of the risks associated with surgery. The average citizen will have no concept that an operation on their spine could lead to paralysis of their legs or incontinence of their bladder or that surgery on one eye might lead to blindness in the other. Various formulae for what should be contained within consent disclosure have been suggested and rejected by English courts, but the most recent still applies. This asserts that '...if there is a significant risk which would affect the judgement of a reasonable patient, then in the normal course it is the responsibility of the doctor to inform the patient of that risk...' [Pearce v UBHT (1999) 48 BMLR 118]. It can be seen that it prescribes wide-ranging disclosure, and pays no attention whatsoever to the numerical incidence of a complication or risk but merely to the effect it could have on the reasonable patient.

Applying this to practice, certain uncomfortable but inevitable conclusions are reached. If you are consenting for a percutaneous central venous catheter insertion, it is unlikely, but foreseeable, that pneumothorax or haemothorax will result and that emergency treatment may be required; these should be disclosed. Equally, loss of the contralateral kidney or the midgut may follow from the attempted resection of a Wilms' tumour and inadvertent intraperitoneal spread of an ovarian germ cell tumour must be acknowledged, as these would clearly constitute the 'significant risks, affecting the judgement of the reasonable patient'. It is accepted that parents may be greatly distressed by the stark realities of the disclosure and have little alternative but to consent despite these fears. However, these legal conclusions are the result of a balancing act between patients' right to control their own fate and the harm that the disclosure might cause. It is our duty to conform to them.

Consent and confidentiality

Consent for treatment operates to protect us from the unwanted touch and in precisely, the same way, operates to protect us from the unwanted disclosure of our personal information. For the purposes of surgical practice, the legal rules governing consent for treatment in children are no different to those controlling the disclosure of their private information. A Gillick competent child may thus defend her information against all comers, including her parents. It will be seen that the General Medical Council asserts circumstances when it may be considered to be in the public interest to disclose information against the wishes of the competent patient or that disclosure is necessary by statute but do this only with extreme caution.

Further reading

Department of Health. Reference guide to consent for examination or treatment, 2nd edn. London: DH, 2009.

Nair R, Holroyd DJ (eds). Handbook of surgical consent. Oxford: Oxford University Press, 2012.

Wheeler RA. The numeric threshold for the disclosure of risk: outdated and inapplicable to surgical consent. Ann R Coll Surg Engl 2012; 94:81–82.

Crohn's disease

Learning outcomes

- To be aware of the intra- and extra-intestinal manifestations of Crohn's disease
- To know when surgery should be considered
- To know what surgical options are available

Overview

Crohn's disease (CD) is a chronic inflammatory disease, which can affect the whole gastrointestinal tract. The inflammation extends transmurally and characteristically has skip lesions, with areas of normal tissue in between.

The most commonly affected sites are the terminal ileum and the colon, and it frequently affects the perineum and anus.

It is a chronic disease with periods of remission and relapse. It has a wide range of symptoms, and extra-intestinal complications are frequent. Surgery is not curative and postoperative recurrence is highly likely.

Epidemiology and aetiology

Prevalence estimates for Northern Europe have ranged from 27 to 48 per 100,000. CD tends to present initially in the teens and twenties, with another peak incidence in the fifties to seventies, but can occur at any age.

Pathologically it shows a transmural pattern of inflammation, with ulceration in highly active disease. Biopsies show mucosal inflammation with focal neutrophil infiltration into the epithelium. Granulomas are present in 50% and are non-caseating. There may also be evidence of chronic mucosal damage, such as intestinal villi blunting, atypical crypt branching and metaplasia.

CD appears to be caused by both environmental factors and genetic predisposition. The chronic inflammation seems to occur when the adaptive immune system tries to compensate for a deficient innate immune system.

Genetic association is primarily with variations of the *NOD2* gene and its protein, which senses bacterial cell walls. Impaired macrophage cytokine secretion contributes to impaired innate immunity and leads to a sustained microbial-induced inflammatory response.

An increased incidence in the developed world indicates an environmental component, and CD is associated with an increased intake of animal and milk protein with an increased ratio of omega-6 to omega-3 polyunsaturated fatty acids. Siblings of affected individuals are at higher risk. Males and females are equally affected with smokers twice as likely to develop CD than non-smokers.

Clinical features

It typically manifests in the gastrointestinal tract and can be categorised by the specific region affected. Ileocolic CD accounts for 50% of cases. Crohn's ileitis accounts for 30% and Crohn's colitis accounts for the remaining 20% and may be particularly difficult to distinguish from ulcerative colitis (UC). Gastroduodenal and jejunal CD can also occur, with the latter showing patchy disease.

Gastrointestinal

Many people with CD have symptoms for years prior to diagnosis. Because of the 'patchy' nature of the gastrointestinal disease and the depth of tissue involvement, initial symptoms can be subtle.

Abdominal pain may occur initially, often accompanied by diarrhoea that may or may not be bloody. Diarrhoea is a common presenting feature in postoperative patients.

In ileitis, the diarrhoea is typically large volume and watery, and colitis may result in smaller volumes, but with higher frequency. Stool consistency ranges from solid to watery, and in severe cases, an individual may have > 20 bowel movements per day and may need to defecate at night. Visible blood in the faeces is less common in CD than in UC, but may be seen in Crohn's colitis. Bloody bowel movements are typically intermittent, and may be bright or dark red in colour. In severe colitis, bleeding may be copious.

The intestinal discomfort may be exacerbated by flatulence and bloating. Intestinal stenoses frequently present with abdominal pain and in severe stenosis, nausea and vomiting may indicate the beginnings of small bowel obstruction.

CD may also be associated with primary sclerosing cholangitis although this is more commonly associated with UC. Perianal discomfort may also be prominent. Itchiness or pain around the anus may be suggestive of inflammation, fistulisation, perianal abscess or anal fissure. Perianal skin tags are also common. Perianal CD may be accompanied by faecal incontinence.

The mouth may be affected by non-healing aphthous ulcers and, rarely, the oesophagus and stomach are involved. Symptoms include dysphagia, upper abdominal pain and vomiting.

Systemic

Among children, growth failure is common, with many first diagnosed based on an inability to grow. Because it may manifest peripubertally, up to 30% have growth retardation. Fever may be present, although fevers > 38.5°C are uncommon unless there is an infective complication.

Amongst older individuals, CD may manifest as weight loss, usually related to decreased food intake, since individuals with intestinal symptoms from CD often feel better when they do not eat so tend to lose their appetite. Those with extensive small intestine disease may also have malabsorption, further exacerbating weight loss.

Extra-intestinal

- Skin – pyoderma gangrenosum, erythema nodosum
- Opthalmic – uveitis, episcleritis
- Rheumatological – seronegative spondyloarthropathy which can lead to ankylosing spondylitis and sacroiliitis
- Haematological – deep venous thrombosis and pulmonary embolism, autoimmune haemolytic anaemia
- Clubbing
- Osteoporosis

- Neurological (in 15%) – seizures, stroke, myopathy, peripheral neuropathy, headache and depression
- Oral – aphthous ulcers, cheilitis granulomatosa, orofacial granulomatosis, pyostomatitis vegetans, geographic tongue, migratory stomatitis

Complications

- Strictures, adhesions, fistulae (enteric, vesicoenteric, enterovaginal, enterocutaneous), abscesses, perforation, haemorrhage
- Small bowel cancer in those with small bowel CD and colon cancer in those with colonic CD (relative risk 5.6); colonoscopy is recommended in those with CD for > 8 years
- Short bowel syndrome

Investigations

- Full blood cell count may show anaemia due to blood loss, vitamin B_{12} deficiency, autoimmune haemolysis or chronic disease
- Erythrocyte sedimentation rate can be useful to gauge the degree of inflammation
- Small bowel follow-through contrast study may suggest the disease and is useful in small bowel CD
- Colonoscopy is performed with biopsies and cannulation of the terminal ileum
- At colonoscopy, 40% have a cobblestone appearance
- MRI is useful for looking for complications such as abscesses, small bowel obstruction or fistulae

Differential diagnosis

- Ulcerative colitis

Treatment

1. Lifestyle – no smoking, elemental diet, proper hydration
2. Medical – antibiotics, corticosteroids, 5-aminosalicylic acid
- **Immunomodulators:** azathioprine, mercaptopurine, methotrexate, infliximab, adalimumab, certolizumab and natalizumab may be useful

- **Surgical options:** surgical principles in CD involve removing as little bowel as possible because the patient may require subsequent bowel resection. After the first surgery, CD usually recurs at the site of resection although can appear in other locations
  - For strictures, stricturoplasty (open or laparoscopic) is performed; the stricture is opened longitudinally and closed transversely
  - For obstruction, open or laparoscopic bowel resection is performed with primary anastomosis
  - For abscesses, surgery is not recommended
  - For fistulae, surgery is not recommended although an SNAP protocol should be followed
    - **S (sepsis):** manage sepsis; e.g. drain abscesses percutaneously
    - **N (nutrition):** ensure proper nutrition, may require parenteral support
    - **A (anatomy):** define anatomy of the fistulae with enteric contrast studies or fistulogram
    - **P (plan):** plan for definitive treatment if spontaneous closure does not occur

Further reading

Gasparetto M, Corradin S, Vallortigara F, et al. Infliximab and pediatric stricturing Crohn's disease: a possible alternative to surgery? Experience of seven cases. Acta Gastroenterol Belg 2012; 75:58–60.

Jakobsen C, Paerregaard A, Munkholm P, et al. Pediatric inflammatory bowel disease: increasing incidence, decreasing surgery rate, and compromised nutritional status: A prospective population-based cohort study 2007–2009. Inflamm Bowel Dis 2011; 17:2541–2550.

Romeo E, Jasonni V, Caldaro T, et al. Strictureplasty and intestinal resection: different options in complicated pediatric-onset Crohn disease. J Pediatr Surg 2012; 47:944–948.

Related topics of interest

- Ulcerative colitis (p. 345)

Cystic hygroma

Learning outcomes

- To understand the underlying aetiology and associated abnormalities
- To highlight the antenatal diagnosis
- To be aware of alternative management options

Overview

Cystic hygromas (CHs) are congenital lymphatic malformations, consisting of multilocular cysts of varying size, arising in any region of the body. The cysts may be uni- or multiloculated and are described as microcystic, macrocystic or mixed, dependent on the cysts being large or < 2 cm in diameter.

Epidemiology and aetiology

CHs affect males and females equally and may arise anywhere in the developing lymphatic system but they classically arise in the posterior triangle of the neck. They occur in approximately 1 in 12,000 live births and up to 65% are diagnosed on antenatal ultrasound. They are associated with a number of chromosomal and structural abnormalities.

CHs tend to form in loose areolar tissue, whereas capillary and cavernous forms of lymphangiomas tend to form in muscle. Studies using cell proliferation markers have demonstrated that lymphangioma enlargement is related to engorgement rather than actual cell proliferation. Molecular studies suggest that vascular endothelial growth factor C and its receptors may play an important role in the development of lymphatic malformations.

The lymphatic system develops during the 5th week of gestation as outgrowths of the venous system. Six primitive lymphatic sacs develop with two jugular sacs draining the head, neck and arms, two iliac sacs draining the legs and two sacs draining the intestine.

CHs are thought to arise due to a failure of lymphatics to connect to the venous system, abnormal budding of lymphatic tissue, and sequestered lymphatic rests that retain their embryonic growth potential. These lymphatic rests can penetrate adjacent structures or dissect along fascial planes and eventually become canalised. These spaces retain their secretions and develop cystic components because of the lack of an outflow tract. The nature of the surrounding tissue determines whether the lymphangioma is capillary, cavernous or cystic.

The result is variable-sized collections of lymphatic fluid, or cysts, which can cause extensive symptoms by their mass effect, often distorting the local anatomy and extending into and around vital structures. In addition to congenital development, CH can arise from trauma (including surgery), inflammation or obstruction of a lymphatic drainage pathway.

Clinical features

Antenatal

Following diagnosis, a thorough ultrasound examination should be performed looking for other anatomical abnormalities or signs of hydrops. Karyotyping should be offered as chromosomal abnormalities occur in 50–75%, with Turner's syndrome the most common. Other anomalies include

- Chromosomal
  - Turner's syndrome (45, XO)
  - Trisomies 13, 18 and 21
- Non-chromosomal
  - Noonans syndrome
  - Multiple pterygium disease
  - Cowchock Wapner Kurtz syndrome
  - Klippel–Feil sequence

Hydrops associated with CH is common (50–90%), and a large persisting CH associated with hydrops carries a very poor prognosis; most will die spontaneously in utero. Prenatal diagnosis may aid planning for a safe delivery by draining the cyst in utero or anticipating a requirement for the ex utero intrapartum treatment procedure.

Postnatal

When not diagnosed antenatally, CHs are usually associated with a good prognosis. At birth 50–65% are evident with 80–90% clinically apparent in the first two years of life. The cysts are typically large and thick walled and have little involvement of surrounding tissue. The overlying skin can take on a bluish hue or may appear normal. Further clinical presentation depends on the site and size of the lesion:

- Stridor and cyanosis due to airway compromise, with suprahyoid CHs usually causing more breathing difficulties than infrahyoid lesions
- Feeding difficulties or failure to thrive
- A rapid increase in size following infection or intralesional bleeding
- Rarely, children with CH display symptoms of new-onset obstructive sleep apnoea; these children usually have a CH or other space-occupying lesion of the supraglottis or paraglottic region
- In the mouth and oropharynx, the microcystic form of lymphangioma predominates over CH; microcystic lymphangiomas commonly appear as clusters of clear, black or red vesicles on the buccal mucosa or tongue

Common sites include
- Head and neck   ~75%
- Axilla   ~20%
- Mediastinum   ~1%
- Abdomen   ~1%
- Other   ~1–2%

Investigations

- Photography – for cosmetic appearance
- Plain X-ray – helpful in delineating gross anatomy
- Ultrasound scanning – demonstrates relationship to surrounding structures
- Magnetic resonance imaging (MRI) – provides the best soft tissue visualisation and details local anatomy
- Computed tomography – inferior images to MRI and carries a significant radiation dose

Differential diagnosis

- Teratoma
- Haemangioma
- Branchial cyst
- Thyroglossal duct cyst

Treatment

Non-operative

CHs are benign and observation using a 'watch and wait' policy may be appropriate; however, spontaneous resolution is uncommon. More invasive management is indicated when symptoms or complications occur.

Sclerotherapy

Varying success has been reported with the administration of a number of sclerosing agents following aspiration of the hygroma fluid in macroscopic CH with a smaller degree of success in microcystic malformations.

The two most commonly used have been bleomycin and OK432, which are injected intralesionally under ultrasound control. Use of doxycycline, absolute alcohol, sodium tetradecyl sulphate and fibrin sealant is also reported.

Bleomycin is a glycopeptide antibiotic produced by *Streptomyces verticillus*. It induces an inflammatory process resulting in fibrosis of cysts. Resolution occurs in 60%, and 30% have a reduction in size. Complications include increasing size of CH, fever and vomiting, cellulitis and pulmonary fibrosis.

Bleomycin should be in stock in most UK hospital pharmacies, is prepared on request and must be prescribed on a chemotherapy chart.

OK432 is a lyophilised product of group A *Streptococcus pyogenes* and penicillin G. It causes migration of inflammatory cells into cysts, damaging the cyst endothelium and increasing apoptosis. Complete or marked shrinkage occurs in 70–80% of affected patients. Complications include local swelling and fever.

Surgical excision

Preoperative planning with appropriate imaging should be performed to determine the extent of the lesion and its relationship to adjacent structures. Simple, superficial CHs should be amenable to complete excision; however, complex CHs may surround or displace vital structures, making their identification and subsequent dissection extremely challenging. In these situations a staged approach to excision or debulking surgery is recommended.

Technical points

- Adequate exposure is very important
- Careful dissection is carried out to avoid rupture of the cyst wall as fluid within the cyst will aid in defining the correct plane for dissection
- Vital structures must be identified and preserved
- Identify and ligate lymphatic channels to prevent accumulation of lymph postoperatively
- Intraoperative placement of a suction or simple drain to reduce the risk of postoperative haematoma or seroma
- Use a nerve stimulator and request the assistance of a maxillofacial or ear, nose and throat colleague if appropriate

Complications and outcome

- Infection and bleeding
- Nerve damage
- Prolonged drainage and seroma
- Laryngeal oedema and airway obstruction (neck dissection)
- Recurrence

Morbidity depends on the anatomic location of the CH and in general is related to cosmetic disfigurement and impingement on other critical structures, such as nerves, vessels, lymphatics and the airway. Mortality has been reported to be as high as 2–6%, secondary to pneumonia, bronchiectasis and airway compromise.

Further reading

Alqahtani A, Nguyen LT, Flageole H, et al. 25 years' experience with lymphangiomas in children. J Pediatr Surg 1999; 34:1164–1168.

Giguere CM, Bauman NM, Sato Y, et al. Treatment of lymphangiomas with OK-432 (Picibanil) sclerotherapy: a prospective multi-institutional trial. Arch Otolaryngol Head Neck Surg 2002; 128:1137–1144.

Muir T, Kessell G, Hampton F, et al. Successful nonsurgical treatment of lymphatic and venous malformations with bleomycin sclerotherapy. Rome: BAPS-EUPSA Joint Congress, 2012.

Related topics of interest

Diabetes mellitus

Learning outcomes

- To have a basic understanding of childhood diabetes
- To be able to recognise and initiate treatment of complications of diabetes
- To understand how to manage diabetic patients requiring surgery

Overview

Diabetes mellitus (DM) is a group of metabolic disorders characterised by chronic hyperglycaemia, arising from defects in insulin secretion and/or insulin action.

Epidemiology and aetiology

- **Diabetes mellitus type 1 (DM1):** This is the third most common chronic disease in childhood, occurring in approximately 1 in 400 children in the UK. It accounts for >90% of paediatric diabetes. There is β-cell dysfunction (autoimmune or idiopathic) leading (ultimately) to absolute insulin deficiency. Numerous genes predisposing to DM have been identified, although environmental factors, such as viral infections, are also implicated
- **Diabetes mellitus type 2 (DM2):** This accounts for approximately 1% of diabetic children in the UK. The incidence has increased, and rising obesity and sedentary lifestyles are implicated. It is caused by insulin resistance and/or a secretory defect
- **Others:** These include genetic defects of β-cell function and insulin action, diseases of exocrine pancreas and drug induced (steroids, tacrolimus)

Clinical features

Clinical features of hyperglycaemia include polyuria (including nocturnal enuresis), excessive drinking (polydipsia), lethargy and weight loss.

Investigations

- **Urine glucose:** A positive test suggests DM1
- **Blood glucose:** A random glucose level of >11 mmol/L or a fasting level of >7 mmol/L is diagnostic
- **Glycosylated haemoglobin (HbA1c):** More than 6.5% is diagnostic and repeat levels aid management
- **Oral glucose tolerance test:** This can exclude DM when hyperglycaemia or glycosuria occurs due to atypical causes or when renal glucosuria is present. Obtain a fasting blood sugar, and then administer an oral glucose load [2 g/kg for children younger than 3 years, 1.75 g/kg for children aged 3–10 years (max 50 g) or 75 g for children older than 10 years]. Check the blood glucose after 2 hours. A fasting level >6.7 mmol/L or 2-hour value >11 mmol/L indicates diabetes. Mild elevations may not indicate diabetes when the patient is asymptomatic and has no diabetes-related antibodies
- **Urinary albumin (if older than 12 years):** Microalbuminuria is an indicator of diabetic nephropathy
- **Islet cell antibodies:** They are non-specific markers of pancreatic autoimmune disease, found in approximately 5% of unaffected children. These may be present, but are not required for diagnosis

Treatment

DM1

Insulin as biosynthetic natural insulin or insulin analogues – a variety of them are available:

- **Short-acting analogues:** onset of action after 15 minutes; duration of action up to 5 hours. (These have largely superseded the short-acting soluble insulins.)
- **Intermediate-acting insulins:** onset of action after 2–4 hours; duration of action 12–24 hours

- **Long-acting analogues:** onset of action after 2–4 hours; duration of action up to 24 hours

Commonly used regimes are as follows:
- **Twice daily:** Free mixing or premixed insulins. Given subcutaneously (sc), e.g. 30% short-acting insulin or analogue, 70% intermediate-acting
- **Multiple daily injections (MDI):** Long-acting insulin or analogue sc once or twice daily. Short-acting insulin or analogue sc before meals and snacks, and correction doses if blood glucose above target range. Most commonly used regime
- **Continuous subcutaneous insulin infusion (CSII):** sc cannula in situ for approximately 3 days to give background basal infusion of insulin and boluses of insulin administered via pump to cover meals and snacks and blood glucose above target range

DM2

- Exercise and weight reduction if raised body mass index
- Oral hypoglycaemic agents, e.g. biguanide metformin
- Insulin therapy often added if poor diabetes control despite the above measures

Complications

The complications of diabetes are potentially life-threatening.

Hypoglycaemia

In diabetic children, blood glucose needs treating if < 3.5 mmol/L (or if < 4 mmol/L and symptomatic).
1. Symptoms
- **Autonomic:** hunger, sweating, shaking, anxiety, pallor, nausea
- **Neuroglycopenia:** dizziness, blurred vision, slurred speech, sleepiness, irritability, weakness, seizures
2. Treatment
- **Awake, orientated and able to swallow:** Give 10–20 g of glucose orally (10 g glucose, approximately two teaspoons of sugar), 50 mL Lucozade, 90 mL Coca Cola (non-

diet), followed by a slice of bread or one or two plain biscuits
- **Awake but disorientated:** Administer Glucogel (10 g/25 g tube). Massage contents of the tube between teeth and cheek, followed by a slice of bread or one or two plain biscuits when orientated
- **Unconscious or fasting:** Give a bolus of 2–5 mL/kg 10% glucose intravenously. Ensure a continuous infusion of 10% glucose/0.45% NaCl with 10 mmol KCl/500 mL is running. If venous access is unobtainable, administer glucagon intramuscularly: < 11 years = 0.5 mg, > 11 years = 1 mg

If on insulin sliding scale (ISS), stop temporarily. If on CSII the infusion may need to be suspended temporarily. Recheck blood glucose 10–15 minutes later and repeat treatment if necessary.

Diabetic ketoacidosis

Absolute or relative deficiency of insulin and the combined effects of counter-regulatory hormones lead to the following biochemical features:
- **Hyperglycaemia:** blood glucose > 11 mmol/L (leads to polyuria, thirst and polydipsia and subsequently dehydration)
- **Acidosis:** pH < 7.3 and/or bicarbonate < 15 mmol/L
- **Ketosis:** raised blood and urine ketones secondary to free fatty acid utilisation

Diabetic ketoacidosis (DKA) can result in significant abdominal pain, gastroparesis or ileus. Consider DKA if a diabetic person describes abdominal pain (or in any patient with symptoms of hyperglycaemia). Patients with DKA are dehydrated with ketotic breath and in the more severe form have Kussmaul respiration. If blood glucose is > 15 mmol/L, check urinary ketones (and if possible blood ketones).
Treatment includes
- Careful fluid resuscitation and insulin infusion
- Regular and careful monitoring of neuro-observations, fluid balance, blood glucose and electrolytes

Elective surgery for patients on insulin therapy

Ideally first on operating lists to facilitate a safe procedure.

1. Preoperatively
- Usual doses of insulin, night before procedure
- First on morning list
  - On the day of the procedure, omit insulin and breakfast (if on CSII continue this)
- First on afternoon list
  - Advise the child to have a normal breakfast no later than 7.30 am
  - Breakfast insulin dose options
    - If on MDI regime, give usual breakfast insulin
    - If on CSII, continue
    - If on a twice daily insulin regime, give one half rapid-acting component of morning dose (as rapid-acting insulin). Liaise with the diabetes team
- Allow clear fluids, including sweet drinks until 3 hours prior to surgery
- Measure and record capillary blood glucose levels (CBGL) hourly once nil by mouth and half hourly during the operation
- If major surgery (unable to eat within 4 hours of start of procedure), start intravenous glucose and ISS infusion in theatre if not on CSII
2. Postoperatively
- Measure and record CBGL in recovery and then hourly for 4 hours and discuss with the diabetes team regarding insulin prescription
- If on ISS, continue intravenous glucose and ISS until taking adequate oral fluids and snacks. The child may eat and drink safely on the ISS. Liaise with the diabetes team regarding restarting sc insulin

Emergency surgery for patients on insulin therapy

Emergency procedures differ from elective ones as children run the risk of developing DKA if unwell. The associated prolonged starvation with delayed surgery poses additional complications.

1. Preoperatively
- Inform the diabetes team immediately
- Check venous urea and electrolytes, glucose and blood gas when the child is cannulated
- If not in DKA, commence a glucose and ISS
- Measure and record CBGL hourly once nil by mouth and half hourly during the operation
- If the patient is ill or diabetes poorly controlled, follow your institution's DKA protocol. Postpone operating until the patient is stabilised
- Operate when
  - Rehydrated
  - Blood pressure stable
  - Serum sodium and potassium within the normal range
  - Blood glucose < 17 mmol/L
2. Postoperatively
- As for elective surgery

Children on CSII

As these systems deliver basal insulin, separate from any bolus insulin. The pump should run on the normal basal setting for the duration of the procedure if the patient is well.

Blood glucose should be checked hourly and the infusion rate altered if necessary. Basal rates can be suspended temporarily to correct mild hypoglycaemia.

Type 2 diabetes and surgery

Due to the increased risk of lactic acidosis, many units stop metformin perioperatively.

Further reading

British Society for Paediatric Endocrinology and Diabetes. Diabetic ketoacidosis guidelines. Bristol: British Society for Paediatric Endocrinology and Diabetes, 2009.

Butler, G Kirk J. Oxford handbook of paediatric endocrinology and diabetes. Oxford: OUP, 2011.

Betts P, et al. Management of children and adolescents with diabetes requiring surgery. Pediatr Diabetes 2009; 10:169–174.

Disorders of sexual development 1

Learning outcomes

- To be able to recognise disorders of sex development
- To be aware of the principles of initial management

Overview

Disorders of sexual development (DSD) are congenital conditions in which the development of chromosomal, gonadal or anatomical sex is atypical.

Epidemiology and aetiology

Normal sexual differentiation is a very complex process, the first step of which is activation of the *SRY* gene (on the Y chromosome of a 46, XY fetus) at 7–8 weeks of gestation to trigger testicular development prior to which the gonad is bipotential (also influenced by *SOX9* and downstream signalling cascade). Failure of this complex chain reaction leads to deficient testicular development and 46, XY DSD.

In some cases, there are chromosomal anomalies, (i.e. mixed chromosomal DSD), instead of either 46, XX or 46, XY. Some of these babies present with asymmetrical external genitalia, where one side is more masculine (often with a descended testis) while the other side is more feminine (with an impalpable gonad, as it is an intra-abdominal non-functional 'streak' gonad, or even an ovary).

Quite commonly the gonadal development is normal, but sex development is perturbed by the effects of abnormal hormones, such as excess androgens in 46, XX females [the most common cause of DSD, with congenital adrenal hyperplasia (CAH)], where excess androgens are produced in the fetal adrenal as a byproduct of a block in the production of cortisol and mineralocorticoids. In 46, XY fetuses there can be mutations in the enzymes that synthesise androgens or Müllerian inhibiting substance [also known as anti-Müllerian hormone (AMH) which leads to the regression of Müllerian structures] produced by the Sertoli cells, as well as mutations in the androgen receptor (AR) producing androgen insensitivity. In severe AR mutations, there may be no androgenic effects at all, allowing the external genitalia to remain feminine, as external genital development requires the androgen dihydrotestosterone (converted from testosterone by 5α reductase) to be masculinised. An overview of normal internal and external genital development is shown in **Figures 12** and **13**. In girls, recent evidence has discovered that ovarian differentiation is a more active process than previously thought, requiring specific factors, including β-catenin, Wnt 4 and RSPO genes.

Clinical features

Babies with DSD present with one or more of the following symptoms:

- Clitoromegaly in an apparent female (easily overlooked: usually CAH)
- Obviously ambiguous external genitalia
- Proximal 'hypospadias' with a bifid scrotum and undescended testes in a presumed male (easily overlooked: usually 46, XY DSD or mixed chromosomal DSD, but could be 46, XX DSD with excessive androgens in CAH)
- Complex morphological anomaly of the external genitalia and adjacent perineum and anorectum (non-hormonal causes of DSD, e.g. cloacal exstrophy)

Later in childhood DSD may present unexpectedly during surgery:

- Inguinal hernia contains discordant gonad or genital tract (e.g. testis in the hernia sac of a girl with complete androgen insensitivity syndrome)
- Uterus or discordant gonad identified at orchidopexy
- Discordant internal genital tracts found at cystoscopy (vaginal cavity in male urethra) or laparoscopy

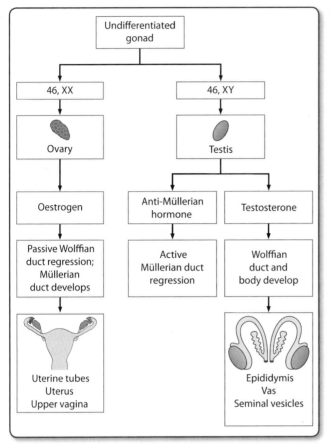

Figure 12 Sexual differentiation of the internal genital ducts is under the influence of testosterone, Müllerian inhibiting substance (or anti-Müllerian hormone) or oestrogen.

The adolescent or young adult with DSD may present with:

- Precocious or delayed puberty (CAH or gonadal dysgenesis defect)
- Abnormal virilisation in a girl (46, XY DSD with deficient prenatal androgen synthesis)
- Primary amenorrhoea or cyclical abdominal pains (obstructed hemivagina)

Investigations

The most important anatomical tests are a thorough physical examination to document:

- Degree of external virilisation
- Position and quality of gonads
- Internal genital tract (rectal examination to feel uterus)

along with ultrasonography, laparoscopy, cystoscopy or retrograde sinogram of the common urogenital sinus.

The hormonal status needs to be determined to diagnose whether the baby has CAH (17-hydroxyprogesterone is elevated, and there may be low serum Na^+ and glucose). The remaining hormonal tests are best done by referral to an experienced endocrinologist. The chromosomal status can be determined by karyotype.

Differential diagnosis

- **46, XX DSD – CAH:** This is the most common (~50%) DSD seen with ambiguous genitalia in infancy
- **46, XY DSD:** These are a heterogeneous group of disorders, including gonadal dysgenesis, gonadotrophin dysfunction, deficient steroidogenesis (enzyme defect), androgen insensitivity (receptor mutation), Müllerian duct persistence and

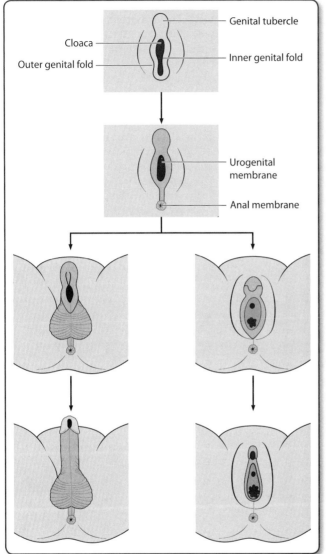

Figure 13 Sexual differentiation of the external genitalia. Androgens in the male cause enlargement of the phallus, masculinisation of the urethra, fusion of the scrotum and inguinoscrotal descent of the testis. Androgens also prevent development of the vagina.

Labels in figure:
- Genital tubercle
- Cloaca
- Outer genital fold
- Inner genital fold
- Urogenital membrane
- Anal membrane

non-hormonal defects, such as cloacal exstrophy
- **Mixed sex chromosome and ovotesticular DSD:** In these conditions, there may be gonadal asymmetry, with one testis and a non-functional 'streak' (45, X/46, XY DSD) or an ovary or ovotestis

Treatment

- The most important management occurs in the labour ward or postnatal ward as soon as a DSD is suspected. Tell the parents that the genital development is incomplete, and that for the moment the gender is uncertain, although once the tests are done, it will be a boy or a girl. The parents should delay naming the baby until after assessment in the quaternary centre. Reassure the parents that gender assignment and a treatment plan will be done at the quaternary centre. Call a meeting of all labour/postnatal ward staff to explain that no one is to give gratuitous advice about gender prior to transfer, and that the baby should not be called 'he' or 'she', but 'the baby'

- Contact the tertiary/quaternary DSD centre for advice about the condition and the timing of transfer
- Urgent referral to a tertiary/quaternary centre with an experienced multidisciplinary team (endocrinologist, surgeon, gynaecologist, geneticist, social worker, psychologist, ethicist)

- Decisions about gender of rearing and medical or surgical treatment are made only after all the DSD team members have assessed the baby and a case conference held to discuss proposed treatment plan
- Ideally, the decisions by medical experts are reviewed by a clinical ethics committee to assess whether the seven ethical principles have been considered:
  1. Minimise physical risk
  2. Minimise psychosocial risk
  3. Preserve potential for fertility
  4. Preserve and promote capacity for satisfying sexual relations
  5. Leave options open for future
  6. Consider views and wishes of child, if old enough
  7. Respect parents' wishes and beliefs

Further reading

Hughes IA, Houk C, Ahmed SF, et al. Consensus statement on management of intersex disorders. Arch Dis Child 2012; 91:554–563.

Hutson JM, Warne GL, Grover SR. Disorders of sex development: an integrated approach to management. Berlin: Springer-Verlag, 2012.

Related topics of interest

- Disorders of sexual development 2 (p. 87)

Disorders of sexual development 2

Learning outcomes

- To be able to determine whether the aetiology is genetic or biochemical
- To show an understanding of the medical management

Classification

Three main groups are as follows:

1. Sex chromosome DSD
- 45XO: Turner syndrome
- 47XXY: Klinefelter syndrome
- 45X/46XY: mixed gonadal dysgenesis; ovotesticular DSD
- 46XX/46XY: chimeric, ovotesticular DSD (de la Chapelle syndrome)

2. 46XY DSD
- Disorders of gonadal (testicular) development
  - Complete gonadal dysgenesis (Swyer syndrome)
  - Partial gonadal dysgenesis
  - Gonadal regression
  - Ovotesticular DSD
  - Ovarian DSD
- Disorders of androgen synthesis/action
  - Androgen biosynthesis defect (e.g. 5α-reductase deficiency, 17-hydroxylase deficiency and StAR mutations)
  - 3-β-hydroxysteroid dehydrogenase 2 deficiency (3βHSD2)
  - P450 oxidoreductase deficiency (POR)
  - Androgen receptor mutations (complete or partial androgen insensitivity syndrome)
  - Luteinising hormone (LH) receptor defects (e.g. Leydig cell hypoplasia/aplasia)
- Anti-Müllerian hormone (AMH)/AMH receptor disorders (persistent Müllerian duct syndrome)
- Other
  - Vanishing testis syndrome
  - Congenital hypogonadotropic hypogonadism (DAX1, KAL1 mutations)
  - Abnormal male genital development, e.g. hypospadias, cloacal anomalies and syndromic (e.g. Robinow and Aarskog)

3. 46XX DSD
- Disorders of gonadal (ovarian) development
  - Gonadal dysgenesis [e.g. SF-1 and follicle-stimulating hormone (FSH) receptor mutations]
  - Testicular DSD (e.g. SOX9 duplication, RSPO1 mutations and SRY+)
  - Ovotesticular DSD
- Androgen excess
  - Fetal [e.g. virilising congenital adrenal hyperplasia (CAH): 21-hydroxylase /11β hydroxylase deficiency; 3βHSD2; POR]
  - Fetoplacental [e.g. aromatase deficiency (CYP19 mutations) and POR]
  - Maternal (e.g. virilising tumours – luteoma; exogenous androgenic drugs)
- Other
  - Müllerian agenesis/hypoplasia (Müllerian duct aplasia, renal aplasia and cervicothoracic somite dysplasia)
  - Cloacal extrophy
  - Vaginal atresia
  - Uterine abnormalities

Assessment

Clinical evaluation

- History (prenatal and family, including history of DSD, parental consanguinity and infertility)
- Clinical assessment
  - Prader staging
    Normal female external genitalia
    ↓
    1. Female external genitalia with clitoromegaly
    2. Clitoromegaly with posterior labial fusion
    3. Increased phallic size with complete labioscrotal fusion forming a urogenital sinus with a single opening

4. Complete scrotal fusion with opening of the urogenital sinus at the base of the phallic clitoris
5. Penile clitoris, urethral meatus at tip of phallus and scrotum-like labia (appear like males without palpable gonads)

↓

Normal male external genitalia

- Presence of chordee
- Location of urethral opening
- Palpable gonads
- Dysmorphic features suggestive of syndromic cause of DSD

In general, DSD patients who have an asymmetrical genital abnormality have a chromosomal disorder and those with symmetrical genital abnormalities have a biochemical aetiology.

Diagnostic evaluation

Initial investigations should include

- **Karyotype:** An initial fluorescent in situ hybridisation for SRY can be undertaken within 24 hours and a formal karyotype follows. DNA should also be stored for further molecular genetic investigations in the future
- **Imaging:** Pelvic ultrasound (in an experienced centre); looking for Müllerian structures and gonads
- **Biochemical:** Androgens (androstenedione, dehydroepiandrosterone and testosterone), 17-hydroxyprogesterone (after day 3 of life), AMH and gonadotropins (LH and FSH). Dependent on these results, further investigations such as urine steroid profile and dynamic endocrine testing (e.g. synacthen and 3-day hCG) may also be required. The possibility of salt-losing CAH with adrenal crisis should be kept in mind with serial electrolyte measurements

Despite advances in genetics and progress made in our understanding of normal sexual development, only 20% of patients with DSD will have an identified molecular genetic diagnosis. Although the majority of 46XX DSD will have a virilising form of CAH, only 50% of patients with 46XY DSD will receive a definitive diagnosis, and this should be borne in mind when counselling families.

Management
Medical

- Generally specific to underlying condition and gender assignment
- Hypogonadism is common to DSD
- Induction of puberty aims to
  - Mimic normal pubertal maturation (secondary sexual characteristics and growth spurt)
  - Mimic bone mineral accumulation
  - Aid psychosexual maturation
1. Treatment options
   - Males
     - Puberty is induced by use of intramuscular depot injection of testosterone esters (monthly)
     - Maintenance in adulthood is done via 3 monthly long-acting esters (e.g. testosterone undecanoate or transdermal preparations, patches or gels), with doses titrated to maintain testosterone within physiological normal range although in partial androgen insensitivity syndrome, supraphysiological levels may be needed for optimum effect
   - Females
     - Oestrogen supplements are required for pubertal induction and menstruation
     - Progesterone is added after breakthough bleeding to prevent unopposed oestrogen action and the risk of long-term endometrial cancer
     - Cyclical progesterone is not necessary in women without a uterus
2. Fertility options – dependent on specific condition

Surgical

- Emphasis should be on functional outcome, including optimising fertility, rather than cosmetic appearance
- In 46XX DSD, evidence suggests that women who underwent feminising clitoral surgery in infancy have significant psychosexual dysfunction. Parents are now less likely to opt for surgery when clitoromegaly is less severe (Prader stages 1–2), and surgery is anatomically based to preserve innervation of the clitoris

and erectile function. In many units, clitoroplasty will only be concealment or recession. A vaginoplasty is often undertaken simultaneously to separate the urethra and vagina. This is based on guidelines from the American Academy of Pediatrics and advocated on the basis of avoidance of potential complications from connection of urinary tract and peritoneum via Fallopian tubes, and the beneficial effects of oestrogen in early infancy. It is likely that surgical reconstruction undertaken in infancy will need further revision at puberty

- In 46XY DSD, there are specific techniques for hypospadias repair, chordee correction and urethral reconstruction. This may be either one stage or two stages, depending on the size of the phallus, urethral plate quality and the degree of chordee. In addition, use of testosterone prior to surgery may be useful to improve operative outcomes. If successful gender assignment is dependent on the procedure, the complexity and likely outcome of the repair must be discussed fully with the family and may well affect the final decision regarding gender assignment
- In patients with streak gonads (e.g. mixed gonadal dysgenesis or females with gonadal dysgenesis and Y chromosome material), bilateral gonadectomy should be performed in early childhood. In patients with a scrotal testis and gonadal dysgenesis, testicular biopsy at puberty is recommended, and if premalignant cells are demonstrated, sperm banking prior to radiotherapy with or without orchidectomy should be carried out

Psychosocial

- Psychosexual development is complex and includes gender identity, gender role and sexual orientation
- Gender identity refers to a person's self-representation as male or female (and some may not identify with either gender completely); gender role refers to sex-typical behaviours (such as toy preference) and is influenced by prenatal exposure to androgens, and sexual orientation refers to hetero-, homo- or bisexuality
- It is influenced by several factors such as exposure to androgens, brain structure, chromosomal and phenotypic sex as well as environmental factors
- Psychosocial management should be an integral part of ongoing care from diagnosis into adulthood and includes decisions regarding gender assignment, disclosure of diagnosis and future fertility to ensure optimal quality of life

Conclusion

- DSDs are a complex and heterogenous group of conditions which require expert multidisciplinary team care throughout life
- Expert surgical assessment is essential for appropriate gender assignment and understanding long-term outcomes

Further reading

Barbaro M, Wedell A, Nordenstrom A. Disorders of sex development. Semin Fetal Neonatal Med 2011; 16:119–127

Biason-Lauber A. Control of sex development. Best Pract Res Clin Endocrinol Metab 2010; 24:163–186.

Hughes IA, Houk C, Ahmed SF, et al. Consensus statement on management of intersex disorders. J Pediatr Urol 2006; 2:148–162.

Related topics of interest

Duodenal atresia

Learning outcomes

- To understand the accepted pathophysiology of duodenal atresia
- To be able to diagnose an infant with this condition
- To be aware of the methods of surgical management

Overview

Calder reported the first case of duodenal atresia (DA) in 1733 although it was not until 1914 that Ernst was successfully able to correct this condition. The standard of care consists of a 'diamond' duodenoduodenostomy via a right upper quadrant incision.

The duodenum is the most common site of neonatal intestinal obstruction. DA, as opposed to stenosis, is a complete loss of intestinal patency resulting in obstruction. If untreated, the patient will die from aspiration and malnutrition. Nearly 50% of infants with duodenal obstruction have a congenital anomaly of another organ system, including Down syndrome (>30%), malrotation (>20%), congenital heart diseases (20%), other gastrointestinal tract anomalies, renal anomalies and annular pancreas.

Epidemiology and aetiology

DA occurs in approximately 1 out of every 2500–5000 live births, with a survival rate of >90%. During weeks 5 and 6 of gestation, there is exuberant growth of the intestinal epithelial lining that completely blocks the small lumen of the developing gut. Excessive epithelial formation versus failure of recanalisation as a cause of atresia remains an issue of debate.

Subsequent degeneration of these cells and recanalisation of the lumen is complete by the end of weeks 8–10 of gestation, and an interruption of this process can lead to loss of lumen in that area.

Another mechanism proposed is vascular infarction, followed by atrophy of the affected segment. Observations of duodenal stenosis in sonic hedgehog mutant mice have suggested that mutations in signalling pathways may play a role in the development of DA. Deletion of fibroblast growth factor 10, which serves as a regulator in normal duodenal growth and development, has been implicated in the pathogenesis of DA.

The obstructed duodenum can range from perforate to stenotic to atretic. Gray and Skandalakis categorised DA into three types:

1. **Type 1 (92%):** Duodenum with a diaphragm formed from mucosa and submucosa. There is no effect on the muscularis
2. **Type 2 (1%):** Fibrous cord connecting the two blunt segments of the duodenum with the mesentery is intact
3. **Type 3 (7%):** No connection between the two blunt segments of the duodenum with a V-shaped mesenteric defect

The aetiology remains unknown.

Clinical features

DA patients present with signs of high intestinal obstruction.

- Bilious vomiting occurs within hours of birth. Vomiting can be non-bilious if the obstruction is above the level of entry of the bile ducts
- Meconium is still passed within 24 hours

Investigations

- A dilated stomach and duodenum during fetal ultrasonography after the 18th week of gestation
- Post-natal abdominal X-ray shows the 'double-bubble' sign, with the first 'bubble' corresponding to the stomach, and the second to the dilated duodenal loop. If this is not visible, injection of air through the nasogastric tube may be used as a contrast medium. Gas in the distal bowel suggests partial obstruction, whereas no gas suggests complete obstruction
- Upper gastrointestinal contrast study demonstrates a smooth, rounded end at

the level of the obstruction in the second portion of the duodenum, whereas a 'beaking' effect in the third portion of the duodenum is seen with volvulus

Differential diagnosis

- Malrotation with volvulus

Management

Patients require surgery. Initial management consists of
- Nasogastric tube insertion
- Search for other anomalies: echocardiogram, renal ultrasound. This should not interfere with definitive surgical management unless the patient is symptomatic from a cardiac defect for example

Open approach

In the open approach, a transverse incision is made above the umbilicus, extending from the midline to 5 cm into the right upper quadrant. The abdominal musculature is divided and the liver is retracted. The ascending and transverse colons are mobilised, and the duodenal obstruction is exposed. The patient should be assessed for other abnormalities.

The level of obstruction is identified and a diamond duodenoduodenostomy is performed. A transverse incision is made on the anterior wall of the caudal end of the proximal duodenum, and a longitudinal incision of the same length is made on the distal segment. The two ends are approximated at the site of the incisions by aligning the distal end of the longitudinal incision to the midpoint of the inferior edge of the transverse incision.

In Type 1 defects with continuity of the muscular wall, it is important to be aware of a 'windsock' deformity. In this situation, bowel dilation may present distal to the origin of the diaphragm, and extra care must be taken to ensure anastomosis of the true defect. The origin of the diaphragm is identified by passing an orogastric tube through the pylorus and into the duodenum. Tenting of the web will cause an indentation of the duodenum at the web origin. The duodenotomy should be performed at the site of indentation. Care must be taken during this part of the procedure as the ampulla of Vater may be in this location. Type 2 and 3 cases are easily identified on dissection due to discontinuity of bowel.

Laparoscopic approach

For the laparoscopic approach, the abdomen is insufflated through a 5 mm umbilical port. In the right lower quadrant and the left midepigastric region, 3 mm ports are placed. The liver is retracted by placing a suture through the abdominal wall, under the falciform ligament, and backed out through the abdominal wall. If this is not sufficient, a liver retractor can be inserted into an additional port at the left upper quadrant.

Once intestinal malrotation is excluded, the colon is mobilised to the left and the proximal duodenum is identified by following the pylorus to the blind-ended duodenum. The distal segment of duodenum must then be identified and mobilised. A transverse incision is made a few millimetres from the end of the proximal pouch, and a longitudinal incision is made on the distal segment, both measuring approximately 1.5–2.0 cm. The first suture for the diamond anastomosis is placed in the lower corner of the incision on the distal duodenum and attached to the midline of the incision on the proximal segment. The back wall of the anastomosis is created with either interrupted or running 4-0 Vicryl suture. The front wall is then closed in a similar fashion.

In the event that the patient has a duodenal web, tenting the web after passing an orogastric tube past the pylorus can help identify its insertion point. A small longitudinal incision is made at this site and the web is partially excised. It is important to be aware of the ampulla of Vater because it is often located near the web, and can be injured during excision.

Further reading

Choudhry MS, et al. DA: associated anomalies, prenatal diagnosis and outcomes. Pediatr Surg Int 2009; 25:727–730.

Dalla Vecchia LK, Grosfeld JL, West KW, et al. Intestinal atresia and stenosis: a 25-year experience with 277 cases. Arch Surg 1998; 133:490–497.

Sweed Y. Duodenal obstruction. In: Puri P (ed.), Newborn surgery, 2nd edn. London: Arnold, 2003:423.

Related topics of interest

- Small bowel atresia (p. 320)

Duplications of the urological system

Learning outcomes

- To understand the embryological process that leads to ureteric duplication
- To recognise the range of clinical scenarios associated with ureteric duplication
- To formulate a management plan for the patient with ureteric duplication

Overview

Ureteric duplication is a developmental anomaly with a range of clinical implications. Many ureteric duplications are asymptomatic. Clinical presentation is usually related to obstruction to the upper moiety or vesicoureteric reflux into the lower moiety. In addition to duplication of the ureter, there are other anomalies of size, position and fusion that affect the renal tract.

Epidemiology and aetiology

There are a variety of anomalies of renal size, position and fusion that can often be completely asymptomatic, so the exact incidence is not known. Horseshoe kidney is a common fusion anomaly, but other variations exist. Horseshoe kidneys are found in approximately 1 in 400 autopsies as an incidental finding. Duplication of the ureter can be complete or incomplete. Triplication of the ureter, though rare, has been reported.

The embryology of the urogenital tract is characterised by complex interrelations. The ureteric bud arises from the Wolffian (mesonephric) duct and migrates cranially to engage with the metanephros to stimulate the development of the kidney itself at around day 32. Thereafter the kidney migrates to its usual location in the renal fossa. Caudally the Wolffian duct between the cloaca and ureteric bud becomes the common excretory duct which is absorbed into the bladder, with migration of ureteral orifices in a cranial and lateral direction. The common excretory ducts fuse in the midline to form the trigone,

and in boys, the Wolffian duct becomes the prostate, seminal vesicles, vas and epididymis. In girls, Wolffian duct remnants guide Müllerian ducts into the midline to form the uterus, Fallopian tubes and proximal vagina. Duplication of the ureteric bud leads to duplication of the ureter. In this process, the upper moiety ureter orifice comes to lie caudal to the lower moiety orifice (Meyer–Weigert law). If a single bud forms then splits, an incomplete or 'Y' duplication occurs. This means that at the kidney there is a duplex configuration but at the bladder there is a single ureteric orifice. Failure of fusion or ascent produces characteristic abnormalities. The most common, horseshoe kidney, is a fusion of the lower poles that results in secondary failure of ascent because the isthmus prevents migration above the inferior mesenteric artery. Pelvic kidneys are a result of failure of ascent, and crossed renal ectopia is a fusion anomaly of upper pole to contralateral lower pole.

Clinical features

There are a variety of clinical presentations associated with duplex kidneys. Many are incidental findings of no clinical importance, especially incomplete duplex systems, because they will typically be associated with a normal vesicoureteric junction. Where there is complete duplication of the ureters, one or both ureteric orifices (UOs) may be ectopic. Lower moiety UOs that are laterally ectopic tend to have shorter, less oblique, tunnels and therefore may have vesicoureteric reflux (VUR). UOs that are medially ectopic are more often associated with ureteroceles, or insert through the bladder neck musculature, and tend to be obstructed. Large ureteroceles can also cause bladder outflow obstruction. This knowledge helps the clinician predict the cause of ureteric dilatation in the setting of duplication.

If the UO is distal to the bulk of the urethral sphincter in girls, incontinence will result. The

UO itself can be difficult to localise because it may open in the urethra, the vagina or on the perineum. This clinical scenario should be suspected in all female patients who present with primary constant dribbling incontinence or dampness despite an otherwise entirely normal pattern of micturition. In the male patient, an ectopic ureter can be a cause of recurrent epididymitis, but as the external urethral sphincter is distal to all of the Wolffian structures, continence is usually preserved. Pelvi-ureteric junction (PUJ) obstruction can occur in duplex kidneys. This tends to affect the lower more than the upper moiety.

Investigations

Duplex kidneys can often be diagnosed on ultrasound scanning (USS). Duplex kidneys are suspected if there is a size discrepancy or a kidney larger than expected for age and weight of the patient, if there is hydronephrosis affecting the upper or lower pole disproportionately, or if two renal pelves or ureters are identified.

When reflux exists into the lower pole, a so-called drooping flower appearance of lower pole calyces can be observed on micturating cystography (**Figure 14**). Where there is poor function in one pole, this can be detected with nuclear medicine scanning. Magnetic resonance urography is the investigation of choice for defining anatomy in girls with wetting, suspected to be related to a small poorly functioning upper moiety ectopic ureter. Intravenous urography and computed tomographic urography can also demonstrate duplex anatomy reliably in experienced hands.

Differential diagnosis

Duplex kidney is suspected on USS when the kidney is larger than expected or if there is asymmetrical hydronephrosis within a kidney. This could be caused by PUJ with a prominent upper pole calyx that is not seen to communicate. A renal cyst or calyceal diverticulum could also cause dilatation confined to one pole. In practical terms,

the presence or absence of asymptomatic duplication is irrelevant. The astute clinician must be aware of the possibilities of duplication, complicating the imaging in the investigation of hydronephrosis or symptomatic renal disease. As mentioned above, the duplex ectopic ureter is an essential differential diagnosis in the female with primary incontinence.

Treatment

Treatment is required for problems relating to infection, obstruction, reflux or incontinence. When there is dilatation and obstruction associated with an ureterocele, the ureterocele can be incised endoscopically or, if there is little function in the upper moiety of the kidney, heminephrectomy may be needed. Residual ureteroceles after heminephrectomy usually only need excision if they cause further symptoms.

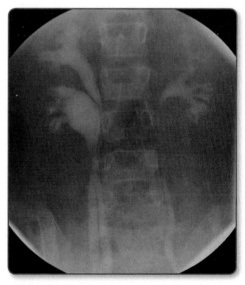

Figure 14 Bilateral vesicoureteric reflux into a right duplex and a left simplex kidney. This is an incomplete or 'Y' duplication, whereas in complete duplications reflux would likely occur into only the lower pole. By comparing the lower moiety with the normal contralateral side, one can appreciate the absence of a normal calyceal pattern. This generates the so-called drooping lily appearance. Courtesy of Starship Children's Hospital Department of Medical Imaging.

Where there is VUR, and this is considered in need of treatment, this should be done in line with standard management of reflux. Reimplantation, if required, can be safely undertaken by a common sheath mobilisation and reimplantation. Heminephrectomy may be indicated if function in the lower moiety is poor.

If PUJ obstruction is identified in a duplex kidney, a standard pyeloplasty can be performed. Anastomosis between the obstructed pelvis and the nonobstructed pelvis or ureter has also been described.

Identification and treatment of an ectopic upper pole ureter causing incontinence is an immensely rewarding process. The usual scenario is that there is a very small and poorly functioning upper pole moiety. The treatment of choice here is upper pole heminephrectomy. This can be safely performed by an open or minimally invasive technique. The distal ureter is by definition not inserted into the bladder and can simply be divided and left to atrophy. If the ectopic moiety is found to have a significant amount of function, the distal ureter can be located outside the bladder and reimplanted or ureteroureterostomy can be performed proximally.

Further reading

Kokabi N, et al. Ureteral triplication: a rare anomaly with a variety of presentations. J Pediatr Urol 2011; 7:484–487.

Park JM. Normal development of the genitourinary tract. In: Wein AJ (ed.), Campbell-Walsh urology, 10th edn. Philadelphia: Saunders, 2012: 2975.

Related topics of interest

Empyema

Learning outcomes

- To understand the aetiology, epidemiology and pathology
- To understand the investigation process
- To understand the treatment options and their indications

Overview

Empyema is the accumulation of infected intrapleural fluid usually arising as a complication of pneumonia.

Epidemiology and aetiology

The incidence of paediatric empyema is about 10 cases per 100,000, with a higher incidence during winter. There is an increasing worldwide incidence. The main predisposing factor is severe pneumonia. The most common organism indentified is *Streptococcus pneumoniae*. The initial effusion (stage 1, 3–5 days) is exudative, resulting in a shift of thin fluid from the lung parenchyma to the pleural space. This then progresses to fibrinopurulent fluid, with septation, loculation and deposition of a layer of fibrin on the parietal and visceral pleura (stage 2, 7–10 days). Further organisation results in a thick fibrous peel which causes lung entrapment, poor chest expansion and loss of thoracic volume and scoliosis on the affected side (stage 3, 2–3 weeks). Empyema can be complicated by lung abscess, bronchopleural fistula and pneumatocoele.

The vast majority of empyemas are secondary to bacterial pneumonia. However, they may occur as a complication of chicken pox or measles. Other causes include penetrating chest trauma, oesophageal leakage, pancreatitis and peritonitis. Patients who are immunocompromised or have chronic respiratory diseases are predisposed.

Clinical features

The patients usually have a background of pneumonia and are already on intravenous antibiotics. Empyema should be suspected when there is worsening respiratory distress and pyrexia. Clinical signs include respiratory distress, poor air entry, tracheal deviation and dullness to percussion.

Investigations

Blood and pleural fluid cultures are negative in the majority of patients. A chest X-ray is sufficient to make the diagnosis in the early stages. This shows the characteristic signs of a pleural effusion, with the fluid going up to the axilla. In some cases there may be a total white-out with mediastinal shift. An ultrasound of the chest gives adequate information in the fibrinopurulent stage. Findings include clear or turbid, septated or loculated fluid. The location of the drainage site can be marked at this time. Computed tomogram (CT) scanning should be reserved for complicated cases: failure of fibrinolysis or surgery, bronchopleural fistula or lung abscess formation.

Differential diagnosis

A thoracic tumour can rarely present as an empyema. Tuberculosis should be suspected if there is a history of tuberculosis contact or a chronic illness. Other diagnoses to consider are haemothorax, lung sequestrations, pulmonary infarction and effusions from other causes.

Treatment

The treatment options include conservative management, drainage (tube or open) only, drainage and fibrinolysis, thoracoscopy or thoracotomy and debridement. Small uncomplicated effusions can be managed conservatively with intravenous antibiotics only. If the effusion is increasing in size then drainage is necessary. Fibrinolysis or surgical debridement is necessary for the fibrinopurulent stage. In the UK, drainage with fibrinolysis has become the first-line intervention. The organised fibrosis stage will respond only to thoracotomy and decortication. The aims of invasive procedures should be to drain the infected fluid and remove as much of the peel as possible to allow lung expansion.

Fibrinolysis

Chest drainage and fibrinolysis with intrapleural urokinase can resolve the loculated effusion in the majority of cases. When compared to drainage only, intrapleural fibrinolysis (urokinase) results in a shorter hospital stay. The use of a small chest drain (10 Fr) for fibrinolysis results in less pain and a shorter hospital stay. The main complication is pain on instillation of the urokinase. Bleeding is not reported. Failure and the need for surgical intervention can occur in 16%.

Intrapleural urokinase administration:

- Chest drain of 10 Fr inserted and connected via a three-way tap to an underwater seal. Effusion aspirated
- Urokinase instilled via a three-way tap into the pleural cavity and drain clamped for 4 hours then opened
  - Patient > 10 kg, dose 40,000U bd for 3 days
  - Patient < 10 kg, dose 10,000U bd for 3 days

Thoracoscopic debridement

Thoracoscopic debridement can be used either as a first-line intervention or for failure of fibrinolysis. General anaesthesia with central endotracheal intubation is maintained. The patient is placed in the lateral position, with the affected side up and a roll under the chest. The first 5 mm port is inserted anterior to the tip of the scapula. The effusion is aspirated and a pneumothorax of 6 mmHg is maintained with a flow of 1.5–2.0 L/min of CO_2. The second 5 mm port is sited either anteriorly or posteriorly, depending on the location of the effusion. The fibrinous peel is removed from the visceral and parietal pleura. Sometimes

minor injuries to the lung surface can occur which can be treated conservatively. At the end of the debridement, the pneumothorax is released, and the anaesthetist is asked to provide manual ventilation. All lobes of the lung should be expanding adequately at this stage. A 16 Fr chest drain is inserted via the 5 mm port and connected to an underwater seal without suction. Minor air leakage will stop as the lung expands. The indications for conversion to thoracotomy include poor vision, excessive bleeding, large air leakage (bronchopleural fistula) and poor lung expansion. The main complications include lung injury, bronchopleural fistula and recurrent empyema. Bronchopleural fistula will require thoracotomy and insertion of a serratus anterior digitation flap to seal the fistula. Recurrent empyema will require thoracotomy and decortication.

Thoracotomy

Thoracotomy should be reserved for advanced or complicated empyema and failure or complications of fibrinolysis or thoracoscopy. It is advisable to request a CT of the chest to look for abscess or bronchopleural fistula. The patient is positioned in the lateral position, with a roll under the chest. The muscle-cutting thoracotomy is performed via the bed of the 4th or 5th rib. The empyema is drained and the fibrous peel is removed from the lung surface. Inevitably, there is significant bleeding and injury to the lung surface. Large tears can be over sewn whist minor injuries can be left alone. Only sufficient peel is removed so as to get the affected lobe expanding. Being overly aggressive can result in unnecessary parenchymal damage. A serratus anterior digitation muscle flap can be sutured into any bronchopleural fistula if present. One or two chest drains are inserted as necessary and connected to an underwater seal without suction. Complications include bleeding, lung injury, bronchopleural fistula and recurrence.

Further reading

Bishay M, Short M, Shah K, et al. Efficacy of video-assisted thoracoscopic surgery in managing childhood empyema: a large single-centre study. J Pediatr Surg 2009; 44:337–342.

St. Peter SD, Tsao K, Harrison C, et al. Thoracoscopic decortication vs tube thoracostomy with fibrinolysis for empyema in children: a prospective, randomized trial. J Pediatr Surg 2009; 44:106–111.

Thomson AH, Hull J, Kumar MR, et al. Randomised trial of intrapleural urokinase in the treatment of childhood empyema. Thorax 2002; 57:343–347.

Endocrine conditions presenting to paediatric surgery

Learning outcomes

- To understand and identify endocrine conditions presenting to paediatric surgery
- To understand pre-existing endocrine problems and their impact on surgery
- To understand endocrine problems that might present to the surgeon
- To understand endocrine problems that might arise due to surgery

Overview

A surgeon may be exposed to endocrine disorders in several ways:

- They may initially present to the surgeon, e.g. bilateral undescended testes and/or hypospadias in undervirilised males or a testis found in a phenotypic female, with an inguinal hernia in disorders of sexual development (DSD)
- They may mimic surgical problems, e.g. abdominal pain and/or vomiting in diabetic ketoacidosis
- Patients with pre-existing endocrine disorders require perioperative surgical management, e.g. diabetes mellitus, diabetes insipidus (DI) (including posthead injury) and adrenal insufficiency
- Patients may develop endocrine disorders as a result of surgery, e.g. DI following surgery to the pituitary and hypothalamus, and SIADH following surgery to the brain

Diabetes mellitus

See also 'Diabetes mellitus' (p. 80). The perioperative management principles are as follows:

- Patients with type 1 diabetes mellitus (T1DM), requiring elective surgery, should be first on morning list
- Regular blood sugar monitoring should be perioperatively
- Short surgical procedures may merely require a delay or change of morning insulin
- Longer procedures require intravenous (IV) insulin and glucose infusion (sliding scale)
- Patients on continuous subcutaneous insulin infusion often only require a background insulin infusion rate
- The diabetes team should be informed of admission well in advance

Patients with type 2 diabetes mellitus (T2DM) may need to omit their oral hypoglycaemic drugs (e.g. metformin) perioperatively.

NB: Patients with newly diagnosed or existing T1DM with diabetic ketoacidosis may present with abdominal pain and/or vomiting, often in association with constipation. Urinalysis reveals glycosuria and ketonuria.

Diabetes insipidus

1. Definition
- Excessive urination (polyuria), usually in association with excessive drinking (polydipsia)
2. Forms
- Arginine vasopressin (AVP) deficiency (cranial DI)
- AVP resistance (nephrogenic DI)
- (Psychogenic)
- May be isolated, or occur in association with other pituitary hormone deficiencies
3. Causes of cranial DI
- Congenital
  - Familial: inheritance autosomal dominant or recessive or X-linked, DIDMOAD (diabetes insipidus, diabetes mellitus, optic atrophy and deafness)
  - Central brain anomaly: septo-optic dysplasia, Laurence–Moon–Biedl syndrome
- Acquired
  - Trauma (closed or penetrating)
  - Neoplasia: craniopharyngioma, germinoma
  - Granuloma: Langerhans cell histiocytosis

- Infection: encephalitis, meningitis, toxoplasma
- Inflammatory: lymphocytic hypophysitis
- Others: vascular, hypoxic, idiopathic
4. Symptoms
- Polyuria: usually day and night, often > 4–5 mL/kg/h
- Polydipsia: will drink any fluids including water
- Dehydration, constipation, fever, failure to thrive, vomiting
- May be features of other pituitary hormone defects
- May be one of several patterns—transient, permanent or triphasic. The latter is the most common after cranial surgery:
  - Polyuric phase: inhibition of AVP, lasting several days
  - Antidiuretic phase (SIADH), following stored hormone release. Hyponatraemia 2° to this, also often concomitant cerebral salt wasting (CSW), see below
  - Permanent DI, when AVP-producing cells are damaged and stores exhausted
5. Caveats
- Not all diuresis postcranial surgery is DI; remember the following:
  - Fluid overload with appropriate diuresis
  - Hyperglycaemia 2° to dexamethasone
- You cannot excrete a water load if you are glucocorticoid deficient
6. Diagnosis
- Because AVP is not secreted under physiological conditions, random or early morning paired osmolalities are only useful if the plasma osmolality is well in excess of normal physiological value of ≤280 mOsmol/kg
- Alternative ways to increase plasma osmolality are
  - Fluid restriction in a controlled fashion for several hours
  - Hypertonic saline infusion with 2.7% saline
- With plasma osmolality > 305 mOsmol/kg and/or sodium > 148 mmol/L; if urine osmolality is
  - < 300 mOsmol/kg, the diagnosis is DI
  - > 750 mOsmol/kg, the diagnosis is not DI

- Levels between these may reflect partial DI
- Desmopressin administration distinguishes between cranial and nephrogenic DI
7. CSW and SIADH
- Occurs independently or concurrently postcranial surgery
- Both produce hyponatraemia and often increased urinary sodium concentration
- Careful assessment of hydration and fluid balance is required because the treatment is very different
  - SIADH: fluid restriction
  - CSW: sodium supplementation

Adrenal insufficiency

1. Causes
- Primary (adrenal)
  - Congenital: adrenal hyperplasia (CAH) and hypoplasia (CAHypo), glucocorticoid deficiency
  - Acquired: autoimmune (isolated/ polyglandular), adrenoleukodystrophy (ALD), drugs (e.g. ketoconazole and cyproterone)
- Secondary (hypothalamopituitary)
  - Congenital: hypopituitarism, septo-optic dysplasia, isolated adrenocorticotropic hormone deficiency
  - Acquired: tumour, surgery, radiotherapy, vascular, trauma, meningitis
  NB: Do not forget prolonged steroid therapy.
2. Symptoms – often not specific
- Neonate: conjugated jaundice, poor feeding, hypoglycaemia, convulsions
- Older children: tiredness, weight loss, increased infections, prolonged recovery period
- Then: vomiting, drowsiness, coma and death
3. Signs
- Pigmentation (buccal, scars, but only in 1° form)
- Hypotension (including postural)
- There may also be features of associated conditions such as
  - Ambiguous genitalia: CAH
  - Micropenis: hypopituitarism, CAH, CAHypo

- Other endocrine problems: hypopituitarism, polyglandular syndrome
- Neurological problems: brain tumour, ALD

4. Steroid replacement
- Glucocorticoid
  - Hydrocortisone 8–15 mg/m^2/day, bd or tds (higher doses given in CAH as suppressive therapy)
- Mineralocorticoid
  - Fludrocortisone 150 µg/m^2/day, once daily
  - Salt supplements ~5 mmol/kg/day, < 18 months
- Adrenal replacement: surgery and also in an adrenal crisis
  - IV hydrocortisone

< 10 kg	~1 year	25 mg
10–20 kg	~5 years	50 mg
> 20 kg	~10 years	100 mg

  - Given intravenously at induction, and repeated qds until eating and drinking
  - May also require increased dose of oral steroids (double or triple) after this

Similar doses of hydrocortisone are required in adrenal crisis, along with IV fluids (saline boluses if required then IV N or saline plus 10% dextrose)

Disorders of sexual development

See the relevant Topics, but DSD can present to the surgeon, in the following situations:
- Testes in a phenotypic female during inguinal hernia repair: 46XY DSD, e.g. due to complete androgen insensitivity syndrome or testosterone biosynthetic defect, e.g. 17-b hydroxysteroid deficiency
- Fallopian tubes and/or rudimentary uterus in phenotypic male during orchidopexy or inguinal hernia repair: persistent Müllerian duct syndrome 2° to anti-Müllerian hormone deficiency or resistance
- Undescended testes associated with hypospadias: partial androgen insensitivity (PAIS), 5α-reductase deficiency or gonadal dysgenesis

If any of these unexpected situations occur, then it is vital to speak to a paediatric endocrinologist from the operating theatre or room to find out what samples (including biopsies) need to be taken, and arrange to speak to the parents and organise follow-up.

Calcium disorders

Causes of hypocalcaemia are:
- Infancy
  - Asphyxia
  - Prematurity
  - Gestational diabetes
  - Hypoparathyroidism (transient or permanent)
  - Hypomagnesaemia
  - Total parenteral nutrition
  - Maternal hyperparathyroidism
- Childhood
  - Vitamin D deficiency
  - Vitamin D-dependent rickets
  - Chronic renal failure
  - Hypoparathyroidism
  - Pseudohypoparathyroidism

Biochemistry tests results in calcium disorders are as follows:

	Calcium	Phosphate	PTH	Vitamin D	Treatment
Vitamin D deficiency	↓ or N	↓	↑	↓	Vitamin D (ergo/cholecalciferol)
Hypoparathyroidism	↓	↑	↓	N	1α-cholecalciferol
Hypophosphataemic rickets	N	↓	N	N	Vitamin D (calcitriol) plus phosphate

Further reading

Butler G, Kirk J. Paediatric endocrinology and diabetes. Oxford: Oxford University Press, 2011.

Raine JE, et al. Practical endocrinology and diabetes in children, 3rd edn. London: Wiley-Blackwell, 2011.

Related topics of interest

Epigastric hernia

Learning outcomes

- To be able to diagnose an epigastric hernia
- To know the indications for surgery and the perioperative requirements

Overview

Epigastric herniae may also be referred to as paraumbilical or supraumbilical herniae and are uncommon in children. Epigastric herniae may occasionally appear away from the midline due to defects in the abdominal wall musculature. Given that they are often asymptomatic and rates of complications are extremely low, expectant management is appropriate for many cases: open or laparoscopic repair is reserved for symptomatic or enlarging herniae.

Epidemiology and aetiology

One study indicates that the incidence in patients is 4% of all abdominal wall herniae in children, although this may be higher. They are usually protrusions of preperitoneal fat, but occasionally contain omentum which appear through a defect in the linea alba and are normally found in the midline between the xiphisternum and the umbilicus.

Based on cadaveric studies, Askar suggests that these herniae are acquired defects, resulting from a unique pattern of aponeurotic decussation in the upper abdominal wall. He further suggests that the occurrence of these herniae in the upper abdomen may be related to traction from fibres originating from the diaphragm that insert into the linea alba between the umbilicus and the xiphoid. Other studies have suggested that these herniae are not acquired, but rather arise in a congenital defect in the linea alba or in an abnormally wide orifice for a blood vessel.

Clinical features

There is a protrusion within the midline of the abdomen between the xiphisternum and the umbilicus. This can sometimes be more evident during physical exercise or when coughing or straining. It may only be evident when the child puts his or her chin onto the chest when in the supine position. Although usually solitary, they can be multiple and have the following features:

- Palpable mass in the epigastrium that may be reducible (65%) or incarcerated
- Symptomatic or enlarging in the majority (55%)
- Pain and/or tenderness due to incarceration of the contents (20%)
- Multiple defects/herniae may be present (10–15%)
- Concomitant abdominal wall defects, e.g. umbilical hernia (10–15%) or rectus diastasis (5%)

Investigations

The diagnosis should be evident on examination. Occasionally, an ultrasound scan may be helpful in confirming the diagnosis and ruling out other causes of a similar swelling.

Differential diagnosis

- Lipoma
- Diastasis of the recti
- Umbilical hernia

Treatment

In contrast with umbilical herniae, the supraumbilical type rarely, if ever, spontaneously close. They do not contain bowel or other intra-abdominal viscera and are thus not at risk of incarceration: preperitoneal fat can occasionally become ischaemic if a large quantity has extruded through the defect, but this is rare. Small asymptomatic herniae can therefore be managed expectantly, with symptomatic or enlarging herniae requiring surgery.

Management should initially consist of reassurance owing to the low risk of incarceration although, if the parents and/or child wish to continue with a surgical procedure, this can be undertaken as a day case. Surgery may exchange a symptomless small swelling for a permanent and occasionally obvious scar.

Prior to the procedure, and with the child awake, the defect should be outlined with a marking pen to prevent the scenario of being unable to locate it once the child is under general anaesthesia.

- A transverse incision is made directly over the previously marked location of the hernia
- The fat that protrudes through the linea alba is isolated and excised once the defect is located
- The linea alba should be cleared of fat to enable the defect to be closed with interrupted absorbable sutures
- Occasionally it is necessary to enlarge the defect in order to be able to close it successfully. Overlapping the defect in a Mayo fashion is rarely necessary
- The skin is approximated using subcuticular sutures

Laparoscopic technique

Described in children by Albanese et al, laparoscopic repair of epigastric herniae can be accomplished with two laterally placed 3 mm trocars, using 'one-handed' suturing and extracorporeal knots that are pushed into place. This approach may be particularly advantageous for managing multiple defects or concomitant umbilical herniae, avoiding the need for multiple incisions. However, a two-trocar technique may not readily permit excision of incarcerated fat or a hernial sac; the use of a Veress needle laterally in the flank, for primary port insertion, is also associated with a risk of intra-abdominal viscera or vessel injury.

There is little published data about complication rates in children: the largest series (n = 38), operated on using the open technique, reported no associated morbidity and no known recurrences, although the length of follow-up was not clear. Similarly, in a series of laparoscopically treated umbilical and epigastric herniae (n = 13), with follow-up duration of 6–35 months, there were no reported recurrences and no associated morbidity.

Further reading

Albanese CT, Rengal S, Bermudez D. A novel laparoscopic technique for the repair of pediatric umbilical and epigastric hernias. J Ped Surg 2006; 41: 859–862.

Askar OM. Surgical anatomy of the aponeurotic expansions of the anterior abdominal wall. Ann R Coll Surg Eng 1977; 59:313–321.

Coats RD, Helikson MA, Burd RS. Presentation and management of epigastric hernias in children. J Pediatr Surg 2000; 35:1754–1756.

Exomphalos

Learning outcomes

- To learn how embryological development leads to the recognised patterns of abdominal wall abnormalities
- To recognise the different types of closed abdominal wall defects and the principles used in planning their treatment
- To recognise the high incidence of associated congenital malformations

Overview

Exomphalos, or omphalocele, is characterised by a defect through the umbilicus covered by a sac, consisting of an inner layer of peritoneum and an outer layer of amnion with Wharton's jelly in between. There is a wide spectrum of severity related to the size of the defect and the size and contents of the sac. Associated congenital abnormalities are common. Repair of smaller defects is simple, but treatment of larger complex defects can be challenging. The prognosis, in terms of survival, depends more on the severity of associated anomalies and comorbidities than the defect itself.

Epidemiology and aetiology

The incidence of exomphalos is approximately 1 in 5000 live births. No primary causative factors have been defined. In experimental models folate deficiency, salicylates and hypoxia have been found to contribute to abdominal wall defects. Exomphalos is not regarded as hereditary although some familial cases have been reported.

Embryology

- The embryo is a flat three-layered disc at 2 weeks. The body cavity forms by a process of elongation and infolding
- Failure of development of the cranial folds results in defects in the upper abdominal and chest wall, including the pentalogy of Cantrell

- Failure of development of the caudal folds is associated with abnormalities of the bladder, hindgut and hypogastrium

Associated anomalies

Other anomalies occur in 30–50% and even in one third of those with normal chromosomes:

- Cardiovascular anomalies occur in about 20%, more commonly in those with an epigastric exomphalos
- Pulmonary hypoplasia
- Pentalogy of Cantrell (epigastric exomphalos, anterior diaphragmatic hernia, sternal cleft, ectopia cordis, cardiac anomaly)
- Genitourinary and hindgut anomalies, particularly lower midline syndrome OEIS (omphalocele, exstrophy, imperforate anus, spinal)
- Gastrointestinal incomplete midgut rotation or non-fixation occurs in 79%
- Testicular maldescent
- Genetic: particularly trisomies 13–15, 18, 21, and Beckwith–Wiedemann syndrome
- Other: VACTERL, EEC (ectodermal dysplasia, ectodactyly, cleft palate), Eagle-Barrett syndrome (prune belly), IVC anomalies, cleft palate, Rieger's syndrome, hydrocephalus

Clinical features

- Most are obvious at birth
- Larger defects can be diagnosed with fetal ultrasonography. Maternal serum alpha-fetoprotein may be raised. Acetylcholinesterase is usually normal, but may be raised in gastroschisis
- Exomphalos is generally classified by the size of the defect and sac, but a number of different terms are used
- Exomphalos major refers to a defect of > 5 cm and exomphalos minor a defect of < 5 cm, but neither refers to the size or contents of the sac. Some exomphalos major may represent failure of development of the abdominal wall

rather than a failure of closure, with extra-abdominal development of foregut and midgut structures

- Giant omphalocele is a term used to describe those with a large sac, particularly containing all or most of the liver and gut
- Hernia of the cord is a type of exomphalos minor in which a small loop of bowel herniates into the umbilical cord

Investigations

Blood glucose should be monitored because there is a risk of hypoglycaemia (Beckwith–Wiedemann syndrome). Investigations are otherwise largely directed to assessment of associated abnormalities (see above) and cardiorespiratory function.

Differential diagnosis

- Gastroschisis
- Umbilical hernia

Treatment

Prenatal

- A search for other anomalies is needed
- Chromosome analysis by amniocentesis or chorionic villus sampling (note potential fetal injury or loss rate of 1%)
- Serial ultrasound scans, echocardiography
- Birth in a centre with tertiary paediatric surgical services is desirable. Some recommend elective caesarean section but there is no consistent evidence in favour of this
- Thorough prenatal counselling for parents and family is essential

Postnatal

- Initial treatment will depend upon the size and contents of the sac and comorbidity
- Ensure adequate resuscitation. Some with lung hypoplasia may need early respiratory support. Monitor for hypoglycaemia particularly if any other features of Beckwith–Wiedemann syndrome are present
- IV access and nasogastric tube drainage are needed unless the defect is small and the baby is very well

- Position the baby so that the contents of the sac do not become kinked or obstruct venous return
- Protect the sac. Placing the baby in a bowel bag up to the level of the chest or wrapping the trunk and defect loosely with cling film are simple effective measures. Moist saline swabs will stop the sac drying out but will cool the baby, with a high rate of evaporative heat loss
- Once stable, thoroughly assess the baby for other anomalies·

Treatment of the exomphalos

- The important factors to consider in the selection of treatment are the size of the defect in the abdominal wall, the size and contents of the sac, and presence of other congenital abnormalities and comorbidities. Emergency exploration is needed only if the sac has ruptured, exposing the viscera, or there is concern about intestinal ischaemia, intestinal obstruction or vessel compression/angulation compromising venous return and organ perfusion
- Conservative treatment is particularly useful for those with a very poorly developed abdominal wall or those unfit for general anaesthesia, owing to heart and lung problems. Also some very small defects, particularly in premature neonates, may not need surgical repair. Usually silver sulphadiazine paste is applied with bandaging to support the sac and its contents. It can take many months for a large sac to epithelialise completely. It should be noted that there has been a recent report of high serum silver levels following silver dressings. A large hernia is left which will need repair later
- Umbilical cord clamp. Very small defects or herniae into the cord can be repaired by the simple application of an umbilical cord clamp across the base of the defect if it can be absolutely certain that the sac is completely empty
- Reduction and primary repair of the abdominal wall. Small or medium size defects amenable to reduction and primary closure of the abdominal wall should be repaired as an urgent elective

procedure when the infant is fully stabilised (see **Figure 15**). For larger defects, prosthetic patches may be needed. Many different patches have been used, including synthetic materials (e.g. Goretex, Silastic, Prolene mesh and Vicryl mesh) or bioprostheses (e.g. bovine pericardium and porcine dermal collagen)

- Staged surgical closure may be needed for giant defects, particularly those with a very narrow unstable stalk that are difficult to position without compromising venous return. The first stage involves application of a silo, and widening of the defect if needed, to reduce and stabilise the bowel and liver. If repair by delayed primary closure cannot be achieved at 10–14 days, the silo can be replaced with a smaller silo or prosthetic patch. Many will still have a large ventral hernia which can be repaired at the age of 1–2 years. If the defect is stable and wide enough, a silo can be sutured outside the sac to enable gradual reduction without exposing the abdominal contents
- The use of tissue expanders to stretch the abdominal cavity or the skin to enable cover has been described

Complications

- Injury to local structures, particularly bowel or liver if attached to the sac

- Ischaemia arising from angulation of intra-abdominal vessels or raised intra-abdominal pressure
- Wound infection, dehiscence, patch infection or dislodgement
- Exacerbation of respiratory problems by increased intra-abdominal pressure and postoperative pain or in those managed conservatively by traction on the chest wall and diaphragm from a heavy pendulous sac
- Residual or recurrent hernia. May need further repair when older, but for many the upper abdominal musculature will always be deficient
- Intestinal obstruction from adhesions or malrotation. With large defects, midgut rotation and fixation may be incomplete. It is difficult to ascertain how likely this is to cause problems in later life, and there is debate about how actively this should be sought and treated in the absence of symptoms

Prognosis

- The long-term prognosis depends more on associated anomalies and comorbidity (e.g. associated anomalies, lung hypoplasia and prematurity) than on the exomphalos itself

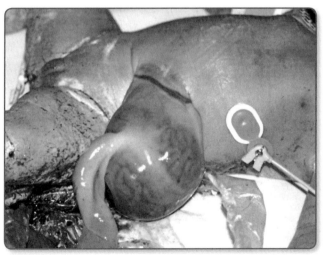

Figure 15 Exomphalos sac containing bowel. The sac has been protected with a bowel bag and the infant has passed meconium. An uncomplicated primary repair was carried out.

Further reading

Christison-Lagay ER, Kelleher CM, Langer JC. Neonatal abdominal wall defects. Semin Fetal Neonatal Med 2011; 16:164–172. ·

Ledbetter DJ. Congenital abdominal wall defects and reconstruction in pediatric surgery: gastroschisis and omphalocele. Surg Clin N Am 2012; 92:713–717.

Van Eijck FC, et al. Past and present surgical treatment of giant omphalocele: outcome of a questionnaire sent to authors. J Pediatr Surg 2011; 46:482–488.

Related topics of interest

- Exstrophy–epispadias complex (p. 109)
- Gastroschisis (p. 137)
- Prenatal diagnosis and counselling (p. 287)
- Umbilical disease (p. 348)

Exstrophy–epispadias complex

Learning outcomes

- To better understand these complex urinary tract anomalies
- To be aware of the principles of surgical management

Overview

Often grouped together as the exstrophy-epispadias complex, these are among the most rare and most severe congenital anomalies of the urinary and genital tracts. In the UK in recent years, their management has been centralised to two main centres, made possible by both central funding and the consent and support of other UK paediatric urologists. This concentration of patients has enabled an improvement in outcomes through a better understanding of the conditions and a concentration of expertise.

Classic bladder exstrophy

Epidemiology and aetiology

Classic bladder exstrophy occurs in approximately 1 in 30,000 live births and is more commonly found in boys with up to a 3:1 ratio. Failure of ingrowth of mesoderm, between the internal and external layers of the cloacal membrane, results in a open pelvic ring and a split between the rectus muscles, with foreshortening of the pubic rami. Rupture of the cloacal membrane results in an open bladder that fills the space in between the layers.

Clinical features

Many cases of bladder exstrophy are now diagnosed antenatally, leading to a decline in numbers of patients in some countries through termination of affected pregnancies. A low-lying umbilical cord, failure to visualise the bladder and a shortened, thickened penis are recognised features. This early diagnosis permits prenatal counselling by the specialist who will undertake the baby's postnatal care and help to give parents a proper future perspective. There is no need to change the mode of delivery or to arrange in utero transfer to deliver nearer the exstrophy centre.

The main features of this lower abdominal wall defect in males are seen in **Figure 16a**. The umbilical cord is low in the abdomen and the exstrophic bladder plate is visible below it. The rectus muscle is split on either side of the bladder and inserts onto the pubis whose symphysis is open (pubic diastasis). The penile corpora are attached to the inferior pubic rami and traverse towards the midline to join below the glans, necessarily giving rise to a significant shortening. Continuous with the bladder plate, the urethra is an open strip on the dorsum of the distal penile corpora and the glans, which is cleft dorsally. The verumontanum can be seen proximally in the midline. In females (**Figure 16b**), the

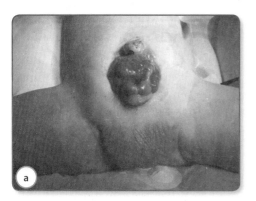
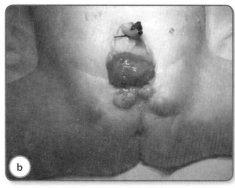

Figure 16 (a) Male bladder exstrophy and (b) female bladder exstrophy.

clitoral corpora and glans are split to either side and the urethral plate is between them in the midline, ending at the vaginal opening inferiorly. There are rarely any associated anomalies in this classic form.

Investigations

- Renal ultrasound
- Routine bloods, a clotting screen and a group and save should be performed on arrival at the exstrophy centre
- One unit of blood is usually cross-matched for the primary bladder closure

Initial treatment

Babies are usually delivered at term and apart from the bladder exstrophy, they are otherwise healthy. After birth and the administration of vitamin K, the lower abdomen should be wrapped in cling film to protect the bladder mucosa, beneath the normal nappy. Feeding (preferably with breast milk) can commence normally and time can be taken to allow the transfer of both the mother and the baby to the exstrophy centre so this and the resultant bonding can continue. There is no need for intravenous fluids or antibiotics, and it is important to safeguard the babies' peripheral veins because they will be needed during the pre- and postoperative management.

Surgical treatment

- Primary closure
  - The first surgical priority in all cases of classic and cloacal exstrophy is to achieve a sound closure of the abdominal wall. Primary bladder closure is preferably done during the first few days of life, but is not an emergency and can be safely achieved later if circumstances dictate. Bilateral, iliac osteotomies are proposed if closure is either late or the diastasis is wider than 4 cm, although experience shows that they are rarely needed in a case of classic bladder exstrophy (They may be needed if a revision repair is undertaken and in all cases of cloacal exstrophy)
  - An epidural cannula is inserted to provide pre- and postoperative analgesia over the first 72 hours.

Ureteric catheters of 4 Fr are inserted for urinary drainage and broad-spectrum intravenous antibiotics administered. A midline incision is made above the umbilical root and continued downwards on either side of the bladder plate, separating it from the abdominal wall skin and rectus muscles laterally. Inferiorly the bladder outlet is defined on either side of the verumontanum in boys or just above the vaginal opening in girls. This dissection can stay extraperitoneal and the umbilical stump is removed, after careful ligation of its vessels. After a full mobilisation of the bladder plate, it is closed with interrupted absorbable sutures around an 8 Fr urethral stent inferiorly. The ureteric catheters are tunnelled and brought out lateral to the rectus muscle

- In boys, inguinal herniae occur commonly after closure, so dissection anterior to the rectus sheath allows a preventative ligation of the patent processus vaginalis at this point
- Large, monofilament, horizontal mattress sutures are used to oppose pubic tissues in front of the bladder and the rectus muscles closed with interrupted sutures. The subcutaneous tissues, skin and the superior introitus are then closed
- Postoperatively the emphasis is on analgesia and feeding and the mother's presence is ideal. Antibiotics can be continued for 2 days, ureteric catheters come out at 7 days, and discharge can follow if the baby is growing and the wound is clean and dry. Follow-up is arranged with an abdominal ultrasound in the first 6 weeks. Long-term prophylactic antibiotics are given because vesicoureteric reflux (VUR) is expected following bladder closure. In the case of upper tract dilatation or urinary tract infection, a narrow outlet may be the cause and clean intermittent catheterisation (CIC) may be needed

- Complete primary reconstruction:
  - For this the primary closure is delayed and a much more extensive

procedure is performed. This comprises radical anatomical reconstruction of the bladder outlet, urethra and penis. Whilst there are significant complications associated with this procedure, it results in voiding continence in some patients

- Secondary procedures:
  - Following a simple primary closure, the patient needs further surgery to address continence and to reconstruct the genitalia
- Modern staged repair:
  - A derivative of the original approach, proposed by Jeffs, first requires an epispadias repair in boys at around 1 year of age using the Cantwell–Ransley technique. The urethral plate and its spongiosum are separated from the penile corpora between the verumontanum and the glans tip. Tubularisation forms the urethra which is brought below the corpora, whose external rotation corrects the dorsal chordee of the penis
  - A subsequent tight repair of the bladder neck follows in both sexes when the bladder has gained capacity, and this provides an obstructed form of continence in a proportion of patients
- Kelly operation:
  - This radical soft-tissue reconstruction restores normal anatomical relations of the bladder outlet, pelvic floor, urethra and penis and is performed at 1 year of age. It requires full mobilisation of the penile corpora from the inferior pubic rami, which in turn requires release of the pelvic floor laterally, including identification and preservation of the pudendal neurovascular bundles running into them. The ureters are reimplanted to prevent VUR and the bladder neck is redefined and closed loosely. The urethra may be either reconstructed using the Cantwell–Ransley technique or completely separated from the glans and brought to a hypospadiac position. Bringing the bases of the corpora together creates penile lengthening and allows the muscle of the urogenital diaphragm to be wrapped loosely around the proximal penile urethra
  - In girls, the same principles are followed, with complete mobilisation of the clitoral corpora, allowing them to be united in the midline. The urethra and vagina remain closely related and both are wrapped in muscle to form a notional sphincter
  - Daytime continence develops over the next 3–4 years and may be achieved in up to 70% of patients. Night-time continence follows as bladder capacity develops
- Continent diversion:
  - This is usually reserved for when the above secondary procedures fail to provide continence, although it used to be the mainstay of treatment 15 years ago. A Young–Dees tight bladder neck reconstruction for outlet resistance, ileocystoplasty for capacity and an appendicovesicostomy (Mitrofanoff) for emptying are tried and tested techniques

Cloacal exstrophy

Epidemiology and aetiology

Cloacal exstrophy is a much rarer and more severe abnormality, more common in boys, with an incidence of 1 in 300,000 live births. It is thought to be due to failure of septation of the cloaca, combined with a lack of mesodermal in-growth into the cloacal membrane.

Clinical features

Many or all of the components can be diagnosed antenatally and termination of pregnancy is frequent. Neonatal mortality is high and remains so if there is a major cardiac or small bowel anomaly. In utero transfer and caesarian section delivery are probably indicated for these babies.

The caecum forms a central portion of the extrophy plate, with the ileum emptying on to it, a distal diminutive hindgut and an imperforate anus being other features (**Figure 17**). The bladder is in two halves on either side and the diastasis is much wider. The penis is much shorter, or may be even in two separate parts. In girls, the vagina is often

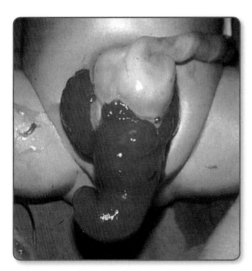

Figure 17 Cloacal exstrophy.

duplicated (with two separate unicornuate uteri) or may be completely absent. The abdominal wall defect is very much larger, and there is usually a large exomphalos superiorly.

There is a high incidence of prematurity and associated congenital anomalies: renal (70%), sacral agenesis (60%), myelomeningocele (50%), limb and spinal deformities (40%), small bowel defects (shortening, malrotation or atresias) (65%) and more rarely cyanotic heart disease (10%).

Initial management

Management of prematurity is needed and time is taken to work up the full extent of the abnormality with urinary and spinal ultrasound, cardiac echocardiography and review by other specialist colleagues. Feeding may commence before closure and is a good way of testing the adequacy of the bowel without formal contrast studies.

Surgical treatment

- Abdominal closure:
  - This may be delayed for weeks or even months to permit conservative treatment and cicatrisation of the exomphalos. Anterolateral innominate osteotomies are essential to allow closure without tension, and even with these, a temporary silo or the use of a prosthetic mesh may be required to achieve closure. The caecum is separated and tubularised, and the hindgut preserved to form an end colostomy on the left side of the abdomen. The bladder halves are joined in the midline and closed into a pelvic container with a narrowed outlet at the base of the corpora. In girls, the vagina may be duplicated or absent, and it is important to note the presence of ovaries and Müllerian structures at this stage
- Secondary procedures:
  - Faecal continence is rarely achieved, so currently an end colostomy remains the best long-term option. The very abnormal and usually neuropathic bladder dictates that bladder neck reconstruction (or closure), combined with a cystoplasty, and a catheterisable conduit are the usual urological options. In addition, spinal and orthopaedic surgeries are often required
- This is characteristically a very demanding group of patients with a very high complication rate and significant long-term issues. Nonetheless the majority survive to adult life. The involvement of nurse specialists and psychologists and a planned transition to adult services are essential

Primary epispadias
Epidemiology and aetiology

Primary epispadias is more commonly found in boys and occurs in 1 in 150,000 live births. Its principal feature is a dorsal deficiency of the urethra.

Clinical features

Many patients present at birth with an obvious external abnormality, although it is not unusual for the diagnosis to be missed in girls and for them to present later with failed potty training. In more distal forms in boys, there may be an intact foreskin, which covers the abnormality, which only becomes apparent either during circumcision or once retraction is possible.

In girls, the clitoris is split on either side, and the bladder neck is invariably involved (**Figure 18a**), so they are all incontinent. In boys (**Figure 18b**), the extent of urethral involvement varies from the distal penis only (in which case continence may develop normally), to more complete and proximal urethral involvement with associated bladder neck abnormality and incontinence.

Investigations

Cystoscopy is usually performed to evaluate the bladder neck in all patients, although the evaluation of continence potential is difficult in baby boys. The bladder neck deficiency is apparent on filling and the verumontanum may be within the bladder. The trigone does appear to be quite abnormal in more severe cases. This observation is borne out during surgical reconstruction, during which the relative lack of muscular development of the trigone and its diminutive size may be noted. The degree of urethral involvement, the appearance of the bladder outlet at cystoscopy and the developed bladder capacity all correlate with bladder neck function.

Surgical treatment

In girls the same continence procedures are used as for classic bladder exstrophy. The Kelly operation has a high success rate and

Figure 18 (a) Female epispadias and (b) male epispadias.

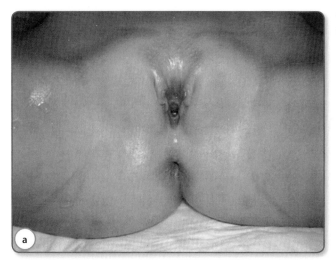

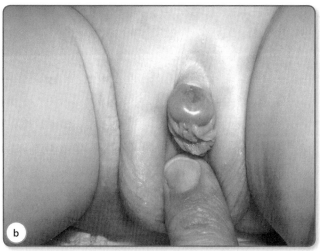

also enables correction of the divided clitoris. Failed and historical cases have often been treated with bladder neck reconstruction, cystoplasty and a Mitrofanoff conduit for CIC.

In boys, the penile abnormality is treated using the Cantwell-Ransley epispadias repair, and this alone is needed where there are no continence issues. The penis may be short and withheld following this procedure, and long-term cosmetic issues are quite common. The Kelly operation may partially address penile length and has been used in patients for whom a bladder neck procedure is also needed. Without the pubic diastasis, however, the penile length enhancement is less than for cases of classic bladder exstrophy. Disappointingly, the results for continence of the various bladder neck procedures may also be poorer than for exstrophy. The bladder neck hypoplasia and dysplasia seen in male epispadias would account for this.

Whilst cystoplasty can provide continence with CIC, urethral voiding continence has become the goal, so newer procedures need to be developed to achieve this.

Further reading

Frimberger D. Diagnosis and management of epispadias. Semin Pediatr Surg 2011; 20:85–90.

Stec AA, et al. The modern staged repair of classic bladder exstrophy: a detailed postoperative management strategy for primary bladder closure. J Pediatr Urol 2012; 8:549–555.

Woo LL, Thomas JC, Brock JW. Cloacal exstrophy: a comprehensive review of an uncommon problem. J Pediatr Urol 2010; 6:102–111.

Related topics of interest

Faecal incontinence and idiopathic constipation

Learning outcomes

- To be able to differentiate between true and pseudo faecal incontinence
- To understand the management options for faecal incontinence and constipation
- To be familiar with surgical management options

Overview

Faecal incontinence is a frustrating and often devastating problem for the child and family. It affects children born with surgical conditions, such as anorectal malformations (ARMs) and Hirschsprung's disease (HD), as well as children with neurological disease or spinal cord injuries.

Constipation is also a difficult issue for patients and parents or carers, who often feel helpless and pursue multiple different options to alleviate the suffering of their children.

Epidemiology and aetiology

Mechanisms of faecal continence are as follows:

- **Voluntary sphincters:** In the normal child, the voluntary muscle structures are represented by the levators, the muscle complex and the parasagittal fibres. They are used only for brief periods when the faecal mass, pushed by the involuntary peristaltic contraction of the rectosigmoid colon, reaches the anorectal area. This voluntary contraction keeps the stool in the rectum by closing the anus. Patients with ARMs have abnormal voluntary striated muscles, with different degrees of hypodevelopment, ranging from good muscle bulk to nearly no voluntary sphincter muscles. Patients with HD may have suffered damage to this sphincter mechanism, and patients with spinal problems may have deficient innervation of these muscles

- **Intact anal canal:** Voluntary muscles are used only when the child has the sensation that determines that it is necessary to use them. To appreciate that sensation, the child needs information that is derived from an intact anal sensory mechanism. Exquisite sensation in normal children resides in the anal canal. Except for patients with rectal atresia, most children with ARMs are born without an anal canal. Therefore, sensation does not exist or is rudimentary. Patients with spinal problems may lack this anal canal sensation as well. Those with HD are born with a normal anal canal, but this can be injured if not meticulously preserved at the time of their colonic pull-through procedure, and patients with perineal trauma may have an injured or destroyed anal canal

- **Motility:** In a normal child, the rectosigmoid colon remains quiescent for varying periods of time (one to several days), depending on defaecation habits or dietary consumption. During that time, sensation and voluntary muscle structures are almost not necessary because the stool, if it is solid, remains inside the colon. The patient can feel the peristaltic contraction of the rectosigmoid that occurs before defaecation. The normal individual can then voluntarily relax the striated rectal muscles, which allows the rectal contents to migrate down into the highly sensitive area of the anal canal. There, the anal canal provides information concerning stool consistency. The voluntary muscles are used to push the rectal contents back up into the rectosigmoid and to hold them until the appropriate time for evacuation. At the time of defaecation, the voluntary muscle structures relax and the stool exits the anus helped by abdominal wall muscles and gravity

Faecal incontinence may be either true or pseudo incontinence. It is important to make the distinction because each entity has its own completely different management strategy.

True incontinence includes a proportion of patients with established surgical diagnoses, such as ARMs and HD, and those with congenital or acquired spinal problems. These children have an underlying structural abnormality that leads to faecal soiling. Pseudo incontinence occurs in patients who have the potential for bowel control but are severely constipated, and this leads to overflow and soiling.

Clinical features

Children are diagnosed with faecal incontinence once they are continent of urine, at an age when the majority of their peers are trained for stool and are ready to start school. The literature has multiple definitions of how many episodes of faecal soiling are considered abnormal. In order to be deemed continent of stool in the spina

bifida population, the child should have less than one soiling episode per month.

Based upon the child's stooling pattern and contrast study findings, the clinician is able to determine if the patient is hypermotile, usually lacking a rectal reservoir and requiring slowing down of the colon, or hypomotile, potentially requiring more stimulation of the colon to empty. Clinical features, combined with results of investigations, are useful indicators of prognosis (**Table 4**).

Investigations

In order to formulate management strategies, a number of studies are useful to help predict what specific enema would be required for bowel management and the potential for bowel control in the future.
- Plain abdominal radiograph (AXR)
- Water-soluble contrast enema
  – Dilated colon (**Figure 19**) – hypomotile, constipated

Table 4 Prognosis for bowel control with anorectal malformations			
Anatomic indicators of good prognosis	Clinical signs associated with good prognosis	Anatomic indicators of poor prognosis	Clinical signs associated with poor prognosis
Normal sacrum	Good bowel movement patterns: one to two bowel movements per day, no soiling in between	Abnormal sacrum	Constant soiling and passing stool
Prominent midline groove (good muscles)	Evidence of sensation when passing stool	Flat perineum (poor muscles)	No sensation (no pushing)
Anatomic indicators of good prognosis		Some types of anorectal malformations: • Rectobladder neck fistula • About 50% of patients who have rectoprostatic fistula • Cloacae with a common channel > 3 cm • Complex malformations	Urinary incontinence, dribbling of urine
Obvious anal dimple			
Some types of anorectal malformations: • Rectal atresia • Rectoperineal fistula • Imperforate anus without fistula • Cloacae with a common channel < 3 cm • Rectourethral bulbar fistula			

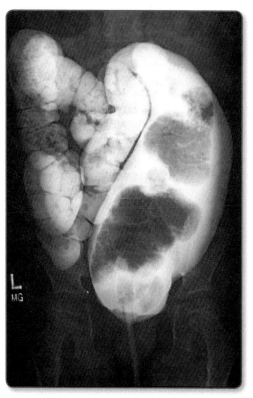

Figure 19 Contrast enema showing a dilated colon. Reprinted from: Peña A, Levitt M. Colonic inertia disorders. Curr Probl Surg 2002; 39:666–730, with permission from Elsevier.

- – Non-dilated colon (**Figure 20**) – hypermotile, tendency towards loose stools
- Sacral radiographs:
  - – Calculation of sacral ratio to help predict potential for continence (especially in ARM)
  - – Normal ratio > 0.7
  - – Currarino triad – sacral defect, ARM, presacral mass – less chance of continence even with mild ARM
- Rule out tethered cord – ultrasound of spine if younger than 3 months, MRI of the spine if older
  - – Presence of tethered cord (or other associated spinal anomaly) decreases chance of potential faecal continence

Differential diagnosis

- Pseudo incontinence secondary to constipation and overflow
- Hirschsprung's disease
- Intestinal pseudo obstruction

Treatment

True faecal incontinence

- Bowel management – daily enemas tailored to the patient's colon to mechanically empty the colon once a day. The child is then free from soiling episodes for 24 hours until the next enema
  - – Tailoring of the enema is done through a week-long program of daily AXRs and patient, parent or carer reports of the presence or absence of soiling episodes
  - – Although some trial and error is involved, an educated guess is made on day one of the program and subsequent daily adjustment of the enema is done by an experienced team after talking with the parents or carers and assessing the amount of stool present on the AXR
- Do not use a combination of enemas and laxatives – the laxatives will provoke a bowel movement prior to the next enema washout

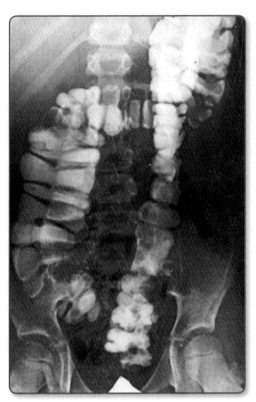

Figure 20 Contrast enema showing a non-dilated colon. Reprinted from Levitt MA, Peña A. Treatment of chronic constipation and resection of the inert rectum. In: Holschneider AM, John M. Hutson JM (eds), Anorectal malformations in children. Berlin: Springer, 2006:415–420. With permission from Springer.

- Enemas are usually composed of 0.9% saline (400–750 mL), glycerine (10–40 mL) and/or soap (10–40 mL)
- Hypermotile patients may require a different management strategy in addition to the enemas – constipating diet (**Table 5**), bulking agents (water-soluble fibres, such as pectin, citrucel and cornstarch) or medical agents (loperamide, co-phenotrope, cholestyramine)
- Consider antegrade colonic enemas (ACE) through a continent appendicostomy if successful on bowel management with enemas to thereby change the route of enema administration to be antegrade and allow for more independence
- If the child requires urologic reconstruction (ARM or spina bifida population), coordinate early with urology colleagues on overall plan of management and surgical strategies and consider timing of ACE at time of urologic reconstruction and discuss splitting the appendix for ACE and Mitrofanoff

Pseudo incontinence and constipation

- If the patient has the potential to be faecally continent, treat with laxatives to provoke peristalsis and overcome hypomotility:
  - Determination of laxative requirement is also done during a week-long program
  - Stimulant laxatives are effective, but stool softeners are not useful in this patient population
  - Laxative dose (senna) is chosen based on stool frequency and findings of AXR. The patient is observed for 24 hours:
    - If no stool, do an enema and then increase laxative dose
    - If stools multiple times and AXR shows minimal stool, decrease laxative dose

Table 5 Constipating diet	
Foods to encourage (foods that bulk stool)	Foods to discourage (foods that loosen stool)
Apple sauce	Milk or milk products
Apples with skin	Fats
Rice	Fried foods
White bread	Fruits
Bagels	Vegetables
Soft drinks (artificially sweetened)	Spices
Bananas	Fruit juices
Pastas	French fries
Pretzels	Chocolate
Tea	
Potatoes	
Jelly (no jam)	
Broiled, boiled, baked meat, chicken or fish	

- Goal is one or two soft bowel movements a day
- Combine laxative with soluble fibre to give the stool bulk so as to avoid potential accidents due to liquid stool
- Determine if and when a colonic resection would benefit the child if an enormous dose of laxatives is required to empty the colon:
  - Rectosigmoid resection for redundant, dilated sigmoid colon
  - Transanal resection if isolated large rectum

Further reading

Bischoff A, Levitt MA, Bauer C, et al. Treatment of fecal incontinence with a comprehensive bowel management program. J Pediatr Surg. 2009; 44:1278–1284.

Malone P, Ransley P, Kiely E. Preliminary report: the anterograde continence enema. Lancet 1990; 336:1217–1218.

Peña A, Levitt M. Colonic inertia disorders. Curr Probl Surg 2002; 39:666–730.

Related topics of interest

Femoral hernia

Learning outcomes

- To recognise the need to identify femoral herniae
- To know the steps in undertaking operative repair

Overview

Femoral herniae are uncommon in paediatric practice and occasionally arise secondary to disruption of pelvic anatomy following orthopaedic surgery. They can be easily misdiagnosed as inguinal herniae unless the bulge is present on examination. Conservative management is contraindicated due to the risk of incarceration and strangulation. These events are rare in children however. There are a number of methods of repair.

Epidemiology and aetiology

There is no difference in incidence between the sexes, and they most commonly occur between 5 and 10 years old. Their aetiology is not well understood, but McVay's theory that a congenitally narrow posterior attachment to Cooper's ligament, resulting in a large femoral ring seems to be the most widely accepted.

Other proposed aetiologies include occurrence secondary to pelvic orthopaedic procedures or following inguinal hernia repair due to the initial diagnosis being incorrect or from iatrogenic disruption of the inguinal canal. Diagnostic accuracy ranges from 33 to 40% in some series. If occurring bilaterally, recurrently or in combination with other abdominal wall herniae, the child may need investigation for connective tissue abnormalities.

Clinical features

The history is similar to that of an inguinal hernia in that the bulge appears when the child is coughing, crying or straining. Its position is classically below and lateral to the pubic tubercle in contrast to the inguinal hernia which is above and medial.

Boundaries of the femoral canal are as follows:

- Anterior: Iliopubic tract or the inguinal ligament (or both)
- Posterior: pectineal ligament (Cooper) and fascia iliaca
- Lateral: a connective tissue septum and the femoral vein
- Medial: the aponeurotic insertion of the transversus abdominis muscle and transversalis fascia or, rarely, the lacunar ligament

Investigations

For infants and neonates, the small differences in location are not appreciable and the bulge may appear at the external inguinal ring. If a sac is not found during a procedure to repair an inguinal hernia, the diagnosis of femoral hernia should be entertained and an exploration undertaken. The femoral hernia sac, if large, can turn upwards and invest in the loose areolar tissue beneath the skin of the groin, further confusing it with an inguinal hernia.

Differential diagnosis

- Inguinal hernia
- Hydrocele
- Lymphadenopathy

Treatment

For an incarcerated femoral hernia, a transinguinal or extraperitoneal approach should be used as the low, infrainguinal approach can lead to difficulty separating the oedematous sac from the surrounding fat. A laparoscopic approach has been used in adults, but there are limited reports in children.

If a concomitant inguinal hernia is present, a transinguinal repair should be undertaken.

Transinguinal (McVay) repair

- Initial approach is the same as for a standard inguinal herniorrhaphy
- Separate the conjoined tendon and transversalis fascia
- Open the internal ring, incising the posterior wall of the inguinal canal towards the pubic tubercle (through the internal oblique aponeurosis and transversalis fascia)
- The spermatic cord is retracted to gain access to the femoral region
- Palpate for the femoral vessels
- Define the space between the femoral vein and the pubic tubercle from lateral to medial
- The sac is identified and delivered avoiding damage to the femoral vein which is in close contact with the sac laterally
- It may be necessary to ligate and divide the inferior epigastric vessels to expose the femoral area from behind
- The contents of the sac are reduced, or if doubt remains the sac is opened and it is subsequently suture-ligated with a fine stitch flush with the peritoneum. If the sac is bulky then it can be inverted and reduced with one or two purse string sutures placed just above the femoral defect
- The defect is then narrowed by approximating the internal insertions of Cooper's and the inguinal ligaments, with two or three fine non-absorbable stitches, taking care not to compress the femoral vessels
- The inguinal canal is reconstructed and the superficial layers and skin are closed

Suprapubic extraperitoneal (Cheatle–Henry) approach

- Suprapubic incision opening the midline and retracting the rectus abdominis muscles laterally, thus gaining access to the femoral ring. This approach was altered by Nyhus who used an incision above and parallel to the inguinal ligament
- The peritoneal sac is retracted cephalad, exposing the femoral ring, with the inguinal ligament above, Cooper's ligament below and the external iliac vein laterally
- The sac should be resected and the femoral ring obliterated by suturing the inguinal ligament to Cooper's ligament with three to four non-absorbable sutures. Care should be taken not to damage the external iliac vein

Infrainguinal (Langenbeck) approach

- A transverse incision is made in a skin crease over the mass from a point just inferior to the pubic tubercle medially and extending laterally past the palpable pulsation of the femoral artery
- Deepen the wound to expose the bulging hernial sac. The sac is covered by cribriform fascia and groin fat, both of which should be incised. It may overlie the femoral vein and extend upwards over the inguinal ligament
- The sac protrudes into the femoral canal medial to the vein, inferior to the iliopubic tract, above Cooper's ligament and lateral to the reflected fibres of the iliopubic tract. It should be carefully palpated for visceral content which should be gently reduced. When this is difficult, for instance following incarceration, the sac can be released by incising the insertion of the iliopubic tract into Cooper's ligament at the medial margin of the femoral ring. The sac can be opened to ensure full reduction
- Hernial repair is initiated with high ligation of the sac using non-absorbable sutures
- The femoral defect is repaired by raising the inguinal ligament to expose pectineus fascia and Cooper's ligament. If this is not performed then the femoral vessels are at risk during suturing. The pectineal fascia and Cooper's ligament should then be sutured together to obliterate the femoral canal medial to the vein
- Finally, prior to closure the remainder of the region should be evaluated to exclude a concomitant hernia

Further reading

Al-Shanafey S, Giacomantonio M. Femoral hernia in children. J Pediatr Surg 1999; 34:1104–1106.

Matthyssens L, Philippe P. A new minimally invasive technique for the repair of femoral hernia in children. About 13 laparoscopic repairs in 10 patients. J Pediatr Surg 2009; 44:967–971.

Tsushimi T, Takahashi T, Gohra H, et al. A case of incarcerated femoral hernia in an infant. J Pediatr Surg 2005; 40:581–583.

Related topics of interest

Gastric and oesophageal foreign bodies

Learning outcomes

- To be familiar with the symptoms of foreign body ingestion
- To understand the indications for the removal of foreign bodies
- To be aware of the potential complications of the ingested foreign body
- To be converse with the therapeutic options for foreign body retrieval

Overview

Preverbal infants and preschool-aged children are at particular risk of foreign body (FB) ingestion, given their tendency to put objects in their mouths. This diagnosis should therefore always be considered in the presence of relevant symptomatology even when a clear history is not available.

Epidemiology and aetiology

In young children, boys and girls are equally affected. Boys ingest FBs more commonly in the older age group. Peak incidence is in the 6-month to 4-year age group. The most common ingested FB is a coin.

In anatomically normal individuals, FBs tend to become impacted at areas of physiological narrowing. In the oesophagus, this is at the level of the cricopharyngeus, at the aortic indentation in the mid-oesophagus or at lower oesophageal sphincter. In the stomach, it is at the pylorus.

In most instances, once the FB has passed through the pylorus, it will eventually exit the gastrointestinal tract in the stool, including sharp objects such as pins. Occasionally, FBs may become impacted at the terminal ileum. Ingested magnets may attract other magnets or other ingested metallic FBs, resulting in perforation or fistula formation.

Impacted disc (button) batteries may cause corrosive necrosis within a few hours. The mechanism of injury is through an external current, leakage of chemical contents or pressure necrosis. Impacted coiled springs may allow passage of oral fluids through their centre, which may result in delayed diagnosis for the unwary.

Certain disorders predispose to FB impaction such as the following:

- Oesophageal stricture secondary to previous oesophageal atresia (OA) repair, gastro-oesophageal reflux disease, oesophageal cartilaginous ring or previous oesophageal replacement
- Oesophageal dysmotility secondary to previous OA repair, fundoplication or achalasia
- Pica

Clinical features

Difficulty with phonation or airway compromise or choking should lead to suspicion of FB ingestion, and the child should be treated as an emergency. Oesophageal symptoms of FB ingestion are sore throat, drooling of saliva, avoidance of feeds or dysphagia. Patients may be able to tolerate oral fluids but not solids. They may point to where they have a sensation of an object being 'stuck' although this seldom gives an accurate indication of the location of a FB and may result from an abrasion to the pharynx or oesophagus. When FB ingestion has been witnessed and the FB has passed into the stomach, the patient is usually asymptomatic.

Delayed retrieval of a FB impacted in the oesophagus may result in life-threatening complications, such as perforation with mediastinitis or peritonitis, tracheo-oesophageal fistula or aorto-oesophageal fistula, with massive haematemesis.

Investigations

Maintaining a low-threshold for considering FB ingestion is important even when no relevant history is initially evident. The standard investigation when considering a FB ingestion is a chest radiograph. Coins in the trachea tend to be orientated in the sagittal plane in contrast to those in the oesophagus, which lie coronally. Oblique orientation suggests perforation or submucosal imbedding. Clinicians should be aware that an accurate history is required to determine whether further investigation is required to exclude the impaction of radiolucent objects, such as wood, glass or plastic. Lateral neck radiographs may be helpful because most fish bones lodge above the level of the cricoid in the tonsillar region. If the FB is noted to be below the level of the diaphragm, it is considered to have passed beyond the oesophagus.

Some emergency departments employ a metal detector to ascertain whether a coin has passed into the abdomen or remains in the chest before requesting a radiograph. It is unusual to have to resort to contrast studies, CT or MRI scans. However, when the diagnosis is delayed and complicated by submucosal imbedding of the FB, retropharyngeal abscess or perforation, a CT scan may be indicated to aid operative planning. Endoscopy is a useful diagnostic and therapeutic modality.

Differential diagnosis

- Oesophagitis
- Oesophageal stricture
- Gastro-oesophageal reflux disease

The clinical history and examination are vital to indicate whether a FB is likely to be in the airway.

Treatment

Oesophageal FBs represent a surgical emergency. With the impaction of foodstuffs, such as bread or meat, some patients, particularly those with dysmotility, have found benefit from carbonated drinks or antispasmodics (Buscopan), but there is no

evidence to support their effectiveness and this should not delay retrieval.

The most common method of FB retrieval is by flexible or rigid endoscopy under general anaesthesia with rapid sequence induction. With radiopaque FBs, it is important to ensure that the interval between the radiograph being taken and the interventional procedure is no more than a few hours as the FB may have moved. Rigid oesophagoscopy may be particularly beneficial for the retrieval of a sharp FB, such as a safety pin or the piecemeal retrieval of an impacted meat food bolus in the upper oesophagus. A 'Roth net' may be helpful to retrieve a gastric FB if graspers are inadequate.

Retrieval of coins or marbles by passage of a Foley balloon catheter is advocated by some clinicians, usually with radiological guidance and occasionally in the awake child. This may place the child at risk of FB inhalation during the procedure unless endotracheal intubation is performed and also fails to allow visualisation of the oesophagus to exclude complications of impaction.

Infective complications include retropharyngeal abscess, mediastinitis and empyema which may require drainage. Longstanding, imbedded FBs may require thoracotomy for retrieval. A right posterolateral thoracotomy gives access to the mid-oesophagus for repair of a perforation or fistula, and a left thoracotomy gives access to the lower oesophagus. In those with a predisposing stricture, consideration should be given to subsequent interventions such as dilatation or antireflux medication.

If asymptomatic, most patients with gastric FBs can be reassured that these will pass in the stools in the subsequent few days. Occasionally, if they develop signs of obstruction, such as vomiting or abdominal pain, they may require retrieval, although it is prudent to repeat an abdominal radiograph to indicate whether the FB remains gastric. Laparoscopy or laparotomy is rarely required for removal.

Further reading

Clarnette T. Esophageal foreign bodies. In: Parikh DH, Crabbe DCG, Auldist AW, Rothenberg SS (eds), Pediatric thoracic surgery. London: Springer-Verlag, 2009:357–361.

Hammond P, Jaffray B, Hamilton L. Tracheoesophageal fistula secondary to disk battery ingestion: a case report of gastric interposition and tracheal patch. J Pediatr Surg 2007; 42:E39–41.

Leopard D, Fishpool S, Winter S. The management of oesophageal soft food bolus obstruction: a systematic review. Ann R Coll Surg Engl 2011; 93:441–444.

Related topics of interest

- Achalasia (p. 5)
- Gastro-oesophageal reflux disease (p. 133)
- Inhaled foreign body (p. 179)
- Oesophageal atresia and tracheo-oesophageal fistula (p. 219)

Gastric volvulus

Learning outcomes

- To understand the axis of rotation of gastric volvulus
- To understand the aetiology of gastric volvulus
- To be aware of a surgical management plan

Overview

Gastric volvulus is a rare clinical entity defined as an abnormal rotation of the stomach > 180° with a resulting closed loop obstruction that can lead to incarceration and strangulation. First described by Berti in 1866, it is thought to be relatively rare in the newborn period and in infancy, although the chronic form is likely to be underdiagnosed. Recognition is essential as it is a surgical emergency.

Epidemiology and aetiology

As many cases are undiagnosed, the incidence and prevalence are unknown. Males and females are equally affected, and 10–20% of cases occur in children.

Normally the stomach is resistant to abnormal rotation, as it is fixed at the gastro-oesophageal junction (GOJ), pylorus and by four gastric ligaments. As a result, congenital gastric volvulus is associated with disruption of one or more of these, although in a percentage it is idiopathic.

Gastric volvulus results from abnormal rotation of one part of the stomach around another, with resulting obstruction at the pylorus or cardia and possible ischaemia and necrosis.

Rotation is one of the following (**Figure 21**):

- **Organoaxial:** The stomach rotates around an axis, connecting the GOJ and pylorus. The antrum rotates in the opposite direction to the fundus. It is the most common type (59%) and is usually associated with diaphragmatic defects. Strangulation and necrosis have been reported in 5–28%

- **Mesenteroaxial:** This axis passes through the lesser and greater curvatures. The antrum rotates anterosuperiorly, so the posterior stomach surface lies anteriorly. Rotation is usually incomplete and intermittent. It comprises 29% of cases and patients usually do not have diaphragmatic defects. They usually have chronic symptoms
- **Combined:** This rare form is a combination of the other two. Again, it normally presents with chronic symptoms

The majority of congenital gastric volvuli are secondary to gastric malfixation (especially at the GOJ) diaphragmatic complications (e.g. congenital diaphragmatic hernia) and absence or laxity of gastric ligaments. Splenic anomalies are common.

It is usually classified as

- Type 1 (idiopathic): 66%; laxity of gastrosplenic, gastroduodenal, gastrophrenic or gastrohepatic ligaments. Cardia and pylorus approximate when the stomach is full. It is most common in adults
- Type 2 (congenital or acquired): 33%; leads to abnormal gastric mobility
  - Associated congenital defects:
    - Diaphragmatic (43%); gastric ligaments (23%); abnormal attachment, adhesion or band (9%);

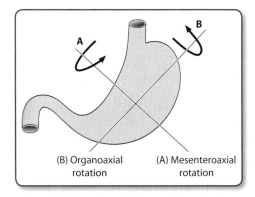

(B) Organoaxial rotation   (A) Mesenteroaxial rotation

Figure 21 Axes of rotation in gastric volvus.

asplenism (5%); bowel malformation (4%); pyloric stenosis (2%); colonic distension (1%); rectal atresia (1%)
- Neuromuscular disorders: poliomyelitis

In adults, the most common causes are diaphragmatic defects.

Clinical features

In children it usually presents within the first few months of life and symptoms depend on the degree of rotation and obstruction. Classic symptoms of Borchardt triad (e.g. unproductive retching, localised epigastric distension and inability to pass a nasogastric tube) may be difficult to elicit in younger children, and the diagnosis should be considered in the presence of other chronic symptoms (e.g. gastro-oesophageal reflux, recurrent vomiting and failure to thrive).

Investigations

Radiographic features are most reliable for diagnosis.
Chest and abdominal X-rays:
- Can show abnormalities in the position and contour of the stomach in the abdomen or chest
- Can also show an abnormal position of the pylorus in relation to the GOJ

Upper gastrointestinal contrast studies may be more informative, although if the stomach is involved at the time of the study, it will not show those intermittent volvuli.

Differential diagnosis

Causes of non-bilious vomiting may be:
- Surgical: pyloric stenosis, achalasia, antral web, preampullary duodenal stenosis, duplication cyst of the antropyloric lesion, ectopic pancreatic tissue in an antropyloric muscle
- Medical: gastroenteritis, increased intracranial pressure, metabolic disorders

Treatment

Acute gastric volvulus, especially intrathoracic, is a surgical emergency.

The aim of surgery is to prevent gastric ischaemia, necrosis, perforation and subsequent cardiorespiratory compromise. Surgery involves:
- An open or laparoscopic technique
- If open, an upper midline or left upper transverse incision can be used
- The diagnosis is confirmed
- The volvulus is reduced, and the viability of the stomach is assessed
- If the stomach is viable, it can be fixed by gastropexy to the anterior abdominal wall, or a Stamm gastrostomy is fashioned. Most authors would recommend a concomitant fundoplication to prevent inevitable gastro-oesophageal reflux
- If the stomach is partially necrotic or perforated, a partial gastrectomy will need to be undertaken with formation of a Stamm gastrostomy
- If the stomach is completely necrotic, a total gastrectomy with oesophagojejunal Roux-en-Y anastomosis will need to be performed
- If this is not possible due to poor anastomotic margins, alternative techniques will need to be employed
- Associated defects, such as a diaphragmatic hernia, should be explored for and repaired if present
- Successful laparoscopic surgery has been reported in acute gastric volvulus

The treatment of chronic cases remains controversial, although surgery is indicated in persistently symptomatic individuals. In cases of chronic symptoms and suspicious or normal contrast studies, a laparoscopic evaluation should be considered. Gradual improvement over time has been reported in conjunction with conservative treatment (e.g. positioning infants in the prone or upright position after meals) in less affected children.

The non-operative mortality rate for gastric volvulus is, reportedly, as high as 80%. Historically, mortality rates of 30–50% have been reported for acute gastric volvulus, with the major cause of death being strangulation, which can lead to necrosis and perforation. With advances in diagnosis and management, the mortality rate is 15–20% from acute gastric volvulus and 0–13% from chronic gastric volvulus.

Further reading

Miller DL, Pasquale MD, Seneca RP. Gastric volvulus
    in the pediatric population. Arch Surg 1991;
    126:1146–1149

Related topics of interest

- Gastro-oesophageal reflux disease (p. 133)

Gastrointestinal bleeding

Learning outcomes

- To be aware of the common causes of gastrointestinal (GI) bleeding
- To be familiar with diagnostic modalities
- To understand the management of specific causes of GI bleeding

Overview

Upper gastrointestinal (UGI) bleeding is defined as bleeding with its source above the ligament of Treitz. Lower gastrointestinal bleeding (LGI) is defined as bleeding with its source distal to the ligament of Treitz.

Epidemiology and aetiology

GI bleeding in infants and children is a fairly common problem, accounting for 10–20% of referrals to paediatric gastroenterologists. Severe GI bleeds are however rare in the general paediatric population.
Causes of UGI bleeding are:
- Vitamin K deficiency in neonates
- Oesophagitis
- Mallory–Weiss tear, with mucosal lacerations at the gastro-oesophageal junction or gastric cardia following forceful retching or vomiting
- *Helicobacter pylori* (*H. pylori*) gastritis
- Peptic ulcer disease
- Non-*H. pylori* gastritis
  - Reactive gastritis secondary to non-steroidal anti-inflammatory drugs, gastropathy, ingestion of caustic agents, trauma caused by the nasogastric or gastrostomy tube
  - Stress gastritis secondary to burns or massive systemic insult, including trauma
- Oesophageal varices
- Vascular malformations
- Haemobilia
- Mucosal lesions
  - Gastrointestinal stromal tumour (GIST)
  - Haemangioma
  - Dieulafoy lesion – a developmental malformation comprising a large submucosal arteriole, usually in the stomach, which bleeds through a mucosal defect

Causes of LGI bleeding are:
- Meckel's diverticulum
- Malrotation and volvulus
- Intestinal ischaemia
- Necrotising enterocolitis (NEC)
- Intussusception
- Inflammatory bowel disease
- Small or large bowel duplication
- Henoch–Schönlein purpura
- Cow's milk protein intolerance
- Polyp
- Haemolytic–uraemic syndrome
- Haemangiomata and vascular malformations
- Rectal prolapse
- Anal fissure

Clinical features

GI bleeding may manifest itself as:
- Haematemesis: vomiting of gross blood
- Haematochezia: passage of bright or dark red bloody stools
- Melaena: passage of tarry black stools, with bleeding source from the proximal GI tract
- Occult bleeding: presenting features being pallor, fatigue, microcytic anaemia

A useful feature to elicit from the history is whether the bleeding is associated with abdominal pain or pain on defaecation. The presence of pain would favour diagnoses such as:
- Anal fissure
- Infective colitis, e.g. *Salmonella*, *Escherichia coli* 0157:H7, *Campylobacter jejuni, Shigella, Yersinia enterocolitica*
- NEC
- Hirschsprung's enterocolitis
- Intussusception
- Solitary rectal ulcer
- Rectal prolapse
- Haemorrhoids
- Beta-haemolytic streptococcal cryptitis
- Inflammatory bowel disease

Painless bleeding is associated with:

- Vascular malformation
- GI polyp
- Mucosal lesion (i.e. GIST)

Occult blood loss may be secondary to:

- Oesophagitis
- Reactive gastritis
- Peptic ulcer
- Coeliac disease
- Inflammatory bowel disease
- Polyp
- Meckel's diverticulum
- Vascular malformation

Investigations

- Full blood count:
  - A low mean corpuscular volume is associated with chronic bleeding but is unreliable in acute severe bleeding
- Liver function tests
- Coagulation profile
- Blood group and cross-match
- Nasogastric tube (NGT) insertion in certain instances (suspicion of oesophageal variceal bleeding is not a contraindication for NGT passage)
  - To ascertain if stomach contains blood
- Testing of vomitus or stool:
  - Guaiac test will confirm presence of gross or occult blood. Rare false-positives may be obtained with haemoglobin in meat or ascorbic acid in uncooked fruit and vegetables

Modalities to consider are:

- Endoscopy
- Double-balloon enteroscopy has a detection rate of 68% for jejuno-ileal bleeding
- Autologous radio-labelled red blood cell scan can detect bleeding if rate > 0.1 mL/min but has significant false-negative and false-localisation rates
- Angiography can detect bleeding if rate > 1 mL/min and may be followed by embolisation
- Diagnostic laparoscopy or laparotomy, with or without on-table segmental enteroscopy:
  - Detects Meckel's diverticulum, small bowel haemangioma or intestinal duplication
  - May have a role in acutely bleeding patients with an unidentified source
- Small bowel imaging capsule:
  - Higher rate of positive findings compared with follow-through studies or push enteroscopy
  - The child must be able to swallow capsule (11×27 mm)
  - Risk of capsule retention
- Contrast studies
- Contrast-enhanced CT of abdomen

Differential diagnosis

- Swallowed blood: epistaxis, dental work, maternal blood in neonates
- Coagulopathy
- Factitious illness

Treatment

The principles of treatment are to assess severity of bleeding, estimate blood loss, provide resuscitation as necessary, using advanced trauma life support principles and stop the cause of bleeding if possible.

Management of UGI bleeding

- Manage underlying conditions and correct clotting abnormalities
- Consider oral or intravenous (IV) inhibitors of gastric secretion:
  - IV proton-pump inhibitors (PPI) have been shown to have improved outcomes in peptic ulcer disease in adults
- Insertion of NGT:
  - No evidence that gastric lavage has a therapeutic role in achieving haemostasis
- Diagnostic yield of barium meal is low
- Emergency UGI endoscopy for patients with continuous bleeding at a rate considered life-threatening:
  - Combination of gastric lavage and IV erythromycin prior to endoscopy may aid visualisation of bleeding point

- Indications for elective early referral for UGI endoscopy are:
  - Uncertain diagnosis or significant pathology suspected
  - Recurrent or significant episodes of haematemesis
  - Persisting or recurrent peptic ulcer disease
  - Suspected portal hypertension

Specific conditions:

- Oesophageal varices
  - Affects up to two-thirds of children with liver cirrhosis
  - IV octreotide (somatostatin analogue) decreases splanchnic blood flow and may stop haemorrhage in 70% of cases. It has fewer side effects than vasopressin
  - Sengstaken–Blakemore tube may achieve temporary control of severe haemorrhage in unstable patients until therapeutic endoscopy is performed
  - Therapeutic endoscopy is performed using:
    - Injection sclerotherapy: carries a risk of stricture formation
    - Ligation of varices: has fewer complications with high rates of survival in adults compared to sclerotherapy
- Peptic ulceration secondary to *H. pylori*:
  - *H. pylori* is a Gram-negative, microaerophilic bacterium
  - Diagnostic CLO test from duodenal and gastric biopsies has 97% sensitivity and 98% specificity
  - *H. pylori* may be visualised in histopathological biopsies
  - Medical treatment is with PPI and two antibacterial agents
  - Acute bleeding may be stopped with endoscopic treatment, using injection with adrenaline diluted in saline or coagulation with diathermy
  - *H. pylori* follow-up testing: stool antigen or breath test

Management of LGI bleeding

- Manage underlying conditions and correct clotting abnormalities
- Insert the NGT to exclude massive UGI bleeding

- In acutely unwell child with abdominal pain and tenderness:
  - Consider plain abdominal radiograph to exclude intestinal obstruction, NEC or perforation
  - Consider abdominal ultrasound or CT, if diagnosis is unclear:
    - Useful if bleeding has stopped
    - May detect small mucosal lesions but poorly identifies vascular abnormalities
- Colonoscopy with similar methods of haemostasis as above

Specific cases

- Cow's milk protein intolerance (CMP) allergy:
  - Enterocolitis due to cow's milk protein or soya milk
  - Eosinophilic infiltration seen on histopathology
  - Treat with exclusion diet with amino acid or hydrolysate-based feeds
  - Most children outgrow CMP intolerance by ages of 2–3 years
- Infective enterocolitis:
  - Three or more stool samples should be obtained for culture
- Haemangiomata and vascular malformations:
  - These lesions are uncommon within the GI tract
  - Exact localisation can be extremely difficult
  - Haemangiomata – steroids, interferon, vincristine, topical imiquimod or beta-blockers may have a role to play in some selected cases
- Anal fissure:
  - Treat underlying constipation
- Gastrointestinal polyps:
  - Juvenile polyps
    - Usually seen at about 4 years of age
    - About 60% are proximal to the sigmoid colon
    - Colonoscopic visualisation of the entire colon is essential
    - If a solitary, benign lesion is encountered, no further investigations are required
  - Juvenile polyposis syndrome
    - Autosomal dominant

- Multiple polyps anywhere in the GI tract
- Malignant change in 15% of patients below the age of than 35 years
- Peutz–Jeghers syndrome
  - Autosomal dominant – mutated genes on chromosome 19p13.3
  - Arise mainly in the small bowel
  - Associated with GI, pancreatic and ovarian malignancy

- Familial adenomatous polyposis:
  - Autosomal dominant
  - Mutation in the adenomatous polyposis coli gene on chromosome 5q21
  - Colonic polyps become malignant in all patients by about 40 years of age
  - Duodenal polyps also have malignant potential

Further reading

Boyle JT. Gastrointestinal bleeding in infants and children. Pediatr Rev 2008; 29:39–52.

Flynn DM, Booth IM. Investigation and management of gastrointestinal bleeding in children. Curr Pediatr 2004; 14:576–585.

Xin L, et al. Indications, detectability, positive findings, total enteroscopy and complications of diagnostic double-balloon endoscopy: a systematic review of data over the first decade of use. Gastrointest Endosc 2011; 74:563–570.

Related topics of interest

Gastro-oesophageal reflux disease

Learning outcomes

- To be aware of the variable presentation of the condition
- To understand its pathophysiology
- To be familiar with the natural progression of the disease
- To be able to request appropriate investigations to aid diagnosis
- To understand the treatment options

Overview

Gastro-oesophageal reflux (GOR) is the reflux of stomach contents into the oesophagus. It may be physiological or pathological. It is pathological when reflux leads to complications. This is termed gastro-oesophageal reflux disease (GORD).

Epidemiology and aetiology

GOR is very common in infants, where it is often benign and only requires attention if it becomes symptomatic. The incidence of GORD has been shown to be 7–20% in the paediatric population. In the absence of an associated underlying condition, symptomatic reflux will improve spontaneously in most cases by 12–24 months. This improvement is seen secondary to a combination of adopting an upright posture, a solid diet and physical development.

The body is naturally predisposed to GOR due to the pressure gradient which arises from the positive intra-abdominal pressure in the stomach and the negative intrathoracic pressure in the oesophagus during inspiration. The physiological mechanisms which counteract this are:

- **Lower oesophageal sphincter:** This smooth muscle has resting tone, which holds the sphincter closed
- **Diaphragmatic crus:** This striated muscle forms a sling around the lower oesophagus, thereby closing the oesophageal lumen because the crus

contracts in respiration, pulling down the gastro-oesophageal junction
- **Angle of His:** The gastric fundus compresses the distal oesophagus. However, when the stomach is full, the angle increases which can facilitate reflux. This angle becomes more acute (90°) as the infant grows, minimising reflux
- **Intra-abdominal oesophagus:** The positive intra-abdominal pressure on the oesophageal wall keeps the lumen closed

Disruption of the normal physiological anti-reflux mechanisms can result in GORD.

- Neurological
  - Transient lower oesophageal sphincter relaxation
  - Cerebral pathology may result in foregut dysmotility, spasticity or a tendency to constipation, which predisposes to GORD
- Mechanical
  - Hiatus hernia: resulting in loss of the diaphragmatic crus sling effect, the angle of His and the intra-abdominal oesophagus
  - Scoliosis: leading to disordered anatomy
  - Previous congenital abnormalities requiring surgery: oesophageal atresia (OA), abdominal wall defects, congenital diaphragmatic hernia. In OA, the oesophagus is short with little or no intra-abdominal portion and there is loss of the angle of His. Abnormal innervation results in disordered peristalsis
  - Distal obstruction: pyloric stenosis, delayed gastric emptying, duodenal stenosis and malrotation

Clinical features

Presentation of GORD in children is very varied and changes with age
- Infants
  - Vomiting
  - Failure to thrive

- Irritability
- Cough, recurrent chest infections, aspiration, respiratory distress
- Acute life-threatening events
- Sandifer syndrome: spasmodic torsional dystonia, with arching of the back without a vertebral or muscular cause
- Older children
  - Retrosternal chest pain
  - Dysphagia (stricture)
  - Respiratory symptoms: asthma, chronic cough, stridor
  - Haematemesis

Investigations

The role of investigations is to identify the presence and severity of GORD, any underlying cause and any resulting complications.

- **Oesophageal pH study:** An oesophageal flexible catheter monitors pH above the lower oesophageal sphincter over 24 hours. A pH reading of < 4 by the probe is considered abnormal. The duration and frequency of recorded abnormal reflux episodes and correlation with symptoms determine whether the reflux is pathological. However, in children, not all symptomatic reflux episodes will be acidic, due to the alkalinity of milk, treatment with proton pump inhibitors and duodenal reflux
- **Impedance study:** This investigation is based upon measuring the resistance to alternating current of the content of the oesophageal lumen and recording the appearance and direction of liquid in the oesophagus. These episodes can be closely related to clinical symptoms
- **Upper gastrointestinal contrast study:** This may detect reflux episodes and will identify anatomical abnormalities, such as oesophageal stricture, hiatus hernia, gastric outlet obstruction and rotational anomalies
- **Oesophageal manometry:** This measures lower oesophageal sphincter tone and peristalsis and can therefore identify transient lower oesophageal sphincter relaxation

- **Endoscopy:** This allows the visualisation of the oesophagus and proximal gastrointestinal tract and enables biopsies to be taken if required

Differential diagnosis

- Overfeeding
- Pyloric stenosis
- Malrotation
- Sepsis
- Achalasia
- Inborn errors of metabolism
- Vomiting of neurological origin

Treatment

The aims of treatment are two-fold: to achieve resolution of symptoms and to prevent complications.

Non-operative management

- In infants, provide more frequent, smaller volume feeds, thicken feeds and nurse in upright position. The left lateral position has been shown to be associated with reduced reflux episodes in infants
- Decrease gastric acid secretion
  - Histamine (H_2) receptor antagonists (ranitidine) reduce acid secretion by competitively inhibiting histamine binding to parietal cells
  - Proton pump inhibitors (omeprazole, lansoprazole) act by irreversibly blocking the H^+/K^+ ATPase of parietal cells
- Increase gastric emptying
  - The dopamine (D_2) receptor antagonist domperidone acts as a prokinetic, thereby increasing gastric emptying and peristalsis
- Neutralise acid: Antacids may relieve symptoms of heartburn and decrease the risk of oesophagitis. However, they play little role in infants, in whom many of the reflux episodes may not be acidic
- Thicken feeds: This may be achieved with several agents, such as sodium alginate (Gaviscon), carob-seed flour, locust bean gum, sodium carboxymethylcellulose or rice cereal. A meta-analysis of 14 randomised controlled trials in infants showed that thickened feeds were

moderately effective in reducing GOR and that no one agent was more effective than another

- Jejunal feeding: Avoiding the presence of food in the stomach decreases the likelihood of aspiration and reduces the production of stomach acid. Administration of the feed via a jejunal tube must be by a continuous rather than by a bolus regimen, which can be impractical for families
  - Nasojejunal (NJ) tube: This is a useful option in the short term. However, an NJ tube is easily pulled out by the child and is therefore less practical for the long-term
  - Gastrojejunal (GJ) tube: This involves the insertion of a jejunal tube through a pre-existing or new gastrostomy site. Compared with gastrostomy tubes, GJ tubes have a higher risk of obstruction, leakage and displacement. The disadvantage of GJ tubes is that replacement requires the use of fluoroscopy, with radiation exposure, or endoscopy under general anaesthesia

Operative management

An operative procedure is only considered when non-operative management has failed.

Surgery in children younger than 2 years is generally best avoided if possible, except for severe respiratory complications.

The options are the following:

- **Surgical jejunostomy:** This requires general anaesthesia but has the advantage of the tube being more difficult to dislodge. However, the risk associated with the operation and replacement of jejunal tubes can be hazardous
- **Fundoplication:** This operation commonly involves reconstruction of the crural sling if a wide crural hiatus is present as well as the wrapping and fixing of the fundus of the stomach around the lower oesophagus, using a laparoscopic or open technique (**Figure 22**). There are a number of different variations of the operation, which involve wrapping the fundus to different degrees either anteriorly or posteriorly around the oesophagus. Fundoplication aims to reconstruct the antireflux barriers, whilst not obstructing the passage of food through the gastro-oesophageal junction. The most common procedure performed is the Nissen fundoplication, which involves a 360° wrap. It offers a more physiological solution and a better quality of life to jejunal feeding. However, there

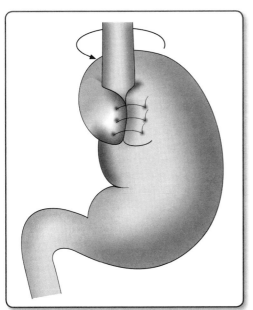

Figure 22 Nissen fundoplication. A 360° wrap is fashioned around the lower oesophagus, using the fundus of the stomach.

is currently no evidence to show that it is superior to jejunal feeding

Studies have shown fundoplication to have a success rate of about 86% in relieving symptoms. Complications include wrap failure and recurrence of symptoms, dysphagia (up to 33%), gas bloat and a decreased gastric volume due to the fundus having been used to form the wrap. The incidence of failure and a redo-operation ranges between 7% and 26%

- **Oesophagogastric disconnection:** This procedure involves division of the gastro-oesophageal junction, closure of the gastric end and anastomosis of the oesophagus to a jejunal Roux-en-Y loop. This procedure has been used as a rescue procedure following failed fundoplication and as a primary procedure, usually in neurologically impaired children, with good outcomes. Careful consideration needs to be given before embarking upon this procedure which can be associated with major morbidity, especially when used as a rescue procedure, and late deaths

Further reading

Campanozzi A, Boccia G, Pensabene L, et al. Prevalence and natural history of gastroesophageal reflux: pediatric prospective survey. Paediatrics 2009; 123:779–783.

El-Matary W. Percutaneous endoscopic gastrojejunostomy tube feeding in children. Nutr Clin Pract 2011; 26:78–83.

Pacilli M, Chowdhury MM, Pierro A. The surgical treatment of gastro-esophageal reflux in neonates and infants. Semin Pediatr Surg 2005; 14:34–41.

Related topics of interest

Gastroschisis

Learning outcomes

- To be aware of the surgical management strategies available
- To understand the recognised risk factors and complications

Overview

Gastroschisis is an anterior abdominal wall defect. The defect is normally to the right of the umbilicus and commonly bowel, but also bladder and genitalia may herniate through the defect. Unlike exomphalos there is no sac. Intestinal atresia occurs in 10%, and there is always abnormal bowel rotation, normally non-rotation. Babies with gastroschisis should generally be born by normal vaginal delivery before 38 weeks gestation, and an urgent surgical review is mandatory. Prognosis is related to the condition of the bowel which is divided into simple and complex. The latter includes atresia, ischaemic bowel, perforation or volvulus, short bowel syndrome and closed gastroschisis.

Epidemiology and aetiology

Gastroschisis is more common in the developed world. Geographic distribution is related to socioeconomic factors. Incidence has been increasing over the past two decades and is currently 4 in 10,000 live births. The reason for this is unknown.

The aetiology has not yet been clearly identified, but several risk factors have been identified:

- Low maternal age (if < 20 years old, tenfold risk) and paternal age
- Exposure to vasoactive substances, such as tobacco, class A and B drugs (four-fold risk)

Likely pathological mechanisms are the following:

- Ischaemic insult (vasoactive substances) to the vitellointestinal artery or involution of the right umbilical vein may cause localised muscular weakness
- Defective mesoderm development

Clinical features

The diagnosis is usually made antenatally, and except in the case of closed gastroschisis, there is an obvious anterior abdominal wall defect with eviscerated bowel.

Investigations

Prenatal

- Ultrasound scanning ('cauliflower' appearance of freely floating bowel)
- Maternal serum alpha-fetoprotein, which is raised
- Amniocentesis not indicated unless associated severe anomalies present

Postnatal

- Simple clinical evaluation, including inspection of bowel for atresia, ischaemia, volvulus or perforation
- Assessment of growth

Associated anomalies

- Intestinal or defect-related anomalies:
  - Atresia 10%
  - Stenosis
  - Non-rotation
  - Hirschsprung's disease (single case report)
- Recognisable syndromes (rare)
  - Non-chromosomal syndrome (0.7%)
  - Chromosomal syndrome (1%)
  - Multiple congenital anomalies (non-defect related) (12%)
    - CNS (4.5%)
    - Cardiovascular (2.5%)
    - Limb (2.2%)
    - Renal anomalies (1.9%)

Treatment

Management comprises postnatal resuscitation, nasogastric tube decompression and IV fluids. Check for hypoglycaemia, respiratory support and broad-spectrum antibiotics. Minimise bowel-related fluid losses with cling film.

Babies with ischaemic bowel should be placed right side down (if the defect is right-sided) in an incubator with a high oxygen fraction. Volvulus of the herniated bowel should be untwisted if present. Principles of surgical treatment are as follows:

- Reduce the viscera
- Close the defect
- Identify associated intestinal or abdominal anomalies
- Support nutrition with parenteral nutrition (PN)
- Recognise and treat complications

Essential surgical options

- Simple
  - Operative primary reduction with early primary fascial defect closure (FDC)
  - Non-operative staged reduction (preformed silo) with delayed primary fascial closure either by operative suturing or by non-operative dressing 'sutureless or plastic closure'
  - Operative staged reduction (custom-made silo sutured to fascia) with delayed primary FDC
  - Non-operative primary reduction (Bianchi) with sutureless defect closure
- Complex
  - Resect perforated or ischaemic bowel, and perform anastomosis or stomas
  - Atresia: immediate or delayed resection of atretic bowel and perform anastomosis or stomas
  - Operative (primary or staged) reduction and primary or delayed FDC
  - Closed gastroschisis: consider tube jejunostomy and bowel tissue expansion programme, followed by delayed anastomosis, with or without autologous gastrointestinal reconstruction (AGIR) (see below)

Complications

- Intestinal
  1. Intestinal ischaemia due to:
     I.   Abdominal compartment syndrome
     II. Necrotising enterocolitis
     III. Volvulus of bowel
  2. Delayed laparotomy for:
     I.   Missed atresia or stenosis or anastomotic stricture
     II. Adhesive small bowel obstruction
  3. Intestinal failure (defined as a requirement for PN > 28 days)
     I.   Slow return of bowel function
     II. Short bowel syndrome
     III. Intestinal dysmotility
  4. Intestinal failure-associated liver disease
- Wound
  1. Dehiscence
  2. Ventral hernia
- Further surgical management options for short bowel or intestinal failure:
  1. Intestinal rehabilitation programme
  2. AGIR
     I.   Longitudinal intestinal lengthening and tailoring
     II. Serial transverse enteroplasty
  3. Organ transplantation
     I.   Liver
     II. Small bowel

Long-term outcomes

1. Favourable – in the majority of cases (simple gastroschisis)
- Median duration on PN or time to full enteral feeds < 28 days
- Hospital stay < 60 days
- Survival > 96% at 1 year
2. Less favourable:
- Complex gastroschisis
- Associated chronic lung disease or cardiac problems
- Syndromic or multiple congenital anomalies
- Hospital stay > 60 days

Further reading

Frolov P, Alali J, Klein MD. Clinical risk factors for gastroschisis and omphalocele in humans: a review of the literature. Pediatr Surg Int 2010; 26:1135–1148.

Marven S, Owen A. Contemporary postnatal surgical management strategies for congenital abdominal wall defects. Semin Pediatr Surg 2008; 17:222–235.

Mortellaro VE, et al. Review of the evidence on the closure of abdominal wall defects. Pediatr Surg Int 2011; 27:391–397.

Related topics of interest

Germ cell tumours

Learning outcomes

- To be able to provide a simple description of the origin and pathology of germ cell tumours
- To recognise the typical clinical presentation of these tumours and their anatomical sites of origin
- To be able to instigate appropriate investigations
- To appreciate the importance of multidisciplinary team-working and to be able to formulate an appropriate management plan
- To be aware of the surgical management options

Overview

Germ cell tumours are a heterogeneous group arising from primordial germ cells broadly considered as 'cranial' or 'extracranial' and can be either benign or malignant. Management is based on:

- Anatomical location
- Resectability, based upon size and involvement of other organs
- Stage
- Evidence of malignancy

Due to their complex nature and the widely differing management plans depending on size, stage and location, it is mandatory to involve the surgical oncology multidisciplinary team (MDT) prior to major surgery.

Epidemiology and aetiology

The incidence of malignant germ cell tumours is about three cases per million population per annum or 3% of all childhood malignancies. Each year, < 45 children develop malignant germ cell tumours in the UK.

There is an association between different locations, age at presentation and clinical features. There are no known causes, but different sites usually present at different ages and the onset of puberty may be a significant event, affecting the biological nature and behaviour of these tumours.

The pathology is complex. A simplified version could be considered as teratoma (which may be mature or immature) or malignant (multiple different subcategories).

Clinical features

Clinical features depend on the anatomical location of the tumour. Only extracranial tumours are considered here, sacrococcygeal teratoma is discussed elsewhere.

- **Ovarian:** They can be found incidentally during ultrasonography or at surgery, or they present with pain which may be severe if associated with torsion or they may manifest with the secondary effects of hormone secretion. For cystic lesions, it is important to distinguish between simple (physiological) cysts and benign or malignant cystic tumours
- **Testicular:** These are usually detected by the patient or parent or carer due to scrotal swelling. The typical appearance is of a non-tender, hard craggy mass, and it is important to exclude a previous history of missed torsion. Testicular tumours that present with precocious puberty due to hormonal secretions are not usually germ cell tumours
- **Anterior mediastinal:** Teratomas are usually benign, very slow growing and relatively asymptomatic. This is in stark contrast to lymphomas which grow very rapidly (days), causing severe symptoms of shortness of breath, inability to lie flat and signs of superior vena caval obstruction
- **Retroperitoneal:** These are either identified incidentally or present due to their pressure effects on adjacent organs

Investigations

- **Tumour markers:** Alpha-fetoprotein (α-FP) and beta-human chorionic gonadotropin (β-hCG) are mandatory preoperative investigations for all suspected germ cell tumours. The result should then be compared with standard age-related charts to show normal values.

It is important to note that mature tumours rarely secrete tumour markers and levels are normally very high in neonates. A high α-FP that drops to normal following surgery is good evidence of complete resection, while a subsequent rise is a sign of recurrence

- **Radiological investigations:** Investigations depend on site. The imaging modality of choice for ovarian and testicular lumps is an ultrasound scan. With ovarian tumours it is important to establish whether there is a simple cyst with a thin wall or a complex cyst with both solid elements and multiple cysts, suggestive of a cystic tumour. If there is a suspicion of a tumour, a chest radiograph should be performed
- **Cross-sectional imaging:** Germ cell tumours from all other sites and ovarian or testicular tumours with evidence of metastatic disease should have detailed cross-sectional imaging. Typical appearance of germ cell tumours, especially teratomas, is a heterogenous mixed cystic solid mass
- **Tumour biopsy:** There is no role for primary destructive surgery, such as bilateral salpingo-oophorectomy, if the tumour appears extensive. In these situations, a biopsy should be taken and the case reconsidered at the MDT meeting

Differential diagnosis

Germ cell tumours should be included in the differential diagnosis for any mass that arises in the locations described.

Treatment

The treatment of choice is complete surgical resection regardless of location, without resorting to mutilating surgery if adjacent essential organs are involved. Resection should avoid any risk of rupture or leakage of cyst fluid. The surgical approach must be carefully considered and depends on location, surgical expertise and clinical status of the patient.

Ovarian tumours

There is no age stratification, radiological features or tumour markers that perfectly define malignancy. If there is a suspicion of a neoplastic ovarian lesion, it should be resected avoiding rupture and spread. Operative technique is as follows:

- **Oophorectomy:** This is the treatment of choice for unilateral ovarian germ cell tumours, which can grow to enormous sizes and, therefore, careful assessment is needed regarding resectability. The author's preference is to use an extended Pfannenstiel incision. The blood supply comes from two primary sources, namely the ovarian artery from the aorta and the uterine artery from the internal iliac artery. These vessels can be sizeable and should be carefully ligated and transfixed before division. Large cystic tumours can be aspirated in a controlled fashion (see later)
- **Salpingectomy:** This is recommended in adult patients when an oophorectomy is being performed, although there is a growing belief that it is unnecessary in young girls under the same circumstances. The Fallopian tube can usually be carefully dissected free and preserved without compromising resection of the ovarian tumour
- **Cystectomy:** Teratomas are usually well encapsulated and may cause the remaining ovary to be stretched over the surface. If there is an identifiable ovary, a very delicate incision can allow a plane to be identified between the tumour and the ovary. Careful blunt dissection will allow the plane to be developed, and the ovary to be separated from the tumour and refashioned with a running absorbable suture. This approach should only be undertaken after detailed imaging, tumour marker studies and review by the MDT suggests a simple cyst or teratoma
- **Laparoscopic approach:** Surgery must be in line with safe oncological principles. A cystic tumour should not be aspirated in an uncontrolled fashion because this leads to microscopic spillage and upstaging of

the tumour. Once the vessels are divided and the tumour dissected away from the Fallopian tubes, it can be manipulated into a specimen bag. A small Pfannenstiel incision or extension of the umbilical incision is made, and the edges of the bag pulled up out of the incision. If there is a cystic portion, controlled aspiration can be done and the entire tumour delivered with gentle traction on the bag, with care taken to avoid rupture of the bag

Testicular tumours

Operative techniques are as follows:
- A large high inguinal orchiectomy is recommended for both localised and metastatic disease, involving testicular and cord removal, without opening the tunica vaginalis, and thus risking scrotal contamination
- The inguinal canal is opened by incising the external oblique aponeurosis and the external inguinal ring is opened
- Prior to tumour delivery, the cord should be mobilised and clamped at the deep ring. The testis should be delivered

within the tunica vaginalis. Gentle scrotal pressure will allow its delivery
- Once delivered the cord should be transfixed and ligated proximal and distal to the soft clamp and divided
- In cases of accidental scrotal incision, it is no longer advised to perform a hemiscrotectomy either at the time or as a subsequent operation

Anterior mediastinal tumours

Teratomas can often grow to an alarming size whilst asymptomatic. Careful preoperative planning is essential. A complete resection may be impossible as it may wrap around essential structures. Sternal and lateral approaches have been used.

Retroperitoneal tumours

Retroperitoneal tumours can present as primary tumours or as metastatic spread. The treatment of choice for metastatic retroperitoneal tumours is chemotherapy. Surgery may have a place for the excision of postchemotherapy residual masses, especially in a postpubertal teenager.

Further reading

Carachi R, Grosfeld JL, Azmy A, (eds) Malignant germ cell tumours. In: The surgery of childhood tumours, 2nd Ed. Heidelberg: Springer, 2008.
Ehrlich PF, Teitelbaum DH, Hirschl RB, Rescorla F. Excision of large cystic ovarian tumours: combining minimal invasive surgery techniques and cancer surgery – the best of both worlds. J Pediatr Surg 2007; 42:890–893.
Mann JR, Gray ES, Thornton C, et al. Mature and immature extracranial teratomas in children: the UK Children's Cancer Study Group experience. J Clin Oncol 2008; 26:3590–3597.

Related topics of interest

Growth disorders

Learning objectives

- To recognise normal growth patterns in children
- To be able to recognise short and tall stature in children
- To be aware of the management options for growth disorders in children

Overview

Growth of a child occurs in three separate phases, which merge into each other, but are under different controls, both hormonal and nutritional:

1. **Infantile phase:** This is first 2–3 years of life, a continuation of fetal growth. This phase is almost completely nutritionally dependent
2. **Childhood phase:** This phase begins from approximately 2 years of life until puberty, dependent on both nutrition and hormones, e.g. growth hormone (GH) and thyroid hormone
3. **Pubertal phase:** From puberty onwards (which starts at an average of 10 years in girls, and 10 ½ years in boys), this phase is under the control of GH and sex hormones acting synergistically

Growth faltering can occur at any of these stages, and timely recognition is vital in order to help the individual achieve their genetically determined target height. Length or height should be measured using appropriately calibrated equipment and in trained hands, accurate to ±3 mm. Shoes should be removed and only thin socks (at most) are worn.

- Supine length is measured up until 2 years of age
- Standing height should be measured from 2 years of age

A standard Frankfurt plane (eyes level with ears) is used for standing height measurements.

Growth and height charts

Height is a normally distributed variable, and therefore can be described either in percentiles or in standard deviations (SDs) from the mean. The current UK Cole 1990 charts combine both. Each of the nine centile lines (0.4th, 2nd, 9th, 25th, 50th, 75th, 91st, 98th, and 99.6th) is two thirds of an SD from the next.

- Short stature is usually defined as height < 2 SDs below the mean for age and sex (i.e. < 2nd centile), or > 2 SDs below the midparental height (MPH)
- Tall stature is usually defined as height > 2 SDs above the mean for age and sex (i.e. 98th percentile)

Repeated height measures, ideally over at least a year to reduce measurement error, and seasonal variation in growth enable a height velocity to be produced, and may give additional valuable information.

Weight velocity is not usually calculated, but weight centile crossing is commonly used, especially in infants. Regression to the mean means that children born small for gestational age (SGA) tend to catch up, and those born large for dates (e.g. the infant of a diabetic mother) tend to catch down.

Genetic influences

Two major sets of genes determine not only final height but also the rate of growth:

1. Final height
- After 2 years of age, there is a correlation between the child's current height centile, final height centile and the parental heights
- MPH or target height is calculated as
  - Boys: [father's height in cm + (mother's height in cm + 13 cm)]/2
  - Girls: [(Father's height in cm - 13 cm) + mother's height in cm]/2
- The target centile range is MPH ± 8.5 cm for both sexes
2. Rate of growth
- The biological as opposed to chronological age is assessed by the 'bone age', calculated by looking at the radiological appearances of the growing ends of the bones (epiphyses). This is characteristically performed using a left wrist X-ray, and assessed how much remaining time

(and therefore remaining growth) there is before the bones fuse, and no further growth will occur
- Puberty is assessed using a standardised staging system, looking at breast development in girls, genital development in boys, and pubic and axillary hair in both sexes. Testicular volume in boys can be measured using an orchidometer

Aetiology

Short stature

1. Normal variation
- Familial short stature (FSS)
- Constitutional delay in growth and puberty (CDGP)
2. Others
- SGA
- Malnutrition
- Endocrine: hypopituitarism (including isolated GH deficiency), hypothyroidism, Cushing syndrome
- Chronic diseases: inflammatory bowel disease, coeliac disease, chronic renal failure, cystic fibrosis, asthma, congenital heart disease
- Skeletal dysplasia: achondroplasia, hypochondroplasia
- Turner's, Down's, Noonan's, Prader–Willi and Silver–Russell syndromes
- Short stature homeobox (SHOX) gene deficiency

Tall stature

- Familial tall stature
- Obesity
- Endocrine causes of precocious puberty, hyperthyroidism, GH secreting pituitary tumours (rare)
- Klinefelter's, Marfan's, Sotos and Beckwith–Wiedemann syndromes

Clinical features

The children may present with one or more of the following features:
- Abnormally short or tall in relation to MPH
- Dysmorphic features, e.g. frontal bossing, midfacial hypoplasia and moon face
- Abnormal body proportions

- Underweight or overweight: the former tend to indicate chronic disease, the latter endocrine disorders
- Puberty – early or delayed, micropenis and/or cryptorchidism (in boys)

Investigations

The diagnostic workup for short stature includes
- Full blood cell count, erythrocyte sedimentation rate, urea and electrolytes, coeliac serology
- Endocrine: thyroid function, insulin-like growth factor (IGF-1), IGFBP-3
- Karyotype in girls (to exclude Turner's syndrome)
- Bone age X-ray to establish skeletal maturity
- MRI head or pituitary (where appropriate)
- GH stimulation tests, with insulin (ITT), glucagon, arginine, clonidine, etc

Investigations for tall stature include
- IGF-1 and/or IGFBP-3
- Androgen levels (where appropriate)
- Karyotype in syndromic causes of tall stature
- Oral glucose tolerance test to suppress GH levels
- Bone age
- MRI head or pituitary

Treatment

Short stature

- Whilst FSS and CDGP usually do not require any medical intervention, short-term therapy with sex or anabolic steroid may be required to kick-start puberty in the latter (especially in males)
- Optimising nutrition is vital and often the only intervention required in children with short stature associated with chronic illnesses
- GH therapy is licensed in children with GH deficiency, Turner's syndrome, Prader–Willi syndrome, chronic renal insufficiency, SHOX deficiency and SGA. However, appropriate patient selection, regular follow-up and good patient

adherence are necessary to achieve optimal final height

Tall stature

- Most familial cases only require reassurance with a predicted final height based on parental height and timing of puberty

- In rare cases, sex steroid therapy to promote early epiphyseal fusion has been advocated
- In GH excess, somatostatin analogue may be used in short term and surgery and radiotherapy for well-defined pituitary tumours

Further reading

NICE. Human growth hormone (somatropin) for the treatment of growth failure in children. TA118. National Institute for Health and Clinical Excellence, 2010.

Nwosu BU, Lee MM. Evaluation of short and tall stature in children. Am Fam Physician 2008; 78:597–604.

Related topics of interest

- Disorders of sexual development 1 (p. 83)
- Disorders of sexual development 2 (p. 87)
- Thyroid and parathyroid glands (p. 338)
- Diabetes mellitus (p. 80)

Haematological malignant disease

Learning outcomes

- To be aware of the range of haematological malignancies in childhood
- To recognise the potential for tumour lysis syndrome (TLS)
- To be familiar with the complications of medical management which are of surgical relevance

Overview

Haematological malignancies account for around 40% of all childhood cancers (leukaemia 32% and lymphoma 10%) and are largely managed by chemotherapy and sometimes by radiotherapy. However, the input of the surgeon is vital to make the diagnosis, to allow the delivery of treatment and to contribute to the management of complications of therapy.

Epidemiology and aetiology

Leukaemias

The cumulative incidence of leukaemia from age 0 to 14 years is 614 per million children in the UK, acute lymphoblastic leukaemia (ALL) 497 per million, and acute myeloid leukaemia (AML) 95 per million. Half of childhood leukaemias occur in the preschool years, with a further quarter in the age range of 5–9 and 10–14 years.

The aetiology of acute leukaemia in childhood is poorly understood. In ALL, hypotheses exist relating to the patterns of viral exposure in early life. Cancer predisposition syndromes, such as Fanconi anaemia, are associated with an increased incidence, as are specific conditions, such as myelodysplastic syndrome and trisomy 21. AML is a recognised late complication of treatment with etoposide for an earlier tumour.

Lymphomas

The cumulative incidence of lymphoma from age 0 to 14 years is 185 per million children (Hodgkin's lymphoma 73 per million, and non-Hodgkin's lymphoma 107 per million). Lymphoma incidence rises gradually throughout childhood, and Hodgkin's lymphoma is virtually never seen in preschool children. There is a male to female ratio of around 2.2:1.

Similarly, for many cases of lymphoma, there is no clear aetiology. There is an association with Epstein–Barr virus (EBV) infection, and in B-cell non-Hodgkin's lymphoma (NHL) (Burkitt's lymphoma) in Africa, it seems that sequential exposure to EBV and malaria may result in mutations in the CMYC gene during tumourigenesis.

Clinical features

Leukaemias

Nearly all leukaemias in childhood are acute leukaemias. The symptoms of leukaemia result from three processes: leukaemic infiltration of the bone marrow, impaired production and function of normal blood cells and leukaemic infiltration of other sites. Symptoms tend to progress rapidly over a period of days to weeks and are varied. Non-specific symptoms, such as fatigue, pallor, abdominal pain, headache, dyspnoea, bruising and mucosal haemorrhage, may be accompanied by more specific features such as hepatosplenomegaly, cutaneous infiltration (leukaemia cutis), bone pain, limp and extensive lymphadenopathy. The diagnosis of leukaemia should be considered in any child presenting with a limp.

Lymphomas

The clinical features of lymphoma are similarly varied and can result from the mass effect of the tumour or from paraneoplastic phenomena. Direct effects of lymphoma include visible or palpable lymph node masses, abdominal visceromegaly, with or without pain, airway compression, with dyspnoea, orthopnoea, stridor or monophasic wheeze and superior vena cava

(SVC) obstruction. Of particular relevance to surgical practice, B-cell NHL is recognised as a cause of small intestinal intussusception and should always be considered, especially in older children. Paraneoplastic features of lymphoma, known as B symptoms, are fever, nocturnal sweating and unexplained weight loss.

Staging

Stage classification of Hodgkin's lymphoma is as follows:

I.   1 lymph node region/structure
II. ≥2 lymph node regions (both on the same side of the diaphragm)
III. Lymph node regions/structures (on both sides of the diaphragm)
IV. Extranodal sites beyond 'E' sites

In addition:
- Absence of B symptoms
- 1 extranodal site contiguous/proximal to the known nodal site
- ≥1 of the following:
  - Night sweats
  - Unexplained persisting/recurrent temperature >38 °C
  - >10% unexplained weight loss in <6 months

2. Staging classification of childhood non-Hodgkin's lymphoma (modified from Murphy, Seminars in Oncology 1980; 332–339) – stage criteria:
   I: A single tumour (extranodal) or single anatomic area (nodal), with the exclusion of mediastinum or abdomen
   II: A single tumour (extranodal) with regional node involvement. Two or more nodal areas on the same side of the diaphragm. Two single (extranodal) tumours with or without regional node involvement on the same side of the diaphragm. A primary gastrointestinal tumour, usually in the ileocaecal area, with or without involvement of associated mesenteric nodes only, grossly completely resected
   III: Two single tumours (extranodal) on opposite sides of the diaphragm. Two or more nodal areas above and below the diaphragm. All primary intrathoracic tumours (mediastinal, pleural and thymic). All extensive primary intra-

abdominal disease. All paraspinal or epidural tumours, regardless of other tumour sites
   IV: Any of the above with initial central nervous system and/or bone marrow involvement

Investigations

Leukaemia

Leukaemia is defined as >20–25% (depending on type) of blast cells on light microscopy of a bone marrow aspirate or trephine biopsy, and this is the definitive test required for diagnosis.

Prior to performing a bone marrow, blood should be obtained for full blood cell count, blood film, coagulation profile, group and save, urea and electrolytes, liver function tests, urate and lactate dehydrogenase (LDH).

A chest radiograph is mandatory prior to the transfer of a child, general anaesthesia or central line insertion, as mediastinal lymphadenopathy may pose a significant risk to the airway and great vessels.

When bone marrow samples are obtained, they are examined with light microscopy, flow cytometry (to establish the immunophenotype) and using cytogenetic and molecular genetic techniques to assist risk stratification and the estimation of prognosis.

Lymphoma

When lymphoma is suspected, the securing of tissue to establish a pathological diagnosis is required. This should be done by biopsy, preferably of a superficial and easily accessible lymph node, for example from the neck, axillae or groins. Fine needle aspiration is not a suitable technique in paediatric lymphoma. Where possible, excision biopsy should be performed. There is no requirement for extensive surgical clearance, as lymphoma is treated mainly by chemotherapy.

Occasionally a more invasive surgical procedure may be required if disease is limited to the thorax or abdomen. In these cases, laparoscopic or thoracoscopic surgical techniques are useful and may limit surgical morbidity.

Staging investigations for lymphoma include chest radiograph, abdominal and pelvic ultrasonography, MRI (or if unavailable, CT) of neck, chest, abdomen and pelvis, echocardiography and in the case of Hodgkin's lymphoma, whole body positron emission tomography CT. Bone marrow aspirates and trephines, and in cases of NHL, lumbar puncture to evaluate the cerebrospinal fluid, complete the staging process.

Differential diagnosis

Haematological malignancy can mimic the features of a diverse range of other conditions:

- Hepatosplenomegaly: infections, storage disorders, metabolic disorders, haemophagocytic lymphohistiocytosis, other cancers, hepatic fibrosis, malaria, osteopetrosis, myelodysplastic syndrome
- Bleeding and bruising: coagulation disorders, sepsis, poisoning, non-accidental injury
- Bone pain: autoimmune and rheumatological conditions, other cancers (bone tumours, neuroblastoma), osteomyelitis, septic arthritis, transient synovitis
- Abdominal presentations: peritonitis, intussusception, mesenteric adenitis, intestinal obstruction, upper or lower gastrointestinal haemorrhage

Treatment

The treatment of childhood leukaemias and lymphomas relies mainly on chemotherapy and for certain tumour types, radiotherapy. This section concentrates on line choice and insertion, recognition and prevention of tumour lysis syndrome (TLS) and some common surgical complications of medical treatment, such as perineal infection, gastrointestinal perforation and typhlitis.

Line choice and insertion

The choice of the central venous access device depends on the diagnosis and treatment intensity, the age of the child, tolerance of the child for insertion of gripper needles and the wider needs of the child outside hospital, such as swimming.

In general, where double lumen access is required, most centres favour Hickman lines but double lumen Portacaths have been used successfully. Where a child or young person has a keen interest in swimming, Portacath insertion is favoured, although with the use of modern drysuits, some patients are able to take part in water-based sport with a Hickman line in situ.

Central venous access is often inserted at the time of biopsy or of staging investigations, such as bone marrow aspiration and lumbar puncture. In the treatment of ALL, the initial induction phase of treatment includes PEG-L- asparaginase, which is a recognised cause of central line-associated deep venous thrombosis, and as such, where possible, the initial phases of treatment should be managed with peripheral venous access. This risk needs to be balanced against the risk of extravasation of chemotherapy and the tolerance of the child for repeated venepuncture.

Central line-associated infection is common in immunocompromised patients. The choice to remove a central line is a difficult one, but in general, infections with organisms forming biofilms, or with *Staphylococcus aureus*, often require the removal of the line. In the case of mediastinal tumours, the choice of line site must be considered, and if there is SVC obstruction, temporary access through the femoral vein may be indicated until the tumour has reduced in size.

Tumour lysis syndrome

TLS is a life-threatening metabolic derangement, which results from the rapid death of tumour cells. Intracellular metabolites and electrolytes are released into the circulation, and the renal threshold for their excretion is exceeded. This leads to accumulation of these substances, renal impairment and potentially serious electrolyte imbalance.

TLS occurs at or shortly after presentation and is usually secondary to treatment with chemotherapy. However, it may also occur spontaneously, or secondary to anaesthesia and surgery.

The tumours at particular risk of TLS are lymphoid malignancies with a high rate of proliferation, such as B-NHL, T-NHL and acute leukaemias, with a high initial white cell count ($> 100 \times 10^9$/L). The presence of raised urate, raised LDH or reduced urine output prior to treatment are risk factors for the development of TLS. Biochemical features include high potassium, urate and phosphate and low calcium.

The general approach to treatment is recognition of risk and avoidance. This includes

- Hyperhydration with 2.5 L/m² of 0.45% saline with 5% dextrose
- Electrocardiogram monitoring
- Absolute avoidance of potassium
- Aggressive treatment of hyperkalaemia
- 6 hourly measurement of serum electrolytes
- Prophylaxis with allopurinol (a xanthine oxidase inhibitor, which inhibits the production of uric acid) or urate oxidase (an enzyme which degrades uric acid)

Urate is relatively water insoluble, hence reduction of formation or metabolism into the extremely water-soluble allantoin is an important means of preventing TLS (**Figure 23**).

Finally, should TLS become established, close liaison with the nephrology team is required, as haemofiltration or dialysis may be indicated.

Surgical complications of medical treatments
Perineal infection
The combination of neutropenia, mucositis and irritation from chemotherapy excreted in urine and stool creates the ideal environment for soft tissue infections in the perineum. Neutropenia ablates the normal inflammatory response, and therefore clinical features, such as rubor, calor and tumour, are no longer reliable indicators of infection. Pain and/or tissue destruction may be the only features of infection.

Many organisms are implicated, but streptococcal, staphylococcal, and particularly pseudomonal infection may result in rapidly progressive infection associated with considerable tissue loss and may require repeated surgical debridement. There is a risk of sphincter loss and of long-term cosmetic, continence, and sexual sequelae.

It is absolutely contraindicated to perform a rectal examination in a neutropenic patient because the coexistent impairment in barrier function of the rectal mucosa may allow translocation of gastrointestinal bacteria, with subsequent life-threatening septicaemia.

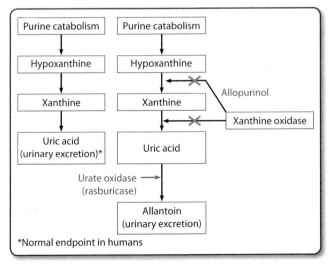

Figure 23 Pathway for purine catabolism and mechanism of action of agents which prevent TLS.

Gastrointestinal perforation

The risk of perforation is worthy of mention because it may present atypically. Treatment protocols with prolonged courses of high-dose steroids can be complicated by perforation, but may also dampen the normal inflammatory response, which results in peritonism. In any oncology patient who is non-specifically unwell or who presents with abdominal pain, however mild, the diagnosis of perforation must be considered and actively investigated.

Typhlitis

Typhlitis, also known as neutropenic enterocolitis, is inflammation of the caecum.

It is a complication of prolonged neutropenia and is presumed to represent bacterial infection in the gastrointestinal mucosa. Patients may present with a selection of features such as abdominal pain, fever, haemodynamic instability, ileus, vomiting as a result of gastrointestinal inflammation, ischaemia or perforation.

Treatment is carried out with gut rest, nasogastric drainage, intravenous fluids and broad-spectrum antibiotic cover, including good anaerobic cover. Laparotomy should be avoided where possible, and should only be undertaken after careful consideration and discussion between senior members of both the surgical and oncological teams.

Further reading

Pinkerton CR, Plowman PN, Pieters R. Paediatric oncology, 3rd Edition. London: Hodder, 2004.

Pinkerton CR, Shankar AG, Matthay K. Evidence based pediatric oncology, 2nd Edition. Malden: Blackwell Publishing, 2007.

Stevens MCG, Caron HN, Biondi A. Cancer in children, clinical management, 6th Edition. Oxford: Oxford University Press, 2011.

Related topics of interest

Haematuria

Learning outcomes

- To recognise that haematuria is not a diagnosis, but a symptom requiring investigation
- To be aware of the possible causes of haematuria
- To be aware of the options for investigating haematuria

Overview

Haematuria is defined as the presence of blood in urine. It may be macroscopic, where the blood is visible to the naked eye, or microscopic. Macroscopic haematuria is an alarming symptom, which causes significant parental concern and therefore is often brought to the attention of doctors urgently. It is not a diagnosis, but a symptom that requires investigation.

Epidemiology and aetiology

Macroscopic haematuria is very uncommon with an incidence of < 0.2%. Microscopic haematuria is more common and has been detected in 0.5–1.6% of asymptomatic school children. It persists beyond 6 months in < 30% of these patients. The presence of microscopic haematuria should be confirmed on repeated testing.

Aetiology includes
- Urinary tract infection (most common)
- Other lower tract causes (e.g. urethritis, polyps, trauma and haemorrhagic cystitis)
- Urolithiasis
- Trauma
- Hypercalciuria
- Glomerulonephritis
- Coagulopathy
- Tumours
- Familial haematurias
- Sickle cell disease

Clinical features

A full history can give clues as to the cause of haematuria.

- Frequency, dysuria, abdominal pain and a pyrexia suggest a urinary tract infection as the cause
- A history of a recent sore throat or skin lesions suggestive of a streptococcal infection point towards glomerulonephritis
- Severe colicky 'loin to groin' pain which precedes the haematuria suggests stone disease
- An obvious history of trauma is usually present when injuries to kidney, ureter or lower urinary tract occur. The presence of haematuria is not indicative of the severity of injury
- Haematuria which occurs at the end of micturation is typical in urethral causes of haematuria. Commonly pain precedes the haematuria. In adolescent boys, this history is classical for posterior urethritis
- History of chemotherapy (especially regimes, involving cyclophosphamide and ifosfamide) or pelvic irradiation therapy is suggestive of non-infectious haemorrhagic cystitis
- Family history of inherited coagulopathy, sickle cell disease (causes renal infarction leading to haematuria) or associated deafness (present in Alport's disease)
- Haematuria which appears after significant exercise and resolves within 48 hours is the classic history in exercise-induced haematuria. It is a benign condition that is due to excess red cell destruction

A full physical examination should always be performed. Specific findings which may help in determining the cause of haematuria include the following:
- Hypertension may suggest glomerulonephritis. If oedema is also present, this may represent acute nephritic syndrome and urgent involvement of a nephrologist is required
- Pyrexia and loin pain are suggestive of pyelonephritis
- Rashes or arthritis may suggest systemic lupus erythematosus or Henoch–Schonlein nephritis

- A palpable abdominal mass or loin mass may be due to hydronephrosis, Wilms' tumour, xanthogranulomatous pyelonephritis or neuroblastoma
- Examination of the penis may demonstrate a meatal ulcer in males who have been recently circumcised or local trauma following forceful retraction of a narrow foreskin

Investigations

The investigation of haematuria can be extensive and invasive. It is important that investigations are tailored to the individual, so that they undergo appropriate timely investigations and, more importantly, they are not subjected to inappropriate investigations. Patients with an incidental finding of microscopic haematuria whilst ill or following exertion should only undergo further evaluation if there is persistent haematuria in two out of three consecutive samples.

The first step is to confirm the presence of haematuria. This should be done by microscopy of fresh urine. If there are any features suggestive of a urinary tract infection, a urine culture from the same specimen should be undertaken. Sterile pyuria in the presence of haematuria raises the possibility of tuberculous infection. Microscopy may also demonstrate the presence of dysmorphic red cells and granular or cellular casts. If these are present or there is proteinuria, the cause may be glomerulonephritis.

If urine microscopy and culture does not reveal a cause for the haematuria, further investigations are required. Initially blood should be sent for urea and electrolytes, creatinine, pH, albumin, ASO titre, complement (C3 and C4), immunoglobulins, anti-nuclear antibodies, anti-DNA antibodies, full blood count and coagulation screen. Urine should be sent for protein–creatinine ratio and calcium–creatinine ratio.

A urinary tract ultrasound should be organised in every case. Ultrasound may demonstrate hydronephrosis, renal calculi or a renal mass which may be due to a tumour or inflammatory in nature (e.g. xanthogranulomatous pyelonephritis). It can also show bladder wall thickening which is present in haemorrhagic cystitis.

Further radiological investigations should be targeted to the suspected cause of the haematuria:

- **Plain abdominal radiograph:** This may demonstrate a calculus in the renal tract or a soft tissue mass
- **Micturating cystourethrogram:** This demonstrates, or excludes, underlying vesicoureteric reflux, bladder or urethral diverticulae or urethral polyps
- **CT scan with contrast:** This can give detailed information regarding renal masses and is the gold standard for imaging urological trauma
- **MRI angiography:** Occasionally this is used to look for rare vascular malformations, and to provide information to plan interventional procedures

Cystoscopy is occasionally utilised. It can demonstrate vesical causes such as small haemangiomas or a diverticulum, as well as urethral causes. Ideally cystoscopy should be performed whilst the haematuria is present. This can also increase the difficulty of the procedure by obscuring the view during the procedure. The decision to perform cystoscopy should not be undertaken lightly, as it can cause urethral strictures in patients with urethritis.

Percutaneous ultrasound-guided renal biopsy is not required routinely; however, it does have a role in persistent or severe cases where other investigations have not led to a diagnosis.

Differential diagnosis

- Haematuria
- Menarche
- Factitious (as seen in factitious disorder by proxy)
- Urine discolouration due to excreted substances, e.g. foods (beetroot, blackberries, red dye additives) or drugs (chloroquine, desferoxamine)

Treatment

The management of haematuria is based upon treating the cause of the haematuria, and is discussed in the relevant Topics.

Further reading

Hutson JM, et al (eds). The child with haematuria. In: Jones' clinical paediatric surgery: diagnosis and management, 6th edn. Blackwell Publishing, 2008:211–214.

Pan CG. Evaluation of gross haematuria. Pediatr Clin North Am 2006; 53:401–412.

Yap H-K, Lau P. Hematuria and proteinuria. In: Geary DF, Schaefer F (eds), Comprehensive pediatric nephrology. Philadelphia: Mosby Elsevier, 2008:179–193.

Related topics of interest

Head trauma

Learning outcomes

- To be able to clinically assess and diagnose the severity of a child's head injury
- To understand the pathophysiology of head injury
- To broadly understand the principles of management of acute traumatic brain injury

Overview

Traumatic brain injury can be classified as primary or secondary. Primary brain injury occurs at the time of impact whilst secondary brain injury occurs as a result of continuing cytotoxic insult to the brain following the initial injury.

Brain injury can also be classified, depending on the intracranial pathology, as focal (localised contusion or haematoma) or diffuse. Focal and diffuse injuries can coexist. Head injury in a child can be closed (without a skull fracture) or open (fracture of skull present). Severity of the injury can be classified based on the Glasgow coma score as minor (GCS 14-15), moderate (GCS 9-13) or severe (GCS <9).

Clinical features

Pathophysiology of head injury: Monro–Kellie doctrine

The brain is enclosed within the rigid skull. The intracranial pressure (ICP) is determined by the volume of the brain tissue, the cerebrospinal fluid (CSF) volume and the cerebral blood volume. Increase in the volume of the intracranial contents, for instance due to cerebral oedema or an extradural, subdural or intracerebral haematoma, results in increased intracranial pressure. Compensation is possible for small rises in ICP by increased CSF absorption and a reduction in intracranial blood volume. If compensatory mechanisms are overwhelmed, ICP will increase rapidly and the brain will herniate through the structures within the skull or the foramen magnum (coning) to cause coma and death.

Infants can compensate better for slow increases in ICP because of their open fontanelles and suture lines compared with children with closed sutures and fontanelles.

Clinical assessment

- **History:** Collateral information from relatives, friends or paramedic crews is vital in the assessment of the child following a traumatic brain injury. A thorough medical history should be obtained with emphasis on the timing and mechanism of injury, seizures and lucid intervals. One should look for any inconsistencies in the history which can hold a clue, especially when dealing with cases of non-accidental injury in children
- **Examination:** The initial assessment of the head-injured child should include examination of the following:
  - Conscious level using the GCS
  - Pupillary response
  - Neurological examination
  - External signs of injury
  - Stigmata of basal skull fracture like bleeding from the ear or nose, black eyes or bruising around the mastoid process (Battle's sign)
- **Assessment of conscious level:** The level of consciousness in a patient following a traumatic brain injury is assessed using the GCS (**Table 6**). The GCS is the sum of the patient's best level for eye opening, verbal response and motor response. The minimum score is 3 and the maximum score is 15
- **Pupillary response:** Testing the direct and consensual pupillary light response is mandatory in the assessment of a head injured patient. In the presence of a rapidly expanding intracranial lesion, such as a haematoma, uncal herniation through the tentorial hiatus causes direct compression on the oculomotor nerve, causing ipsilateral papillary dilatation. This is an important localising sign
- **Neurological examination:** Assessment of limb power also provides useful information in lateralising intracranial pathology following a traumatic brain

Table 6 Glasgow coma scales		
	Original	**Modified for infants**
Best eye response	1. Does not open eyes	1. None
	2. Opens eyes to painful stimuli	2. Opens eyes to pain
	3. Opens eyes to verbal command	3. Opens eyes to shout/loud noise
	4. Opens eyes spontaneously	4. Opens eyes spontaneously
Best verbal response	1. No response	1. None
	2. Incomprehensible sounds	2. Grunt or agitated
	3. Inappropriate words	3. Inconsolable screams
	4. Disoriented and confused	4. Consolable, cries
	5. Fully oriented and converses	5. Smiles, coos
Best motor response	1. No motor response	1. None
	2. Extension (decerebrate posture)	2. Extension to pain (decerebrate)
	3. Flexion (decorticate posture)	3. Flexion to pain (decorticate)
	4. Withdraws from painful stimuli	4. Withdraws to pain
	5. Localises painful stimuli	5. Localises pain
	6. Obeys verbal commands	6. Normal movement

injury. This is usually performed by determining limb response to a painful stimulus. Hemiparesis typically occurs in the limbs contralateral to the lesion. Ipsilateral hemiparesis and pupillary dilatation occur if there is sufficient compression to cause indentation of the contralateral cerebral peduncle by the edge of the tentorium. This is known as Kernohan's notch phenomenon

- **External signs of injury and stigmata of basal skull fracture:** External signs of head injury must be carefully assessed and documented. The presence of bilateral periorbital or retromastoid ecchymosis as well as CSF rhinorrhoea or otorrhoea may signify a skull base fracture

Investigations

Computerised tomography

Computerised tomography (CT) scanning of the head (**Figure 24**) is the investigation of choice following a head injury whenever there is history of loss of consciousness or amnesia. If an associated cervical spine injury is suspected or the mechanism of injury

suggests that the spine is at risk, a CT scan of the cervical spine should also be performed.

Magnetic resonance imaging

Magnetic resonance imaging is an investigation which is helpful in identifying

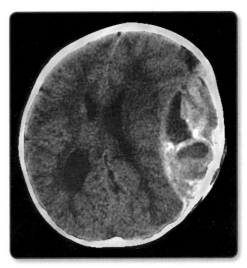

Figure 24 CT scan of head showing left-sided hyperacute extradural haematoma with shift of midline structures.

lesions, such as small diffuse contusions, which may not be identified on CT scan but is a complementary investigation to prognosticate the head injury and should not be used as a first-line investigation of choice.

Skull radiograph

Plain radiographs are useful in identifying a skull fracture. It has no significant role in the management of the head-injured child but should be performed as part of skeletal survey in non-accidental injuries.

Management

The primary aim of treatment is to prevent secondary damage to an already injured brain. As such, head-injured children should initially be managed using established advanced trauma life support protocols. The guidelines recommend:

- Universal supplemental oxygen
- Identification and rapid correction of hypotension, hypoxia, hypoventilation and hypercarbia
- Timely administration of isotonic fluid to maintain systolic blood pressure in (age-specific) normal range
- Airway control when GCS is ≤ 8

- Sedation, analgesia and neuromuscular blockade may be considered to facilitate safe transport
- Neither mannitol nor mild hyperventilation should be considered prophylactic measures but can be useful when there are signs of acute cerebral herniation in a child who is euvolemic and adequately resuscitated
- If the patient is kept intubated and ventilated, a continuous ICP-monitoring device in an intensive care setting should be considered so that the cerebral perfusion pressure can be maintained in the current recommended range (45–60 mmHg).
- Keeping the patient normothermic, normotensive and normocarbic, with serum electrolytes within normal range until such time that the ICP is stabilised

The immediate neurosurgical management strategy depends on the initial CT findings. Any expanding mass lesion should be immediately surgically evacuated. Intravenous mannitol (0.5 g/kg) or hypertonic (3%) saline infusion should be considered if the patient's GCS score is rapidly deteriorating.

Further reading

Debono P, Agius S, Ansari S. Paediatric head inury – a review. ACNR 2011; 10:30–35.
Forbes ML, Adelson PD, Kochanek PM. Critical care management of traumatic brain injury. In: Leland

Albright A, Pollack IF, Adelson PD (eds), Principles and practice of pediatric neurosurgery, 2nd edn. New York: Thieme Medical Publishers, 2007: 833–847.

Related topics of interest

Hepatoblastoma

Learning outcomes

- To be aware of the epidemiology and postulated aetiology
- To be familiar with the clinical presentation and staging
- To understand the basis of the investigations
- To be aware of the management strategy

Overview

Hepatoblastoma is the most common malignant liver tumour of childhood. Nevertheless, it is a rare diagnosis. The majority of tumours are highly curable but require a skilled and careful multidisciplinary approach to management.

Hepatoblastoma can be cured in the majority of children with a combined strategy involving surgery and chemotherapy. The careful selection of patients for surgical resection is paramount, and the results of liver transplantation in appropriately selected children are excellent. New risk stratification will allow further reduction in therapy for standard risk patients without compromising survival. For a small proportion of children with adverse biological factors, failure to clear metastatic disease or who have unresectable tumours, there is still a pressing need to find new, novel chemotherapeutic agents to improve outcomes.

Epidemiology and aetiology

The incidence of hepatoblastoma is in the order of 1 per million. In the UK, this equates to approximately 10–15 newly diagnosed cases per year. Hepatoblastoma is a disease of young children, the majority of cases occurring in infancy, and it is an unusual diagnosis over the age of 4 years.

Whilst the majority of children presenting with hepatoblastoma have no obvious underlying condition, there are a number of known associations which result in a higher than normal predisposition to the disease. The best described of these are children with congenital overgrowth syndromes, typified by Beckwith–Wiedemann syndrome (also responsible for a predisposition to Wilms' tumour). Other important genetic causes of hepatoblastoma include familial adenomatous polyposis (FAP) coli, in which the tumorigenic drive is mediated through a Wnt-signalling pathway, leading to an accumulation of intracellular beta-catenin, resulting in the stimulation of a number of downstream oncogenic signalling pathways. It has been estimated that up to 10% of cases of hepatoblastoma may be associated with FAP, which has long-term implications for future screening of these patients for bowel polyps and carcinomas.

Clinical features

The clinical presentation comprises abdominal swelling (71%), weight loss (24%), anorexia (22%), pain (18%), vomiting (13%) and jaundice (7%). Children may rarely present with features of sexual precocity, secondary to the release of human gonadotrophic hormones by the tumour. Some children also display signs of osteoporosis, with bone fractures and vertebral compression. Between 10–20% of children with hepatoblastoma present with metastatic disease in the lung.

Clinical staging

A preoperative staging system (PRETEXT) (**Figure 25**) has been developed by the International Society of Paediatric Oncology Epithelial Liver Tumor Group (SIOPEL). PRETEXT aims to assess the resectability of tumours based on anatomical distribution, presence of extrahepatic disease and vascular involvement. The staging is based on Couinaud's segmental anatomy of the liver and the distribution of the hepatic veins, which divide the liver into four sectors: PRETEXT I tumours have three sectors free of tumour, PRETEXT II tumours have two adjoining sectors free of tumour, PRETEXT III tumours have one sector or

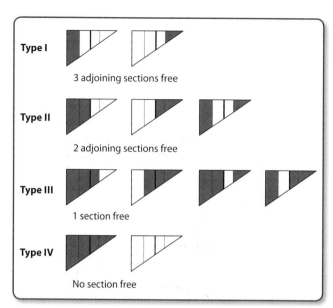

Figure 25 PRETEXT staging system.

two non-adjoining sectors free of tumours and PRETEXT IV tumours have all sectors involved. Evaluation of metastatic disease (M), extrahepatic disease (E), tumour focality (F) and involvement of the caudate lobe (C), portal vein (P), inferior vena cava and hepatic vein (V) and lymph node (N) are all included in the final staging assignment. This has formed the historical basis for risk stratification of treatment into two groups: standard risk (PRETEXT I–III) and high risk (PRETEXT IV and/or the presence of any other adverse features).

Recently, a further iteration of the European risk stratification has been published which is likely to form the basis for future clinical trial design. In this analysis, the presence of metastatic disease, low alpha-fetoprotein (AFP) ($< 100\,\mathrm{ng/mL}$) and small cell undifferentiated histology all confer a particularly poor outcome. Older patients > 5 years, high AFP ($> 1.2 \times 10^6\,\mathrm{ng/mL}$), multifocality and PRETEXT IV tumours have an intermediate prognosis and PRETEXT I–III tumours without any other risk factor continue to have the best outcomes.

Investigations

- **Liver function tests:** These are usually normal in hepatoblastoma
- **Full blood count:** This may reveal thrombocytosis, with platelet counts $> 1000 \times 10^9/\mathrm{L}$ not being unusual
- AFP: The typical biochemical hallmark of hepatoblastoma is an elevated AFP, seen in over two-thirds of patients. Most laboratory analytical methods report an artificially low or normal AFP when levels are $> 1,000,000\,\mathrm{ng/mL}$, and the laboratory should be instructed to make serial dilutions of the serum sample if hepatoblastoma is clinically suspected in the presence of an apparently normal AFP level
- **Radiology:** The imaging modality of choice for the liver is MRI. Timing of contrast-enhancement is important in order to delineate the hepatic and portal venous systems, which have implications for staging, risk stratification and potential surgical resectability. The MRI scan will also allow assessment of extrahepatic disease and evaluation of the risk of

tumour rupture. It is important, but sometimes hard, to distinguish true tumour invasion of vessels from tumour compression, and further information about the involvement of hepatic and portal blood vessels can be gathered by Doppler flow studies at an ultrasound examination

- Plain chest radiography will fail to detect metastatic disease in 50% of patients, and CT scanning is mandatory in all new cases of hepatoblastoma

Differential diagnosis

- Infantile haemangioendothelioma
- Mesenchymal hamartoma
- Focal nodular hyperplasia
- Hepatocellular carcinoma

Treatment

Accurate clinical staging of hepatoblastoma is essential for adopting a risk-stratified management plan, which exposes children to appropriate chemotherapy intensity and surgical technique. The interaction of the oncologist, surgeon, pathologist and radiologist in planning treatment is therefore vital.

The use of adjuvant cisplatin-based chemotherapy in the 1980s revolutionised the outlook for children diagnosed with hepatoblastoma, at a time when overall survival was < 15%. Over the past 30 years, clinical trials have further refined chemotherapy options for these children, alongside improved surgical techniques and liver transplantation options. Today, children with standard-risk hepatoblastoma experience survival rates > 90%.

The SIOPEL group has focused on intensive use of cisplatin as the main strategy to improve the outcome for hepatoblastoma. The SIOPEL 3 study randomised standard-risk patients to receive chemotherapy, with 3-week cycles of cisplatin and doxorubicin (PLADO) versus cisplatin monotherapy, given at 2-week intervals. The results of this study demonstrated that cisplatin monotherapy was equivalent to PLADO in terms of survival. Importantly, avoiding the use of the

potentially cardiotoxic drug, doxorubicin, in these young patients is a huge advance.

For high-risk patients, SIOPEL has attempted to further dose-intensify cisplatin in a weekly schedule, in combination with doxorubicin in their SIOPEL 4 study. Early results have been presented at international congresses, and results appear very exciting, even in the very high-risk patients with metastatic disease. Publication of these results is expected soon.

The surgical management of patients with hepatoblastoma is key to success. Patients with unresectable tumours or those with macroscopic residual disease after surgery have a universally fatal outcome. Complete tumour excision is therefore required to effect cure. Although the SIOPEL approach for many years has been to advocate preoperative chemotherapy prior to surgery for all patients, the Children's Oncology Group in the United States has encouraged primary resection for small, localised tumours. This approach has allowed the recognition of a small subgroup of patents with pure fetal histology (PFH) to be identified and who appear to need no adjuvant chemotherapy with 100% survival. In addition, the complete resection of small primary tumours may further allow a subset of children to be identified with non-PFH tumours who may require minimal adjuvant chemotherapy.

The majority of children with hepatoblastoma however currently receive neoadjuvant chemotherapy and delayed surgery. In the UK, early referral of these children to specialist liver transplant centres, where surgical expertise exists for both major resection and transplantation, is advocated. PRETEXT staging at diagnosis often provides an accurate assessment of the likely surgical procedure necessary. Liver transplantation should be considered for all PRETEXT 4 patients irrespective of their response to chemotherapy. The other main group of tumours to consider for transplantation are those central tumours involving the hilar structures. These are often the most challenging cases where the options for partial liver resection can sometimes be entertained following a good response to chemotherapy. This must be balanced against the excellent outcome for liver transplantation in this group of children.

The main contraindication to transplantation is the presence of intra-abdominal extrahepatic disease. In patients with lung metastases, a complete response to preoperative chemotherapy and/or rendering the lungs free of disease by surgical metastasectomy is not a contraindication to transplantation, and these patients have an excellent outcome. A review of worldwide experience reported long-term survival in 82% of patients undergoing transplantation, an excellent result given these patients in the main would have presented with 'high-risk' features.

Further reading

Maibach R, Roebuck D, Brugieres L, et al. Prognostic stratification for children with hepatoblastoma: the SIOPEL experience. Eur J Cancer 2012; 48:1543–1549.

Perilongo G, Maibach R, Shafford E, et al. Cisplatin versus cisplatin plus doxorubicin for standard-risk hepatoblastoma. NEJM 2009; 361:1662–1670.

Roebuck DJ, Aronson D, Clapuyt P, et al. 2005 PRETEXT: a revised staging system for primary malignant liver tumours of childhood developed by the SIOPEL group. Pediatr Radiol 2007; 37:123–132.

Hirschsprung's disease

Learning outcomes

- To recognise signs and symptoms of Hirschsprung's disease
- To be familiar with the underlying pathology
- To be aware of the methods of diagnosis
- To understand management principles – before and after surgery
- To be familiar with the surgical options available

Overview

Hirschsprung's disease is a congenital condition characterised by the absence of intramural ganglion cells in the rectum and colon. The aganglionic segment varies in length, which results in the spectrum of manifestations of the disease.

Epidemiology and aetiology

Hirschsprung's disease occurs in approximately 1 in 5000 births. Males are more frequently affected than females. Inheritance is multifactorial. Approximately 5–32% of patients have an associated congenital anomaly, with trisomy 21 being a common association. Other known associations are with *MEN2*, and a mutation in the *RET* proto-oncogene.

Pathologic diagnosis is based on confirmation of the absence of ganglion cells and the presence of hypertrophic nerve trunks in the rectum. The acetylcholinesterase staining on histology is also increased.

It is believed that the aganglionic segment is a result of the failure of migration of the neurenteric ganglion cells (originally from the neural crest) down from the upper gastrointestinal tract, down the vagal fibres and along the distal intestine. The ganglion cells are missing from the Auerbach, Henle and Meissner plexi.

Absence of these cells results in uncoordinated contractions of the affected bowel, leading to spasm and lack of propulsive peristalsis. In addition, there is lack of relaxation and spasm of the internal sphincter.

There have been recent developments in determining the associated genetic defects. A mutation in the long arm of chromosome 6 has been identified. In addition it is known that a mutation of the *RET* proto-oncogene is also associated with Hirschsprung's disease.

Clinical features

Hirschsprung's disease typically presents within the first few days of life. There are occasional children who present later, who have had less severe, intermittent episodes of symptoms.

Constellation of symptoms is abdominal distension, delayed passage of meconium, vomiting, spontaneous or induced explosive bowel movements and gas. Clinicians must be aware of the possibility of enterocolitis – prolonged distension and faecal stasis, with liquid and foul-smelling stools. Children can quickly become ill due to bacterial translocation from the stasis leading to sepsis, hypovolemia and shock.

Investigations

Plain abdominal radiograph may show a distal bowel obstruction. A normal appearance does not exclude Hirschsprung's disease. If there is evidence of colonic distension on the abdominal film (**Figure 26**), the clinician must be wary of enterocolitis.

A water-soluble contrast enema is the most important imaging study (**Figure 27**). The presence of a transition zone or an inverted rectosigmoid ratio is suspicious of Hirschsprung's disease.

Confirmation of the diagnosis is based on the absence of ganglion cells and presence of thickened nerve trunks ($> 40\,\mu m$) from a rectal biopsy. The biopsy should be taken at least 1.5 cm proximal to the pectinate line. In neonates, a suction rectal biopsy is usually adequate; however, in the older infants or child, a full-thickness rectal biopsy

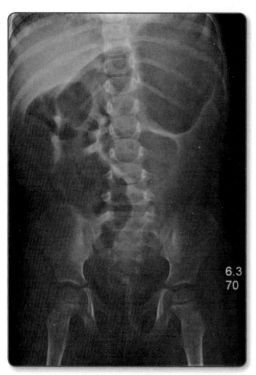

Figure 26 Abdominal radiograph showing colonic distension, in a patient with with enterocolitis.

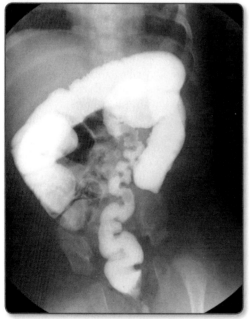

Figure 27 Contrast enema with proximal sigmoid transition zone.

done under general anaesthesia is needed for sufficient tissue for diagnosis. The rectal biopsy specimens should include mucosa and submucosa.

Additional immunohistochemistry that may be performed to confirm the diagnosis includes increased acetylcholinesterase staining and absence of nicotinamide adenine dinucleotide phosphate diaphorase-containing neurons.

Anal manometry is used by some to confirm the diagnosis of Hirschsprung's disease. This physiologic study will demonstrate failure of internal sphincter relaxation, which is pathognomic of Hirschsprung's disease. However, a rectal biopsy is sufficient to make the diagnosis and manometry is not required.

Differential diagnosis

- Meconium plug syndrome
- Meconium ileus
- Small left colon syndrome
- Colonic Ileus secondary to metabolic disorders – hypothyroidism
- Idiopathic chronic constipation
- Distal small bowel obstruction – atresia or stenosis

Treatment

Treatment of the patient with Hirschsprung's disease is variable, depending on the symptoms and length of colon involved. In typical disease, the segment involved includes the rectum and the sigmoid colon (70–80%).

Bowel irrigation

Bowel irrigation is done in the newborn period to manage distension prior to surgery. Enterocolitis is managed by decompressing the bowel and halting the cycle of faecal stasis, distension and subsequent sepsis.

An irrigation should not be confused with an enema. An enema is a larger volume of fluid instilled into the rectum and colon, which is later spontaneously expelled. An irrigation is used when small amounts of saline solution (10–20 mL) are used at a time to wash the colon. A large rectal tube is used to instill the fluid and drain the fluid. The tube is rotated and moved, instilling the small amounts of saline, to allow for evacuation of stool and gas. In treating enterocolitis, a combination of irrigation plus metronidazole is used.

Surgery

Definitive management has transitioned, in most institutions, in uncomplicated Hirschsprung's disease from a three-stage approach to a single-stage operation. Faecal diversion may still be necessary if a child is severely ill with enterocolitis or has distension that does not improve with irrigations. The stoma should be made above the transition zone. A stoma should also be done if there is no paediatric pathologist to help with the diagnosis, or in very ill or low-birth-weight infants.

Surgery

Technical options of the pull-through procedures can include a transanal and laparoscopic or laparotomy component.

- **Swenson:** This involves full-thickness excision of the rectum and remaining aganglionic bowel
- **Soave:** This involves distal removal of the mucosal layer from the rectum (endorectal dissection), and full-thickness resection of more proximal bowel
- **Duhamel:** This procedure has been devised to avoid extensive pelvic dissection. The distal aganglionic rectum is preserved anteriorly; the normal intestine is pulled through a presacral space created by blunt dissection and connected to the original rectum, leaving the anal canal intact

Further reading

De la Torre-Mondragon L, Ortega-Salgado JA. Transanal endorectal pull-through for Hirschsprung's disease. J Pediatr Surg 1998; 33:1283–1286.

Kim AC, Langer JC, Pastor AC, et al. Endorectal pull-through for Hirschsprung's disease – a multicenter, long-term comparison of results: transanal vs transabdominal approach. J Pediatr Surg 2010; 45:1213–1220.

Levitt MA, Martin CA, Olesevich M, et al. Hirschsprung disease and fecal incontinence: diagnostic and management strategies. J Pediatr Surg 2009; 44:271–277.

Related topics of interest

- Colonic atresia (p. 62)
- Faecal incontinence and idiopathic constipation (p. 115)
- Long segment Hirschsprung's disease (p. 188)

Hydrocele

Learning outcomes

- To understand the developmental anatomy and natural history of a hydrocele
- To assess, diagnose and formulate a treatment plan for a patient with a hydrocele
- To appreciate the merits of conservative and surgical management and their outcomes

Overview

A hydrocele is a common cause of scrotal swelling in infants and children. A congenital hydrocele is caused by failure of the processus vaginalis (PV) to obliterate, resulting in a patent processus vaginalis (PPV). Fluid accumulates in the PPV, resulting in a swelling in the scrotum or groin.

Epidemiology and aetiology

A hydrocele is present in approximately 5% of term male newborns. The natural history is of spontaneous resolution, and by the age of 2 years, 90% will have resolved. However, the PV is not entirely obliterated in up to 90% of term male newborns, therefore, the relationship between a patent deep inguinal ring, seen at laparoscopy, and a hydrocele is not fully understood.

Hydroceles are rare in female infants and are described as hydroceles of the canal of Nuck.

Hydroceles may be congenital or acquired. Acquired causes include:

- Trauma
- Tumours of the testis or local structures (rhabdomyosarcoma, teratoma, lymphoma)
- Infection (systemic or local, viral or bacterial
- Torsion of the testis or of the hydatid of Morgagni
- Iatrogenic, occurring after reduction of an incarcerated inguinal hernia or after varicocele surgery

They can be exacerbated by unusual volumes of liquid (cerebrospinal fluid, dialysate and ascites) in the peritoneal cavity, because of ventriculo-peritoneal shunts, peritoneal dialysis and liver failure.

A neonatal gastrointestinal perforation may present with meconium staining of hydrocele fluid (a meconium hydrocele), and intra-abdominal bleeding following trauma may present with a haematoma within the hydrocele.

Hydroceles occur as a result of altered embryogenesis. The PV is an evagination and elongation of the peritoneal lining of the abdominal cavity. The PV develops during the inguinoscrotal phase of testicular descent and allows transmission of the testis from the abdominal cavity to the scrotum. The gubernaculum (rudder) is a key component in testicular descent.

Once testicular descent has occurred, obliteration of the potential space between the visceral and parietal layers of the PVs occurs, sealing the channel between the abdominal cavity and scrotum. Calcitonin gene-related peptide (CGRP) has been shown to be involved in the obliteration of the PVs and hernia sac.

Clinical features

Hydroceles are usually noticed by parents. In infants there is often a preceding viral illness.

In boys a hydrocele most often presents as a scrotal swelling. They are much less common in girls and present as a groin swelling. The swelling may be tense, making it difficult to palpate the testis, causing a diagnostic dilemma as to whether the testis is normal.

The ability to distinguish between a hydrocele and an incarcerated inguinal hernia is crucial, since the management and outcome of the conditions is different.

Inspection of a patient with a hydrocele usually reveals a bluish tinge to the scrotal skin. Unless the infant is starved, the patient is usually comfortable and the swelling is non-tender to palpation. The key discriminating factor between a hydrocele and a hernia is the ability to 'get above the swelling'. Since a hydrocele is usually limited by the obliteration of the layers of the tunica vaginalis as the PV passes into the inguinal canal, the examining thumb and index finger palpating 'above' the hydrocele will meet, with only the skin and cord structures between them. In contrast, when examining an incarcerated inguinal hernia, the examining thumb and index finger will not be able 'to get above the swelling'. lateral to the pubic tubercle, as the swelling continues into the inguinal canal. The examining thumb and the index finger are separated by the skin, cord structures and contents of the hernia (usually bowel). A hydrocele can be made to trans-illuminate brightly in a darkened room with a pen torch. Trans-illuminate is not a good discriminating tests because bowel in an incarcerated inguinal hernia in an infant may also trans-illuminate. Variants of the classic type of hydrocele described above include:

- Encysted hydrocele: These occur during closure of the PV when fluid is trapped within its layers and compartmentalised. They are often difficult to distinguish from an inguinal hernia, but the main distinguishing feature is the ability to get above them and feel normal spermatic cord, thus excluding a hernia
- Scrotal hydrocele: These non-communicating hydroceles occur predominantly in adolescent boys either primarily or following varicocele surgery
- Abdomino-scrotal hydrocele: These unusual variants are purported to occur following normal closure of the PV at the internal ring. One theory is that there is a long PV which is patent down to the scrotum. Fluid is produced within the patent part of the PV and enlarges the hydrocele proximally. A retroperitoneal portion forms as this enlarging hydrocele passes through the internal ring as there is limited or no growth potential within the scrotum or inguinal canal. The retroperitoneal portion continues to enlarge. Clinically there is a large hydrocele with a palpable pelvic mass. Pressure on the pelvic side causes enlargement of the scrotal component
- A hydrocele of the canal of Nuck

Presents with a cystic ovoid swelling of the groin in girls, which can be difficult to differentiate from an inguinal hernia, containing an ovary.

Investigations

In the majority, the diagnosis is clinical.

Ultrasound scan (USS) is useful if doubt exists about whether a swelling is an inguinal hernia or a hydrocele (in both sexes). USS is important to confirm the structure of the testis because the hydrocele may be secondary to testicular tumour), if the testis cannot be adequately palpated.

USS or magnetic resonance imaging is useful in determining the extent of an abdominoscrotal hydrocele.

Differential diagnosis

- Inguinal hernia
- Coexistent hydrocele and inguinal hernia
- Varicocele
- Torsion
- Tumour
- Infection

Treatment

Since the majority resolve spontaneously, an explanation of the natural history of the condition to parents is all that is necessary.

If a hydrocele persists beyond the age of 2 years, most centres carry out PPV ligation as day-cases because the PPV is no longer expected to resolve and enlargement of the hydrocele is likely. There is speculation about the long-term effects of hydroceles, particularly on fertility. Surgery may be open or laparoscopic.

- Open surgery
  - Skin crease groin incision
  - Delivery of the cord structures into the wound (with or without opening the external oblique)
  - Careful separation of the PPV from the testicular vessels and vas deferens
  - The PPV is ligated proximally, to close a potentially communicating hydrocele, and opened distally to allow drainage of hydrocele fluid

- Laparoscopy involves circumferential suture ligation of the deep inguinal ring and drainage of hydrocele fluid
- The non-communicating hydrocele requires a scrotal approach and involves either excision of excess PV and imbrication of the free edge (Lord procedure) or marsupialzsation of the free edge (Jaboulay procedure)
- Management of the abdominoscrotal hydrocele consists of complete excision of all components of the sac, usually via a generous groin incision or laparotomy
- Surgical complications are wound infection, bleeding, injury to the vas deferens and recurrence

Further reading

Hutson JM, Hasthorpe S. Testicular descent and cryptorchidism: the state of the art in 2004. J Pediatr Surg 2005; 40(2):297–302.

Spitz L, Coran AG. Rob & Smith's operative surgery: paediatric surgery, 5th edn. Boca Raton: CRC Press, 1998.

Standring S. Gray's anatomy, 40th edn. Philadelphia: Churchill Livingstone, 2008.

Related topics of interest

Hypospadias – distal

Learning outcomes

- To understand the aetiology of hypospadias
- To recognise the indications for surgery and cosmesis
- To understand the common surgical techniques
- To be aware of the outcomes and complications of surgery

Overview

Distal hypospadias (DH) is a common anomaly, generally amenable to day-case surgery that can be performed early in life. Those with more minor anomalies without significant functional or cosmetic disturbance do not need surgical correction.

Epidemiology and aetiology

Hypospadias has an incidence of 1 in 250–300. DH represents 85% of hypospadias cases with a recurrence risk of 7% and 14%, respectively, for sons and brothers.

During urethral fold fusion, the distal urethra develops by tissue differentiation, involving cellular signalling of endoderm and ectodermal tissues under the influence of 5alpha-reductase, activated androgens and androgen receptors. Most cases of DH are sporadic with familial polygenetic influences and endocrine disruptors, such as maternal or environmental oestrogen exposure and environmental chemicals, including insecticides influencing the reported increasing incidence. Premature and low-birth-weight infants have an increased incidence.

Clinical features

The classification of hypospadias is no longer based on the site of the preoperative urethral meatus alone (**Figure 28**).
Assessment includes:

- Predicted meatal site after chordee correction
- Prepuce (hooded or complete)
- Glans (size and cleft depth)
- Urethral plate (quality and width)
- Degree of penile rotation or torque
- Degree of scrotal transposition and testicular descent
- Assessment of chordee

Hypospadias is considered to be glanular or distal where the defect affects the glans or distal urethra only. This excludes cases with a distal meatus but a poor urethra with loss of spongiosus more proximally or significant corpora cavernosa-based chordee (**Figure 27**).

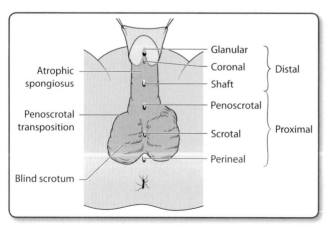

Figure 28 Hypospadias classification and assessment of distal chordee and post chordee correction – meatal position, testicular position and scrotal development.

Labels: Atrophic spongiosus; Penoscrotal transposition; Blind scrotum; Glanular; Coronal; Shaft — Distal; Penoscrotal; Scrotal; Perineal — Proximal

Treatment

Timing of surgery

The practice of delaying surgery for phallic growth is now considered unnecessary and potentially emotionally harmful. Children become increasingly sensitive to hospitalisation after 18 months of age and are phallic aware from the age of 2 years. Phallic growth from the age of 2 years until early puberty is slow. Most surgeons would therefore choose to complete surgery by the age of 2 years, and DH surgery may be undertaken from the age of 3 months.

Indications for surgery

- Degree of chordee
- Angle of urinary stream deviation
- Cosmetic appearance

In DH it can be difficult to assess the presence of chordee, and history of urinary stream strength and direction may be absent. If needed, an artificial erection test and stream test under general anaesthetic may be undertaken. Warmed normal saline is injected into the tourniqueted corpora cavernosa, and the site and angle of chordee, if present, is assessed. The bladder is filled with warm saline via a small-gauge polyurethane catheter which is then removed and the bladder then gently expressed until the urine stream direction is confirmed.

An anatomically abnormal glanular meatus without stream deviation is likely to be asymptomatic in adulthood and may not therefore warrant intervention, but some families request correction, including foreskin management to improve cosmesis.

Management of foreskin

The options are:
- Circumcision
- Repair in layers
- No intervention
- Use as reconstructive graft for urethroplasty

Because there is no perfect answer, most surgeons offer parents a choice regarding foreskin reconstruction. It is successful in roughly 90% of DH cases, and it has been suggested that fistula outcomes may be improved with simultaneous preputial repair.

However, long-term phimosis rates are not yet clear.

Principles of urethral reconstruction in distal hypospadias

The aims of surgery are to achieve a straight phallus, with a terminal meatus, unrestricted coherent urinary flow and good cosmesis with minimal morbidity for the child and his family.

The most commonly used techniques are:
- Urethral mobilisation (MAGPI, urethral mobilisation)
- Distal flap graft
- Urethral plate retubularisation (e.g. Snodgrass tubularised incised plate (TIP) urethroplasty)

Catheter drainage in DH repair remains an individual surgeon's preference, but there is a gradual trend against catheters for the distal TIP. There is no agreement on many aspects of techniques. Surgery is recommended, including the use of a tourniquet, bipolar diathermy or adrenalin to reduce bleeding.

Example techniques

- Foreskin reconstruction (**Figure 29a**)
  - Patients are assessed intraoperatively by approximation of the foreskin in the midline at the level of the coronal groove. The foreskin is suitable for reconstruction if there is no tension and the cosmetic effect is good
  - The hooded prepuce wings are displayed between tension sutures at the natural ventral limits, and the foreskin is incised. Closure is performed without tension in two to three layers with absorbable sutures
  - Dehiscence or phimosis may occur if the repair is under tension or there is a lot of oedema
- Mavis–Mathieu technique (**Figure 29b**)
  - A U-shaped incision is made from the meatus proximally for the required flap length, allowing a perimeatal margin to give a good blood supply, and the flap is elevated. The incision line is continued along the edges of the urethral plate to the proximal margin of the planned neomeatus which may

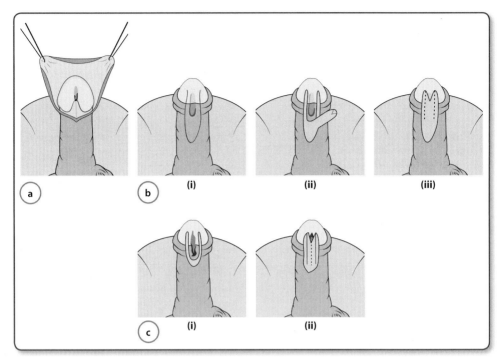

Figure 29 (a) Foreskin reconstruction; (b) Mathieu repair: (i) distal-based flap is marked, (ii) flap elevated and 'V' notch excised, (iii) bilateral continuous suture lines before closure in layers; (c) tubularised incised plate (TIP) repair: (i) lateral plate margins incised, deep midline urethral plate incision widens plate, (ii) single midline anastomosis, meatus closed to midglans.

be advanced by V-Y meatoplasty. The neourethra is formed using continuous 7/0 subcuticular suture. A 'V' notch is excised from the distal margin of the flap to improve the vertical appearance of the meatus, and this is incorporated into the glans closure. The glanular wings are approximated with mattress, or two layers of sutures. Foreskin reconstruction is an option in most cases. The use of stents and dressings varies between surgeons

- Complications – stenosis is rare but fistula occurs in 2–5% of patients

- Tubularised Incised Plate (**Figure 29c**)
  - In DH the urethral plate may be widened by a midline incision into the urethral plate. This may be sufficient for urethroplasty without stricture where the urethral plate is >6 mm in diameter. A tension suture is placed at the apex of the glans, and most surgeons use a tourniquet. The margin of the urethral plate is incised, leaving a 2 mm margin around the hypospadiac meatus, and the shaft skin is degloved to the penoscrotal junction. The glans wings are mobilised, preserving the urethral plate. An incision is made through the urethral plate in the midline from within the hypospadiac meatus to the neomeatus. The neourethra is constructed over a 10 cm stent using continuous absorbable 7-0 monofilament suture. Care is taken not to over-close the glans. Local or dorsal dartos tissue is mobilised to cover the anastomotic lines. The glans is sutured and foreskin reconstructed if appropriate
  - A compressive dressing and stent may be used for 3–7 days

- Outcomes
  - There is a surprising variation in reported outcome of DH surgery, with 20-year adult reviews suggesting

complications of up to 50% and individual authors suggesting complications of < 1%. DH outcomes with < 10% morbidity are, however, reported regularly with each of the techniques described above. Urethral mobilisation requires a good-quality urethra, and some authors are concerned about meatal regression, with the MAGPI technique in particular. The Mathieu repair may have the highest fistula rate, but stenosis is uncommon and the 'Mavis' technique – 'V' incision of the distal flap – improves the otherwise poor meatal appearance. The TIP technique is now the worldwide-preferred technique for distal shaft and coronal hypospadias giving a good meatal cosmesis and facilitating foreskin repair. Stenosis rates of up to 20% have been reported, but the importance of not over-closing the urethra is now stressed

Further reading

Baskin LS. Hypospadias and urethral development. J Urol 2000; 163:951–956.

Snodgrass W. Tubularized, incised plate urethroplasty for distal hypospadias. J Urol 1994; 151:464–465.

Springer A, Krois W, Horcher E. Trends in hypospadias surgery: results of a worldwide survey Eur Urol 2011; 60:1184–1189.

Related topics of interest

Hypospadias – proximal

Learning outcomes

- To recognise and understand aetiologies, associated conditions and syndromes
- To be familiar with the indications for and principles of available surgical techniques, including one- and two-stage repairs
- To be aware of the outcomes and complications of surgery

Overview

Proximal hypospadias (PH) includes cases with a meatal position located anywhere along the penile shaft, but more severe forms of hypospadias have a urethral meatus located at the scrotum or perineum. In comparison with distal hypospadias (DH), other abnormalities are more common and repair is much more complex with a much higher complication rate.

Epidemiology and aetiology

PH represents 10–15% of hypospadias cases with an increased familial risk. American and Swedish studies have identified significant increases in the incidence of PH between three- and eight-fold over the last decade. This cannot be a change in reporting alone, and it is largely assumed to be associated with environmental changes, as yet unknown.

Cryptorchidism in boys with PH has an incidence of up to 30%, suggesting a strong association between PH and a spectrum of endocrinopathy. Chromosomal anomaly is present in 22% of patients with PH and undescended testis. A disorder of sex development (DSD) is identified in 27% of such cases, but others may represent a spectrum of these disorders.

Clinical features

As discussed in the Topic on DH, the classification of PH is based on a full assessment of the urethral plate width and quality, predicted meatal site after chordee correction, size and quality of the glans

and cleft, the severity of available penile skin, chordee and torque in addition to the degree of scrotal transposition, and testicular descent. Undescended testis, micropenis and asymmetrical hypovirilisation are particularly suggestive of DSD. An enlarged prostatic utricle may be present in 57% of patients with perineal hypospadias and 10% of penoscrotal hypospadias cases. This Müllerian remnant is occasionally the cause of urinary tract infection, stone formation or post-void incontinence but commonly causes difficulty with catheterisation. Herniae occur in up to 15% of cases.

Investigation

All patients with perineal hypospadias or associated undescended testis will require investigation for DSD, including ultrasound scan, karyotype and testosterone and DHT in addition to careful examination, exclusion of cardiac defects and associated syndromes. Follow-up until puberty is recommended.

Treatment

Surgery of PH is challenging and multiple alternative approaches have been proposed. However, the principles include:

- Reconstruction of the urethra
- Reconstruction of the glans
- Correction of the chordee
- Minimisation of scarring with hair-free skin cover of the phallus

Unlike DH, when the urethra may be reconstructed using local skin in all primary cases, deficiency of ventral skin formation and severe curvature restrict this option in many infants. Single-stage lateral-based skin flaps, preputial pedicle flaps as an onlay to the existing urethral plate or as a tubularised substitution for the urethral plate, forms the main alternative to free grafting as part of a two-stage procedure. Where preputial skin is insufficient, bladder or buccal mucosa or postauricular free grafts are used. These patients are complex and severe penoscrotal transposition, orchidopexy or hernia may require correction as a further procedure. Micropenis, particularly associated with partial androgen insensitivity syndrome, is a challenge, and in some the glans is too small to be reconstructed over an adequate urethra and the meatus is brought to the coronal sulcus.

Meticulous technique, magnification and non-reactive fine-gauge suture material are essential for these approaches. In all techniques, the interposing layer between skin and neourethra constructed from adjacent fascia is thought to reduce fistula formation.

Urethroplasty

Two-stage free graft (Figure 30)

If the urethra is assessed to be insufficient for single-stage reconstruction or when the surgeon prefers the two-stage approach, the urethral plate and atrophic corpora spongiosus tissue is excised and the chordee is corrected. This is confirmed with an artificial erection test. The glans is deeply incised, and the shaft cleared of residual tissue overlying Buck's fascia to form a vascularised bed for the free graft. The graft is selected: preputial skin is preferred but defatted buccal mucosa and postauricular skin are options. Bladder mucosa is generally considered to have a higher morbidity rate. The 15 mm wide graft may be sewn in place in one or more pieces and is usually fenestrated and sutured to the plate bed to prevent haematoma, lifting the graft. Bladder catheter drainage is then obtained,

and mild graft compression is established for 7–10 days.

The second stage is performed after full vascularisation of the graft at least 6 months later. The margins of the graft are incised, and generous mobilisation of adjacent tissues is performed to minimise tension. The neourethra is then formed, and the anterior edges are approximated using 7-0 polydioxanone (PDS) suture. Dartos fascia is used as a third layer and the skin edges are closed over this layer. A stent is left through the anastomosis for at least 7 days.

Island onlay flap repair (Figure 31)

Duckett (1980) identified that the urethral plate did not require division in the majority of penoscrotal hypospadias cases and that chordee could be corrected with the urethral plate in place. The in situ urethral plate could then act as the base of a neourethra constructed from an onlay pedicle graft formed from transverse inner preputial skin on a vascularised dartos pedicle. This approach reduces the higher stricture rate of fully tubularised pedicle grafts. The graft width and urethral plate should jointly measure 15 mm, and it is important to excise any poor-quality proximal urethra and replace this with graft. The glans is reconstructed over an 8 Ch catheter which is left in place for 14 days.

Correction of chordee

Ventral curvature (chordee) is evaluated by artificial erection test and may be:

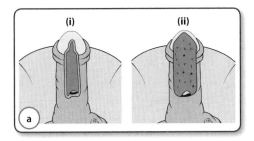
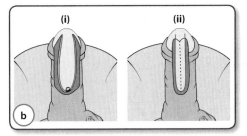

Figure 30 Two-stage urethroplasty. (a) First stage: (i) urethral plate and atrophic spongiosum excised, (ii) fenestrated free graft sutured into plate bed. (b) Second stage, 6 months later: (i) graft edges mobilised widely, (ii) midline continuous anastomosis and closure in layers.

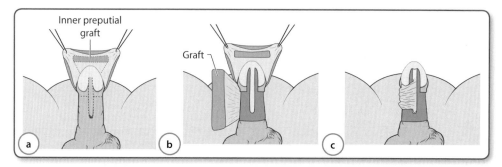

Figure 31 Single-stage onlay pedicle graft urethroplasty. (a) Degloved and plate preserved and post chordee correction graft length assessed; (b) inner preputial skin graft mobilised on vascular pedicle; (c) pedicle windowed or wrapped: continuous suture anastomosis of onlay graft.

- **Skin or subcuticular tissue based:** This is released by proximal mobilisation of the skin and atrophic remnants of the corpora spongiosum distal and lateral to the hypospadiac meatus
- **Corporal disproportion:** This is treated by dorsal plication, such as the Nesbit corporoplasty, or in severe cases by ventral inlay grafting with local tissue such as tunica vaginalis, dermal or biosynthetic grafts

Penoscrotal transposition

It is important to identify the margin of potentially hair-bearing scrotalised skin, although in the very undervirilised infant this may be difficult; rotation flaps move this tissue ventrally but may narrow the available phallic skin base, encouraging two-stage correction. It is important that the shaft and the urethra are free of hair-bearing skin.

Outcomes

Complications

Complications are more common than for DH and increase with length of follow-up, and this contributes to the variability between series. A 20-year follow-up suggests that two thirds of all major complications

present over 12 months postoperatively, and thus prolonged follow-up is recommended for these patients. However, combined complication rates in most series are 5–25% rising to > 50% at 20 years.

Complications include:
- Oedema, bleeding and haematoma
- Urethral stent displacement or blockage, bladder spasm
- Wound infection
- Skin or flap necrosis
- Fistula or repair dehiscence
- Persistent or recurrent chordee
- Meatal or urethral stricture, balanitis xerotica obliterans
- Urethral diverticulum or megalourethra

Long-term functional outcomes

Despite this long list of complications and a significant risk of revision surgery, the long-term psychological and sexual outcome of PH surgery is surprisingly good. Moriya has reported similar levels of concern about penile appearance and sexual performance between hypospadiac and normal men, with the majority of complaints in both groups relating to phallic size – 40% dissatisfaction compared to 34% dissatisfaction for non-hypospadiac men.

Further reading

Kraft KH, Shukla AR, Canning DA. Proximal hypospadias. Scientific World Journal 2011; 11:894–906.

Moriya K, Kakizaki H, Tanaka H, et al. Long-term cosmetic and sexual outcome of hypospadias surgery: norm related study in adolescence. J Urol 2006; 176(Suppl 1):1889–1893.

Moursy EE. Outcome of proximal hypospadias repair using three different techniques. J Pediatr Urol 2010; 6:45–53.

Duckett JW Jr. Transverse preputial island flap technique for repair of severe hypospadias. J Urol 2002; 167:1179–1182.

Related topics of interest

Inguinal hernia

Learning outcomes

- To recognise the presentation of an inguinal hernia in an infant
- To describe the appropriate technique to reduce an inguinal hernia
- To describe definitive surgical treatment options

Overview

Inguinal hernia repair is one of the common paediatric surgical procedures, and the indirect variety accounts for 99%. Of the 20% with incarceration at the time of initial presentation, 75–80% can be reduced with proper technique.

Epidemiology and aetiology

The incidence of inguinal herniae is highest in the first year of life, and the male-to-female ratio is 4:3. Infants born before 37 weeks also have a higher rate of indirect herniae (3–5%) than those born at full term (1–3%).

An indirect inguinal hernia results from persistent patency of the processus vaginalis, an opening between the peritoneal cavity and the scrotum that allows for the descent of testicles before 37 weeks' gestation. When it remains patent, abdominal viscera can protrude through this opening, passing both the internal and external rings of the inguinal canal (**Figure 32**).

Clinical features

Inguinal herniae in infants present as a bulge in the groin or scrotum. The contents of the hernia sac may spontaneously retract, and the mass will not always be detectable on examination. If the hernia is not present, parents will often confirm a swelling lateral to the base of the penis that increases in size with crying or straining. On examination, there may only be a thickened cord to palpate.

If contents are present in the sac and not easily reducible, it is an incarcerated hernia. When an incarcerated hernia is associated with signs of a bowel ischaemia, such as fever, skin colour changes, obstruction or a toxic child, the hernia is strangulated and immediate surgical intervention is required.

Investigations

The diagnosis of an incarcerated inguinal hernia is based on history and examination. Plain abdominal films are rarely helpful, but ultrasound may be useful to identify fluid or vascular compromise. In patients with a strangulated hernia, an elevated white count or lactate may be seen, but these are often late features.

Differential diagnosis

- Hydrocele
- Varicocele
- Testicular torsion
- Testicular malignancy
- Femoral hernia

Treatment

If a child presents with an incarcerated hernia, it is appropriate to attempt reduction. Applying pressure to the hernia

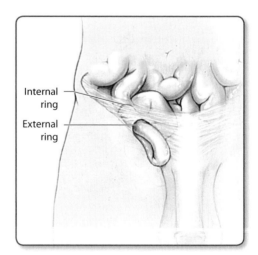

Internal ring

External ring

Figure 32 Anatomy of the inguinal canal including the internal and external rings. Courtesy of Rainbow Babies and Children's Hospital, Division of Pediatric Surgery in Cleveland, Ohio.

contents with one hand often fails because the contents slide above the top of the external ring as opposed to through it (**Figure 33a**). The correct approach is to apply pressure with one hand above the external ring while simultaneously using the second hand to push bowel contents slowly toward the abdominal space (**Figure 33b**). This significantly decreases the chance of pushing bowel over the external ring. If the hernia is reducible, it may take up to 10 minutes and can be performed with or without sedation.

The definitive treatment is surgical, and the timing of the procedure is based on the hernia being reducible, incarcerated or strangulated. If the hernia is not reducible, immediate surgical repair is advised. In reducible herniae, the optimal time for semielective repair is between 12 and 72 hours after reduction.

Open repair

The principle is to achieve a high ligation of the hernial sac. Key steps of the open procedure are described as follows:
- An incision is made superior and lateral to the pubic tubercle and continued laterally along Langer's skin lines

- Dissection in layers until external oblique muscle is identified and incised, staying above the inguinal ligament
- The cremasterics are grasped and separated revealing the hernia sac behind. The sac has a characteristic glistening, white-like appearance and lies anteromedially to the cord structures
- The spermatic fascia is bluntly opened, allowing the vas deferens and vessels to be dissected away from the hernia sac
- The sac is divided and the proximal end raised vertically, and cord structures are dissected down to the internal ring
- High ligation is achieved by twisting the sac and placing two absorbable sutures at the base. The distal sac is left in situ as resection increases the risk of ischaemic orchitis and haematomata

In female patients, there is no spermatic cord, although often a gonad, tube or mesosalpinx may exist within the sac.

Laparoscopic repair

Several techniques for the laparoscopic repair exist including:
- Percutaneous, preperitoneal ligation
- Laparoscopic division of the sac, with or without suture closure

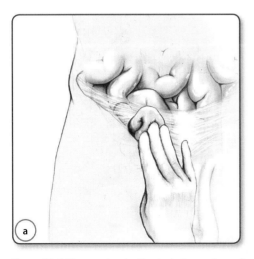 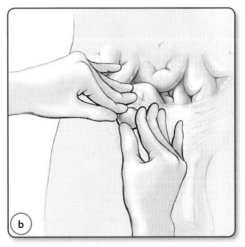

Figure 33 (a) Incorrect reduction technique using only one hand; (b) appropriate reduction technique using the two-hand approach. Courtesy of Rainbow Babies and Children's Hospital, Division of Pediatric Surgery in Cleveland, Ohio.

- Laparoscopic, intracorporeal suture ligation

At our institution, we utilise the percutaneous, preperitoneal approach that begins by placing a 3 mm camera through the umbilicus, followed by hydrodissection of the peritoneum from the cord structures, with a 25-gauge needle.

- An 18-gauge spinal needle is then passed from the 12 o'clock position around the lower half of the ring preperitoneally between the peritoneum and the cord structures and is maintained superior to them
- The tip of the needle is then punctured through the peritoneum and into the preperitoneal space on the other side
- A looped non-absorbable suture is passed through the needle sheath so that the loop emerges into the peritoneal space, with the free ends maintained extracorporeally
- The needle is removed and passed in a similar fashion preperitoneally in the upper half of the inguinal ring. The tip of the needle is punctured into the same peritoneal opening as the previous needle pass
- The suture is then brought out of the abdomen by a loop wire or looped suture

through the needle sheath and tied extracorporeally

In animal models scoring the interior surface of the hernia sac laparoscopically creates a more durable repair.

Open versus laparoscopic

While the laparoscopic approach to inguinal hernia repair has increasingly been adopted in adult patients, this is not the case in paediatrics. Observed benefits in adults include less pain, better cosmesis and easier repair of recurrent herniae.

Early paediatric laparoscopic series raised concern about cord structure damage, but recent studies have been more promising. Chan and Tam reported a series of 79 hernia repairs, with one recurrence and no cord damage. A contralateral open ring was detected laparoscopically in 28% of patients, suggesting added benefit to this approach, although repair of these is the subject of debate. Proponents of the laparoscopic approach note that there is a theoretical advantage of no-touch of the cord structures during the repair.

Further reading

Chan KL, Tam PK. Technical refinements in laparoscopic repair of childhood inguinal hernias. Surg Endosc 2004; 18:957–960.

Fitzgibbons RJ Jr, Filipi Charles J, Quinn Thomas H. Inguinal hernias. In: Brunicardi FC, Andersen DK, Billiar TR, et al. (eds), Schwartz's principles of surgery, 8th edn. New York: McGraw-Hill Medical, 2004.

Sato T, Oldham K. Pediatric abdomen. In: Muholland M, Lillemoe K, Doherty G, et al. (eds), Greenfield's surgery scientific principles and practice, 4th edn. Philadelphia: Lippincott Williams & Wilkins, 2006:1882–1883.

Related topics of interest

Inhaled foreign body

Learning outcomes

- To understand the epidemiology of inhaled foreign bodies
- To know when to suspect an inhaled foreign body
- To know how to remove an inhaled foreign body

Overview

The inhaled foreign body (FB) is a common problem in childhood despite improvements in toy manufacturing and legislation to prevent this.

Epidemiology and aetiology

Inhaled FB commonly occurs between 1 and 3 years of age, but no age is excluded. The FB can not only occlude the distal airway but also set up a local inflammatory reaction which may worsen the obstruction. Peanuts produce a severe inflammatory reaction in the mucosa which worsens the oedema and obstruction. Acutely there may be a ball valve mechanism which results in hyperinflation. A chronic FB can result in granulation tissue formation. The lung lobes distal to it become atelectatic with eventual bronchiectasis.

Inhaled FB may become lodged anywhere from the larynx to the bronchus. In children they consist mainly of food, but small parts of toys are also common

Clinical features

The typical presentation is of a previously well toddler who suddenly develops coughing, choking and cyanosis. A high index of suspicion must be maintained in the at-risk group even if the symptoms and signs are mild. Laryngeal obstruction may present with hoarseness, stridor, coughing and cyanosis. Tracheal impaction may present with stridor, wheezing, coughing, dyspnoea and cyanosis. Bronchial impaction may present with fixed wheezing, or absent air entry in the affected lobes.

Investigations

The mainstay of radiologic investigation is the chest X-ray. X-rays of the neck may also show a laryngeal FB. Radiologic signs include hyperinflation in expiration, collapse of a lobe or visible FB. Bronchoscopy is mandatory if the X-rays are normal but the clinical suspicion remains high. Computed tomography (CT) of the chest is useful for investigating the chronic FB (e.g. hyperinflation, consolidation and bronchiectasis).

Differential diagnosis

In the chronic cases, it may very difficult to distinguish from other chronic airway or lung problems. These patients may have to undergo CT as well as rigid or flexible bronchoscopy in order to reach a diagnosis.

Treatment

Bronchial foreign body removal

It is important to check that all the equipment is available and in working order before the patient is anaesthetised. A ventilating rigid bronchoscope with an optical grasping forceps is the instrument of choice. General anaesthesia is preferred with the patient breathing spontaneously. The patient is positioned supine with a roll under the shoulders to extend the neck. Once the bronchoscope is introduced, the ventilation channel is connected and the FB is located. The telescope is then removed and the optical forceps is introduced. Solid objects can be grasped and either removed together with the bronchoscope or pulled into the bronchoscope and removed. A McGill's forceps should be at hand to remove the FB if it gets stuck in the larynx or falls into the pharynx. Peanuts can be challenging specially if they have been there for a few days since they can disintegrate. A flexible suction catheter can be used to suck up the tiny peanut particles. A Fogarty catheter can be passed distal to the FB and inflated and withdrawn to pull the FB into the bronchoscope. Postoperatively, if the patient is still symptomatic or there are persisting radiologic signs, a repeat bronchoscopy is indicated.

Complications are more frequent if the FB is chronic: failure to remove, trauma, persistent atelectasis and bronchiectasis.

Further reading

Ashcraft K, Holcomb GW, Murphy PJ. Pediatric surgery, 4th edn. Philadelphia: Saunders, 2005:137–145.

Parikh DH, Crabbe DCG, Auldist AW, et al. Pediatric thoracic surgery. 2009:365–371.

Related topics of interest

Intussusception

Learning outcomes

- To understand the aetiology and pathology of intussusception
- To appreciate the difference between primary and secondary intussusception
- To gain a clear understanding of the clinical features and the initial management of children with intussusception
- To be familiar with the management techniques

Overview

Intussusception is a relatively common cause of bowel obstruction. The classical definition of intussusception is full-thickness invagination of proximal bowel (forming the intussusceptum) into distal bowel (intussuscipiens).

Epidemiology and aetiology

In a 3-year population-based surveillance of intussusception in Switzerland, the yearly mean incidence was 38, 31 and 26 cases per 100,000 live births in the first, second and third years of life, respectively.

Approximately 60% of children are younger than 1 year and 80–90% younger than 2 years. It occurs less commonly before 3 months and after 3 years of age. Approximately 80–95% of cases are ileocolic, with other forms, including ileoileal, caecocolic, colocolic and jejunojejunal being increasingly rare.

The invagination of the proximal bowel into the distal bowel causes the bowel mesentery to become compressed and the arterial supply to the bowel is eventually compromised. Failure to recognise the diagnosis can lead to prolonged ischaemia, bowel wall necrosis, bowel perforation, sepsis and death.

Primary intussusception is the most common type. It is idiopathic and is common after a viral illness. It occurs typically at ages 5–10 months. It is characterised by a lack of pathological lead point. It is associated with hypertrophied Peyer's patches in the ileal wall (**Figure 34**) and is typically ileocolic.

Secondary intussusception is noted in a slightly older age group and occurs secondary to a defined pathology which acts as a lead point. Common lead points are Meckel's diverticulum, intestinal polyps, intestinal duplications and appendiceal stump, usually after inversion appendicectomy.

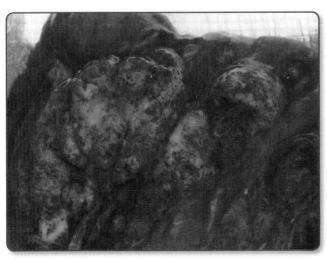

Figure 34 An operative specimen of terminal ileum showing grossly enlarged Peyer's patches as the lead point for the intussusceptum.

Other conditions which predispose to the development of intussusception are Henoch–Schönlein purpura, leukaemia, cystic fibrosis and haemophilia.

Postoperative intussusception is responsible for 3–10% of cases of postoperative bowel obstruction. Approximately 90% of cases occur within 14 days of initial laparotomy. Retroperitoneal dissection, as is performed during Wilms' nephrectomy, seems to predispose to this type of intussusception.

Clinical features

The classical features described in many textbooks are intermittent cramping abdominal pain, vomiting which may be bilious, redcurrant jelly stools and a palpable mass on examination. However, only 25% of patients will present with all these features. The older child may present with features to suggest a pathological lead point: perioral pigmentation in Peutz–Jeghers syndrome and the classical purpuric rash over the buttocks and the extensor aspects of the arms and legs in Henoch–Schönlein purpura. Pathological lead points are increasingly common, the older the child.

Typically the child will have an episode of severe abdominal pain, causing updrawing of the legs to the chest and inconsolable crying. Accompanying attacks of pallor are common. This may be followed by an episode of vomiting and apparent resolution, with the child falling asleep. This may become cyclical, with increasing abdominal distension and lethargy becoming more prominent.

Finally, the child passes blood per rectum, which is a relatively late feature, indicating bowel wall ischaemia and necrosis. At this stage, the child is at significant risk of overwhelming sepsis. Children in the UK still die from intussusception as a result of their profound illness being underestimated.

On examination, the child may be well or unwell, depending upon the stage of the disease at presentation. Late presentation is associated with dehydration, lethargy, abdominal distension and tenderness. There may be a palpable sausage-shaped abdominal mass and blood in the nappy. With ileocolic intussusception the ileum will have invaginated into the caecum and right ascending colon. The mass is palpable in the right upper quadrant, leaving the right lower quadrant empty, and this is known as the 'dance' sign.

Investigations

- Full blood count
- Serum electrolytes, urea and creatinine

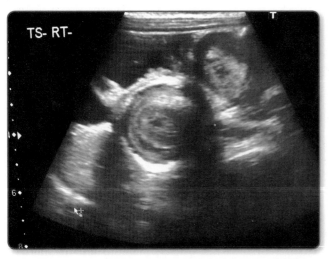

Figure 35 An ultrasound revealing the doughnut sign – multiple rings indicating bowel within bowel.

- The radiological investigation of choice is abdominal ultrasound which shows a classical 'doughnut' or 'target' sign appearance (**Figure 35**)
- An abdominal radiograph is not indicated. However, an abdominal radiograph will not infrequently have been performed prior to the child being seen by the surgical team. It may show paucity of gas in the right lower quadrant

Differential diagnosis

- Gastroenteritis
- Malrotation
- Appendicitis
- Incarcerated inguinal hernia
- Meckel's diverticulum
- Bowel obstruction secondary to a congenital band or adhesive obstruction

Treatment

Initial resuscitation

- The child is resuscitated using the 'ABC' principle
- Intravenous cannulation
- Correction of dehydration with normal saline and KCL (20 mmol/L); an initial bolus of 10–20 mL/kg is often appropriate, followed by a slower rate of infusion
- Maintenance intravenous fluid therapy
- Passage of a large-bore nasogastric tube to decompress the stomach, followed by regular aspiration
- Replacement of nasogastric losses millilitre for millilitre, with intravenous normal saline and KCL (20 mmol/L)
- Broad-spectrum antibiotics
- Analgesia
- Group and save blood sample for blood transfusion if needed later
- Non-operative reduction
  - The established standard is non-operative pneumatic reduction by a radiologist with expertise in this area
  - Younger children will tolerate air reduction awake. However, the older child will require a general anaesthetic
  - A large catheter is inserted per rectum and air is instilled under fluoroscopic control to a maximum pressure of 80 mmHg in infants and 120 mmHg in older children. The intussusception is seen to reduce, and air is seen to enter the previously obstructed (dilated) segment of bowel
  - Hydrostatic reduction uses a similar technique except contrast is instilled again under fluoroscopic control
  - The success rate is 75–85%
  - False-positive reductions are known to occur, and a high index of suspicion is required in the child that fails to improve or has ongoing symptoms despite previous non-operative reduction
  - In a subgroup of infants, only a partial reduction is possible initially. If the clinical condition allows, a second attempt is made 4–6 hours later during which time ileocaecal oedema may subside and successful reduction is achieved
  - An absolute contraindication to non-operative reduction is peritonitis, suspected or confirmed perforation and failure to respond to fluid resuscitation
- Operative reduction (laparoscopic or open) if pneumatic or hydrostatic reduction fails or there are contraindications
- Bowel resection
  - If the bowel at laparotomy fails to reduce, or is frankly ischaemic, the bowel is resected and a primary anastomosis is performed

The recurrence rate for intussusception is 10%. A third of cases will recur within 24 hours and the majority within the first 6 months of the primary episode. It is important to counsel carers about recurrence.

Further reading

Bonnard A, Demarche M, Dimitriu C, et al. Indications for laparoscopy in the management of intussusception. A multicentre retrospective study conducted by the French Study Group for Pediatric Laparoscopy. J Pediatr Surg 2008; 43:1249–1253.

Niramis R, Watanatitan S, Kruatrachue A, et al. Management of recurrent intussusception: nonoperative or operative reduction? J Pediatr Surg 2010; 45:2175–2180.

Somme S, To T, Langer JC. Factors determining the need for operative reduction in children with intussusception: a population based study. J Pediatr Surg 2006; 41:1014–1019.

Related topics of interest

Long gap oesophageal atresia

Learning outcomes

- To be able to make a clinical diagnosis of long gap oesophageal atresia
- To understand the variation of management compared with standard types of oesophageal atresia
- To understand the alternatives for therapy and their long-term outcomes

Overview

No universally accepted definition exists for long gap oesophageal atresia (LGOA). Some authors describe a gap of over three to four vertebral bodies. A more simple definition would be the inability to anastomose the two ends of the oesophagus in the neonatal period. There is usually no fistula associated with LGOA. The term 'wide gap' is used when there is inability to perform primary anastomosis in the presence of a distal fistula.

The premise of many surgeons has been to preserve the native oesophagus at all costs although this has frequently resulted in a poor quality childhood through chronic illness and prolonged hospitalisation.

Epidemiology and aetiology

Long gap accounts for around 6% of all cases, with similar patterns of associated abnormalities and theories of aetiology. A fistula to the upper pouch is seen more commonly in the presence of LGOA than any other form of oesophageal atresia (OA).

Clinical features

Clinical features are antenatally similar to those of other forms of OA. If anything, the presence of polyhydramnios and absent stomach bubble is more likely to represent a fetus with LGOA, owing to no fistulous connection to distend the stomach. Postnatally the specific diagnosis of LGOA is suspected by the typical clinical features of OA along with the absence of any visible gas pattern under diaphragm (**Figure 36**).

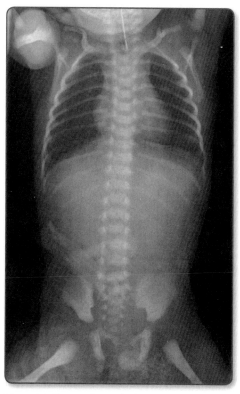

Figure 36 Chest radiograph showing a nasogastric tube in upper oesophagus and no bowel gas under diaphragm.

Investigations

A chest and abdominal radiograph reveals the presence of the arrested nasogastric tube in the upper mediastinum along with no gas evident under diaphragm (**Figure 36**). Other investigations are conducted along the lines of children with other forms of OA.

Differential diagnosis

Blockage of a distal fistula through thick secretions could potentially be mistaken for LGOA, but in clinical practice this is very rare.

Treatment

The infant is stabilised and intravenous access is established. Absence of a fistula renders the infant safe until planned elective surgery can be performed even in the presence of respiratory distress and ventilation.

Definitive treatment is surgical. The principles of surgery are as follows:

- **Establishing a route for enteral nutrition:** This is usually achieved through a small midline laparotomy and Stamm gastrostomy. It can be a difficult procedure due to the small size of the stomach, and it is rarely possible to be able to attach the stomach to the back of the anterior abdominal wall.
- **Establishing the distance between the two ends of the oesophagus:** This so-called gap assessment is performed by inserting a radio-opaque structure into the proximal oesophagus via the mouth and the distal oesophagus via the gastrotomy. An X-ray is taken to document the distance between the two ends of the oesophagus. (**Figure 37**)

Full enteral feeds are established via the gastrostomy, and upper pouch secretions are controlled with continuous suction through a replogle tube. After a period of 4–6 weeks, the infant is returned to theatre and a further 'gap assessment' is performed. Potential outcomes following this assessment are as follows:

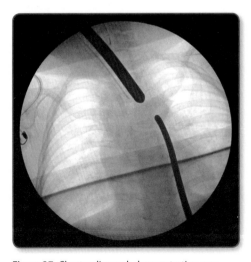

Figure 37 Chest radiograph demonstrating gap assessment.

- If the gap is less than three vertebral bodies in length, then delayed primary anastomosis via a right-sided thoracotomy or thoracoscopy is performed. The anastomosis is often tight under these circumstances but the ends of the oesophagus are more robust and hold stitches well. A period of postoperative sedation and paralysis in intensive care unit for 5 days helps to ensure a very low rate of anastomotic leak and disruption.
- If the gap remains long, then a further period of waiting may be undertaken before reassessing the gap.
- If the gap remains significant, the oesophagus can be abandoned and a cervical oesophagostomy is performed via a right-sided collar incision, bringing the upper pouch to the skin surface medial to the carotid vessels. Replacement of the oesophagus is undertaken at a later stage, but while waiting the child can be allowed home to feed via the gastrostomy and sham feed orally to maintain oral skills.

Complications

Continued respiratory symptoms prior to definitive repair should prompt microlaryngobronchoscopy to exclude an upper pouch fistula. Failure to resolve can lead to the need for cervical oesophagostomy to divert the salivary stream.

Rates of anastomotic stricture and gastro-oesophageal reflux are higher in cases of delayed primary anastomosis. This is secondary to the tension at the time of repair. Techniques employed to achieve primary anastomosis include:

- Regular bouginage of the oesophageal ends
- Traction of the oesophageal ends (e.g. Foker and Kimura techniques)
- Myotomy or flaps of the upper pouch (e.g. Gough flap)

Such techniques have not filtered into regular practice although proponents of the Foker technique claim good results.

Techniques for oesophageal replacement include:

- Gastric transposition

- Gastric tube based on greater or lesser curve
- Transverse colon
- Jejunum (either pedicled or free graft)

The most commonly used graft remains the whole stomach interposition. There is increasing experience with minimally invasive techniques to perform this procedure.

Long-term outcomes

Long-term results show no significant difference in outcome between gastric and colonic transposition. Good quality of life is seen in children after gastric transposition. Barrett's oesophagus has been reported in the proximal oesophagus following gastric transposition.

Further reading

Arul GS, Parikh D. Oesophageal replacement in children. Ann R Coll Surg Engl 2008; 90:7–12.

Ludman L, Spitz L. Quality of life after gastric transposition for oesophageal atresia. J Pediatr Surg 2003; 38:53–57.

Ron O, De Coppi P, Pierro A. The surgical approach to esophageal atresia repair and the management of long-gap atresia: results of a survey. Semin Pediatr Surg 2009; 18:44–49.

Related topics of interest

- Oesophageal atresia and tracheo-oesophageal fistula (p. 219)

Long segment Hirschsprung's disease

Learning outcomes

- To recognise differences between typical and long segment diseases
- To understand pre- and postoperative management strategies
- To be aware of the surgical options available

Overview

Hirschsprung's disease is a congenital condition characterised by the absence of intramural ganglion cells in the rectum and colon and sometimes the small intestine. The aganglionic segment varies in length, which results in the spectrum of manifestations of the disease. Long segment Hirschsprung's is defined as aganglionic bowel, extending to and proximal to the hepatic flexure.

Epidemiology and aetiology

Long segment disease is treated as a separate entity compared to typical disease because it has a higher mortality and complication rate. It is difficult to manage these patients with irrigations prior to surgery and they often do not present with the classic symptoms of Hirschsprung's disease. Long segment Hirschsprung's disease seems to be more frequent in females.

Clinical features

Neonates and children with long segment Hirschsprung's disease may or may not present with the classic symptoms of abdominal distention, delayed passage of meconium, vomiting, spontaneous or induced explosive bowel movements and gas.

Investigations

A water-soluble contrast enema is the most important imaging study (**Figure 38**). Confirmation of the diagnosis is based on the absence of ganglion cells and the presence of thickened nerve trunks ($>40\,\mu m$) from a rectal biopsy. The biopsy should be taken at least 1.5 cm proximal to the pectinate line. The rectal biopsy specimens should include mucosa and submucosa.

Differential diagnosis

- Meconium plug syndrome
- Meconium ileus
- Small left colon syndrome
- Colonic ileus secondary to metabolic problems – hypothyroidism
- Idiopathic chronic constipation
- Distal small bowel obstruction – atresia or stenosis
- Typical Hirschsprung's disease

Treatment

Treatment of the patient with long segment Hirschsprung's disease differs from typical Hirschsprung's disease. Instead of a primary pull-through, infants are managed with an initial ileostomy or hepatic flexure colostomy, followed by the definitive pull-through procedure, at 2–3 years of life. This is often due to the inability to irrigate and decompress the entire colon effectively prior to a primary pull-through and potentially leading to faecal stasis and sepsis from bacterial translocation.

To limit severe perineal excoriation secondary to frequent liquid stools, the pull-through is delayed until the child is continent for urine and out of diapers. All patients and families should be adept at irrigations prior to closing the ileostomy, since there may be a higher tendency to have enterocolitis in the long segment Hirschsprung's patient after the pull-through procedure.

Definitive management in long segment Hirschsprung's disease can be either a straight ileoanal pull-through or a Duhamel pouch. If a Duhamel pouch is created, the pouch should be limited in size since leaving large pouches of aganglionic bowel can cause problems with obstruction secondary to the inability of the pouch to empty.

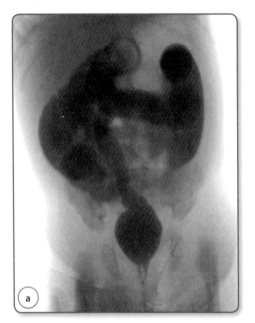
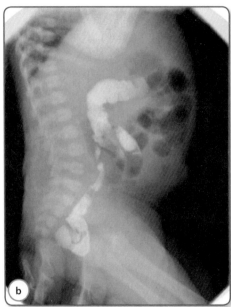

Figure 38 (a) Lower gastrointestinal (GI) contrast study in a patient with total colonic Hirschsprung's disease. There is no obvious transition zone and the flexures are curved. (b) Lateral view of a lower GI contrast study in a patient with total colonic Hirschsprung's disease.

Further reading

Amiel J, Lyonnet S. Hirschsprung disease, associated syndromes, and genetics: a review. J Med Genet 2001; 38:729–739.

Levitt MA, Dickie B, Peña A. Evaluation and treatment of the patient with Hirschsprung disease who is not doing well after a pull-through procedure. Semin Pediatr Surg 2010; 19:146–153.

Ruttenstock E, Puri P. A meta-analysis of clinical outcome in patients with total intestinal aganglionosis. Pediatr Surg Int 2009; 25:833–839.

Related topics of interest

Lymphadenopathy

Learning outcomes

- To be aware of causes of lymphadenopathy
- To be able to decide on appropriate investigations
- To understand when surgical intervention is indicated

Overview

The patient with presumed abnormal lymph node enlargement is a common clinical problem. Whilst the lymphadenopathy may be present in any area, cervical lymphadenopathy is perhaps the most common and challenging situation. Whilst the cause of the lymphadenopathy is frequently benign, the child and family are often anxious because of a presumed diagnosis of cancer.

Lymphadenopathy can arise from multiple causes, and it is important to obtain a clear history of the length of time the adenopathy has been present, whether it was associated with any infection or exposure to infective agents, local symptoms (pain and tenderness) and general symptoms, including the 'B symptoms' associated with lymphoma (e.g. fever, night sweats, weight loss and pruritis). It is also important to conduct a thorough examination of the adenopathy to assess the lymph node group involved, to determine whether the adenopathy is localised or generalised, to assess for the presence of erythema, for the presence of a local cause or trigger, for enlargement of the liver and spleen and for the presence of other masses.

Epidemiology and aetiology

Approximately 50% of healthy children develop palpable peripheral lymphadenopathy. Lymph nodes are generally considered normal when they are < 1 cm in size. The most common cause of acute bilateral cervical lymphadenopathy is a viral upper respiratory tract infection or streptococcal pharyngitis. In cases of acute unilateral cervical lymphadenopathy, 40–80% cases are due to a streptococcal or staphylococcal infection. Cat scratch disease, mycobacterial infection and toxoplasmosis are the most common causes of chronic or subacute lymphadenopathy. Anterior cervical lymphadenopathy is much more likely to be associated with a benign diagnosis than supraclavicular or posterior cervical lymphadenopathy. Malignant pathologies may include neuroblastoma, leukaemia, rhabdomyosarcoma and non-Hodgkin's lymphoma in the child younger than 6 years. In the older child or adolescent, Hodgkin's lymphoma is the most common tumour presenting with cervical lymphadenopathy (**Table 7**).

Clinical features

- Palpably enlarged lymph nodes
- Enlarged liver and/or spleen
- Weight loss
- Signs of generalised condition
- Local cause – red, enlarged tonsils; dental caries; infected eczema

Table 7 Causes of lymphadenopathy	
Viral infection	Viral upper respiratory tract infection
	Epstein–Barr virus
	Others such as cytomegalovirus
Bacterial infection	*Staphylococcus aureus*
	Group A β-haemolytic streptococci
	Bartonella henselae (cat scratch disease)
	Mycobacteria: tuberculosis and atypical
Protozoal infection	Toxoplasmosis
Malignancies	Neuroblastoma
	Leukaemia: acute lymphoblastic leukaemia
	Lymphomas: non-Hodgkin's, Hodgkin's
	Rhabdomyosarcoma
Miscellaneous	Kawasaki disease
	Drugs
	Post vaccination
	Rosai–Dorfman disease

Investigations

Often the clinical history and examination will allow a diagnosis to be made and exclude the need for further investigations. In some instances, observation for a 4- to 6-week period, with or without a course of antibiotics, will allow reactive causes to be more obvious. Investigations need to be tailored to the presumed diagnosis but may include:

- **Blood tests:** Full blood count, with differential white blood cell count, urea and electrolytes, liver function tests, lactate dehydrogenase (LDH) level, C-reactive protein
  - LDH is often raised in lymphoma
- **Radiological investigations:** Chest radiograph, ultrasound of lymphadenopathy, with or without abdominal ultrasound, contrast-enhanced CT scan
  - If mediastinal lymphadenopathy is present, it is essential to obtain information about the mediastinal mass and tracheobronchial encasement. Under a general anaesthetic, the airway may collapse with disastrous results
- **Microbiological:** Blood culture and titres, microscopy and culture of lymph node material
  - Samples should be sent fresh, and if mycobacteria or other notifiable organisms are suspected, hazard warnings should be applied to the specimen and the laboratory should be alerted
- **Histology/cytology:** Biopsy of the largest or most abnormal node should be performed either by fine-needle aspiration (FNA), core biopsy; formal incisional or excisional biopsy
  - Samples should be sent fresh and promptly to the laboratory. Both standard and immune stains are used to characterise tumours
- **Cytogenetics:** Samples should be sent fresh or in cytogenetic media for assessment
  - Cytogenetic information is sometimes essential for diagnosis and in some cases for prognostic information (N-Myc in neuroblastoma)
- **Haematological malignancy diagnostic service:** Fresh samples are sent for flow cytometry, immunohistochemistry, tissue imprints or fluorescent in situ hybridisation
- Despite the majority of causes of peripheral lymphadenopathy being benign, malignant causes are frequent enough to justify biopsy, in a large number of cases. Because up to 77% of lymph node biopsy findings were benign in one series and the therapeutic yield was only 20% in another, many have tried to identify clinical factors that can predict the diagnosis and need for lymph node biopsy. In a retrospective review of 60 patients undergoing lymph node biopsy, increasing size of the lymph node, number of sites of adenopathy and increasing age were all associated with an increasing risk of malignancy. In addition, the presence of a supraclavicular node, an abnormal chest radiograph and fixed nodes were also independently associated with malignancy. Others have found the ratio of maximal width to maximal length of the largest cervical node as measured by ultrasound to be predictive of malignancy. The presence of nodes in multiple cervical regions and the largest node in the jugular or posterior triangle were also associated with an increased risk of malignancy.

Differential diagnosis

- Thyroglossal cyst
- Branchial cyst
- Dermoid cyst
- Sternomastoid tumour
- Haemangioma
- Lymphangioma and cystic hygroma
- Inguinal hernia

Treatment

Treatment is governed by the underlying diagnosis:

- In reactive lymphadenopathy due to acute viral infection, no treatment is necessary
- For acute bacterial infection, appropriate antibiotic therapy, possibly helped by FNA of the affected gland, is necessary

- If the nodes become fluctuant, either repeated aspiration or formal incision and drainage is indicated
- In cases of atypical mycobacterial lymphadenopathy, formal excision of the affected glands is curative
- In those situations where excision is not possible or desired, treatment with clarithromycin may be effective
- Cat scratch disease is usually benign and self-limiting, with resolution of the lymphadenopathy over 6–8 weeks
- Rosai–Dorfman disease (RDD) is a benign histiocytosis that presents with massive, bilateral, painless lymphadenopathy associated with fever, night sweats and weight loss. Treatment of RDD is rarely necessary
- The diagnosis of a malignant condition necessitates referral to the paediatric oncology or haematology team for completion of staging investigations and appropriate treatment according to appropriate protocols

Further reading

Leung AKC, Robson WLM. Childhood cervical lymphadenopathy. J Pediatr Health Care 2004; 18:3–7.

Nield LS, Kamat D. Lymphadenopathy in children: when and how to evaluate. Clin Pediatr 2004; 43:25–33.

Wang J, Guanghua P, Qiang J, et al. Unexplained cervical lymphadenopathy in children: predictive factors for malignancy. J Pediatr Surg 2010; 45:784–788.

Related topics of interest

Malrotation

Learning objectives

- To understand the normal embryological process of midgut rotation and fixation
- To recognise the different clinical presentations of abnormalities of midgut rotation
- To understand the principles of surgical management of malrotation and its complications, recognising the urgency of relieving midgut ischaemia

Overview

Intestinal malrotation is a developmental anomaly affecting the position and peritoneal attachments of the intestine during organogenesis in fetal life. Malrotation is defined as incomplete or abnormal rotation and fixation of the embryonic midgut around the axis of the superior mesenteric artery (SMA). Patients often present acutely with bilious vomiting and management is by a Ladd's procedure.

Epidemiology and aetiology

Malrotation occurs in approximately 1 in 500 births, 50–75% of patients become symptomatic in the first month of life and 90% of patients before 1 year of age.

Intestinal development begins around 5 weeks' gestation as a process of elongation, rotation and fixation. During elongation the bowel lengthens so rapidly that it is extruded into the umbilical cord, forming a temporary physiological hernia. As the bowel returns to the abdomen, it rotates 270° anticlockwise around the SMA. During the tenth week, the rotation is completed with the SMA contained within a broad mesenteric base attachment. The distal duodenum extends across the midline towards the left upper quadrant; the duodenojejunal flexure is pushed into a position below and to the left of the root of the mesentery while the caecum and the colon are forced to the right side of the abdominal cavity, thus crossing over the mesenteric root. The caecum moves caudally from the upper quadrant of the right abdominal cavity into the right iliac fossa and becomes fixed to the posterolateral abdominal wall.

The spectrum of rotational abnormalities is as follows:

- **Non-rotation:** An abnormally lax umbilical ring has allowed the midgut to return without rotating. The third and fourth parts of the duodenum descend vertically caudally along the right side of the SMA. The small bowel lies to the right and the colon doubles on itself to the left of the midline
- **Reversed rotation:** The caecum and colon are behind the superior mesenteric vessels and the duodenum crosses anterior to it
- **Malrotation:** The normal process of rotation is arrested at any part of the rotational phase. Often the caecum lies in a subhepatic or central position. This may also be associated with anomalous fixation of the gut, usually with dense fibrous bands (Ladd's bands), extending from the caecum and right colon across the duodenum to the retroperitoneum of the right upper quadrant (**Figure 39**)

Clinical features

Bilious vomiting is an important sign, and the diagnosis of malrotation and volvulus must be considered when assessing any infant or child with such a history. Due to bowel volvulus and ischaemia, the patient can rapidly develop a metabolic acidosis and hypovolemic shock. Abdominal wall erythema, haematemesis and melaena are late signs and represent intestinal ischaemia and peritonitis. Diagnosis in older children becomes more difficult, as the differential diagnosis for abdominal pain, vomiting, and a disturbance of stooling pattern is much wider. Pain and bilious vomiting are the most frequent symptoms although vomiting can be initially non-bile-stained in up to 50% of cases.

Bowel obstruction due to volvulus leads to mesenteric venous and lymphatic obstruction and subsequently impairment of drainage.

Chylous ascites can be a subsequent finding often at laparotomy (**Figure 40**).

Presentation can be with:

- Signs of duodenal obstruction
- Midgut volvulus, resulting in ischaemia or necrosis of the bowel
- Chronic symptoms such as abdominal pain, constipation and/or weight loss
- Incidental discovery in an asymptomatic patient (e.g. diaphragmatic hernia and atrial isomerism)

Associated anomalies occur in 30–62% of affected patients. Rotational anomalies of the bowel are often present in children with exomphalos, gastroschisis and congenital diaphragmatic hernia. Malrotation can also occur in association with other gastrointestinal abnormalities, such as biliary atresia, Hirschsprung's disease, oesophageal and other intestinal atresias, and anomalies involving other organ systems (e.g. atrial isomerism).

Investigations

- **Plain abdominal radiograph:** Features suggestive of malrotation and/or volvulus are a paucity of gas shadows and a dilated stomach although a plain X-ray can be often normal. A gasless abdomen is also possible because the compromised bowel may be filled with fluid alone.
- **Upper gastrointestinal contrast study:** This is the optimal investigation for any child presenting with bilious vomiting. Abnormal findings include
  - Duodenum failing to cross the midline and duodenojejunal flexure lying inferiorly to the duodenal bulb on the right of the spine. The normal position of the duodenojejunal flexure is to the left of the left-sided pedicles of the first lumbar vertebrae
  - Obstruction of the duodenum
  - 'Coiled spring' or 'corkscrew' appearance of the obstructed intestine suggesting volvulus (**Figure 41**)

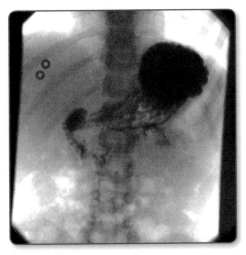

Figure 39 Upper gastrointestinal contrast study showing normal rotation.

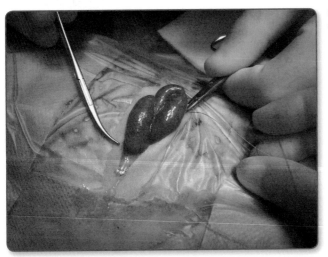

Figure 40 Operative photograph of chylous ascites.

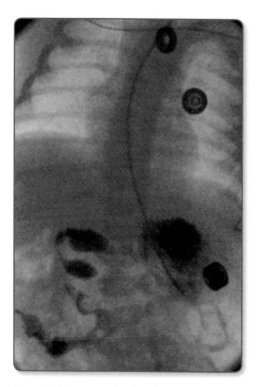

Figure 41 Upper gastrointestinal contrast study showing malrotation and volvulus manifest by a duodenojejunal flexure to the right of the midline and a corkscrew appearance to the distal bowel indicating volvulus.

- **Abdominal ultrasound:** This is to examine SMA and superior mesenteric vein (SMV) orientation. The SMV is normally located to the right of SMA on axial views, but the relative positions of the vein and artery are reversed in 60% of patients with malrotation

Treatment and management

Patients with confirmed symptomatic malrotation and volvulus should be appropriately resuscitated with intravenous fluid and nasogastric decompression, given intravenous broad-spectrum antibiotics, and taken to the operative theatre for emergency laparotomy. If the diagnosis is highly suspected and the patient is unstable, resuscitation and surgery should be considered without the need for radiological confirmation because this will increase the bowel ischaemia time. If resuscitated and stable, the diagnosis can be confirmed, or excluded, by performing an upper gastrointestinal contrast study.

Surgical management and operative repair

Once the diagnosis has been made, a laparotomy is performed through a right upper quadrant transverse incision. After delivery of the intestine from the wound, the fundamental steps of the procedure are

- Devolving of the bowel (if volvulus exists), most commonly in an anticlockwise direction
- Assessment of bowel for vascular compromise with a period of warming if necessary
- Division of the fibrous bands of peritoneal tissue (Ladd's bands) that attach the caecum to the lateral abdominal wall compressing the foregut
- Broadening the base of the small bowel mesentery
- Considering appendicectomy (as the appendix will no longer lie in the right lower quadrant following derotation)
- Returning the bowel to the abdomen in a non-rotation position

If ischaemic bowel is found at laparotomy, every attempt should be made to preserve bowel length because short bowel syndrome is a significant long-term complication. If any doubt exists about viability, a second-look laparotomy can be done 24–48 hours later, without initial resection or with very conservative resection, to allow the demarcation of obviously necrotic segments.

Recurrence is reported, but it is rare and may be due to an incomplete derotation of the bowel. Adhesive bowel obstruction is not uncommon and requires surgical management in most cases.

The procedure can also be performed laparoscopically using three to four ports though advanced skills are required. Adhesions may be reduced using the laparoscopic approach.

Further reading

Bax KMA, van der Zee DC. Intestinal malrotation. In: Bax KMA, et al (eds). Endoscopic surgery in infant and children. Heidelberg: Springer-Verlag, 2008:299–304.

Little DC, Smith SD. Malrotation. In: Holcomb GW III, Murphy P (eds), Ashcraft's pediatric surgery, 5th edn. Philadelphia. Saunders Elsevier, 2010:416–424.

Pierro A, Ong EGP. Malrotation. In: Puri P, Höllwarth ME (eds), Pediatric surgery. Heidelberg: Springer-Verlag, 2006:197–202.

Related topics of interest

- Congenital diaphragmatic hernia (p. 65)
- Duodenal atresia (p. 90)
- Gastric volvulus (p. 126)
- Gastrointestinal bleeding (p. 129)
- Necrotising enterocolitis (p. 211)
- Short bowel syndrome (p. 312)
- Small bowel atresia (p. 320)

Management of the wetting child

Learning outcomes

- To know some basic normal parameters of urinary control and to understand the normal bladder cycle
- To have an approach for assessing the wetting child and to have an understanding of the differing causes of urinary incontinence
- To be able to plan appropriate treatment for the wetting child

Overview

Urinary incontinence in children is common. Anatomical causes of wetting account for < 1% of cases. Bladder dysfunction and the neurogenic bladder are dealt with in Topic Bladder dysfunction (p. 31). The foundation of managing a wetting child is a full history and examination and understanding the normal bladder filling and emptying cycle.

Epidemiology and aetiology

The normal bladder cycle is under both voluntary and involuntary controls. On filling, bladder sensory receptors provide efferent impulses to the spinal cord, which are then modulated by impulses from higher levels to give inhibition of detrusor contraction via parasympathetic pathways (S2–4) and urethral sphincter contraction via sympathetic pathways (T10–L2) and voluntary somatic control (S2–4).

Emptying occurs by voluntary S2–4 urethral sphincter relaxation, voluntary S2–4 pelvic floor relaxation and involuntary parasympathetic S2–4 detrusor contraction. Once the bladder is empty, there is then voluntary contraction of the urethral sphincter (S2–4). Often the pathophysiology of childhood wetting is due to a poor bladder cycle having developed.

It is important to understand the normal fluid requirements and bladder capacity of a child, and some simple formulae and normal values are given here:

- Bladder capacity (mL): If age < 2 year = weight (kg) × 7; if age > 2 years = age × 30
- Urine production: 2–3 mL/kg/h
- Approximate fluid intake needs: < 5 years = 500 mL; 7 years = 750 mL; 10 years = 1000 mL; 12 years = 1250 mL; 15 years = 1500 mL
- Childhood frequency of micturition during waking hours is between three and seven per day

To help understand childhood wetting better, the International Children's Continence Society (2006) classifies childhood urinary incontinence as follows:
Urinary incontinence
- continuous
- intermittent
  - daytime
  - night time (enuresis)
    - non-monosymptomatic
    - monosymptomatic

The term enuresis is reserved for night-time urinary incontinence.

Those children with continuous urinary incontinence usually have a structural abnormality (ectopic ureter, female epispadias). Non-monosymptomatic enuresis gives daytime symptoms as well and is usually due to a functional or neurogenic problem. Monosymptomatic enuresis is a result of a failure of arousal with a full bladder at night, nocturnal polyuria or a small bladder capacity.

Clinical features

With continuous urinary incontinence, there is never a dry day or night and urinary leaks occur minute by minute constantly. Children with an ectopic ureter may be less wet at night as they are horizontal during sleep.

With intermittent urinary incontinence, there is often urgency (the sudden and unexpected experience of an immediate need to void), urge incontinence (not getting to the toilet on time) and frequency. This may be due to bladder overactivity or pure sensory urgency. Giggle incontinence specifically occurs only during laughter or giggling.

The remaining history should elicit substantial information about the following: drinking volume, types of drinks (known bladder stimulants are tea, coffee, hot chocolate, cola drinks and blackcurrant squash), drinking frequency and timings, bowel habit, presence of stress incontinence, urinary tract infections, urinary stream (hesitancy, flow characteristic, postmicturition dribble), other relevant medical history (especially neurological and gastrointestinal) and family, social and drug history.

Examination should include the abdomen, external genitalia, back, spine and lower limbs, including reflexes and palpation to rule out any of the following:

- In the female – fused labia minora, imperforate hymen, urogenital sinus anomaly, female epispadias
- In the male – foreskin scarring and balanitis xerotica obliterans, meatal stenosis, primary epispadias
- In both females and males – back abnormalities such as hairy patches, skin discolouration over the spine, sacral agenesis and neurological deficits

Investigations

All children should record a complete fluid input and output chart for 48 hours and include details of bowel actions using a Bristol stool chart. Urinalysis to exclude glycosuria or a urinary tract infection is essential. A renal and bladder ultrasound scan to look for a duplex kidney and at bladder wall thickness and post micturition residual is a good non-invasive investigation. Urine flow rate and ultrasound measurement of post-void residual urine volume enable assessment of urine outflow.

More invasive and complex investigations include videourodynamics and rarely intravenous urography or magnetic resonance urography. Occasionally sleep studies identify nocturnal hypoxia that reduces nocturnal arousal in children with enuresis.

Differential diagnosis

- Bladder dysfunction
- Neurogenic bladder

Treatment

Simple emphasis on regular voiding, regular and appropriate timing of fluid intake, and avoidance of constipation and urinary infections is good for all children.

Monosymptomatic enuresis is treated either with a night-time alarm to help with arousal, or vasopressin analogue (desmopressin), to reduce urine output or both in combination. Improving sleeping patterns and occasionally tonsillectomy have been shown to help children with enuresis.

A demonstrably overactive but normally compliant bladder may respond to anticholinergic medication (oxybutynin, tolterodine, solifenacin), to TENS (transcutaneous electrical nerve stimulation) or to intravesical botulinum toxin injection, although the latter has a significant risk of producing urinary retention and a paralysed bladder, requiring clean intermittent catheterisation for emptying until the botulinum toxin wears off after about 6 months.

Behavioural therapy and cognitive biofeedback therapy to teach children to normalise their bladder cycle and the associated sensations are labour and time-intensive but are producing good outcomes for many with a functional cause for their incontinence. Very rarely more invasive measures, such as sacral neuromodulation or bladder reconstructive surgery, are required to treat children with long-standing functional urinary incontinence that does not respond to anything else and where the child is desperate to be dry.

Further reading

Nevéus T, von Gontard A, Hoebeke P, et al. The standardization of terminology of lower urinary tract function in children and adolescents: Report from the Standardisation Committee of the International Children's Continence Society. J Urol 2006; 176:314–324.

Wright A. Evidence-based assessment and management of childhood enuresis. Pediatr Child Health 2008; 18:561–567.

Related topics of interest

Meatal stenosis

Learning outcomes

- To be able to recognise meatal stenosis
- To know the underlying aetiology
- To be aware of the management options, including when to recommend surgery
- To be aware of the surgical options available

Overview

Meatal stenosis occurs when the meatal orifice of the glans penis is narrowed.

Epidemiology and aetiology

Meatal stenosis is most common following a neonatal circumcision or as a complication of a hypospadias repair, but can be secondary to balanitis xerotica obliterans. The symptoms can rarely be the presenting features of a stenotic hypospadiac opening.

There is a high incidence of meatal stenosis following neonatal circumcision (1.5–11.0%), which is thought to be due to meatal ulceration secondary to chemical and ammonaical irritation in the nappy, loss of meatal epithelium, and fusion of its ventral edges. This results in a pinpoint orifice at the tip of the glans and a meatal web. Other theories include ischaemia secondary to division of the artery in the frenulum.

Following hypospadias repair, meatal stenosis can occur due to ischaemia of the glans flap or urethra at the apex of the meatus or secondary to an inadequately mobilised glans wrap. Meatal stenosis secondary to balanitis xerotica obliterans occurs following chronic inflammation and fibrosis of the glans and meatus which leads to scarring and web formation. There is also a report of meatal stenosis secondary to junctional epidermolysis bullosa.

Clinical features

The child may present with one or more of the following symptoms:
- Difficulty voiding
- Narrowed and forceful urinary stream
- Spraying
- Urinary tract infections secondary to incomplete bladder emptying
- Spotting haematuria (usually terminal in nature)

The stenosis is always on the ventral aspect of the meatus and causes dorsal deflection of the urinary stream.

Investigations

The diagnosis should be evident on examination alone, which should include watching the child void. Occasionally, the history can represent a urethral stricture, and if doubt exists then an examination under anaesthesia, cystoscopy and calibration can be performed along with any required definitive treatment. If the stream is not narrowed and/or there is no or minimal dorsal deflection ($< 30°$ angle), then it would be appropriate to pursue non-surgical management options.

Differential diagnosis

- Balanitis xerotica obliterans
- Postsurgical complication
- Non-Herlitz junctional epidermolysis bullosa

Treatment

- Steroid creams, e.g. betametasone 0.05%
- Intervoiding dressings (for the epidermolysis bullosa type)
- Serial dilatation – this option is not recommended because dilatations lead to further scarring and recurrence of the stenosis
- Redo glanular hypospadias surgery
- Meatotomy
  - Under general anaesthesia, the ventral web is clamped for 1 minute then divided. The clamp should not extend more than halfway toward the corona
  - The meatus should be able to accept an appropriately sized catheter for the age of

the child. If not then the ventral incision should be extended using the above steps

- There are then a number of options
  (a) Parents spread the meatus and apply ointment several times daily for a prescribed time period
  (b) A meatoplasty in which the meatal urethral mucosa is sutured to the glans with absorbable monofilament sutures (6/0) and postoperative care is as for (a). This approach has shown to be beneficial in postcircumcision meatal stenosis, with no episodes of postoperative recurrence

Further reading

Persad R, et al. Clinical Presentation and pathophysiology of meatal stenosis following circumcision. Br J Urol 1995; 75:91–93.

Rubin AI, et al. Urethral meatal stenosis in junctional epidermolysis bullosa: a rare complication effectively treated with a novel and simple modality. Int J Derm 2007; 46:1076–1077.

Van Howe RS. Incidence of meatal stenosis following neonatal circumcision in a primary care setting. Clin Pediatr 2006; 45:49–54.

Related topics of interest

- Balanitis xerotica obliterans (p. 24)
- Hypospadias – proximal (p. 172)
- Hypospadias – distal (p. 168)

Meckel's diverticulum

Learning outcomes

- To understand the embryological origin of Meckel's diverticulum
- To be familiar with its clinical presentation and methods of investigation
- To be aware of management options

Overview

Meckel's diverticulum is a true diverticulum arising from the antimesenteric border of the distal ileum. The 'rule of 2s' is often used for Meckel's diverticulum: within 2 feet of the ileocaecal valve, 2 inches in length, occurring in about 2% of the population, two times more symptomatic in males, symptomatic by 2 years of age and potentially containing two heterotopic tissues, gastric and pancreatic.

Epidemiology and aetiology

The first known description of Meckel's diverticulum was made in 1598 by Hildanus. In 1809, the anatomist and physician Johann Friedrich Meckel identified the origin of the diverticulum as the vitellointestinal duct. Heterotopic pancreatic tissue in the diverticulum was identified in 1861 by Zenker and gastric mucosa in 1904 by Salzer.

Meckel's diverticulum is the most common vitelline duct abnormality and the most common congenital anomaly of the gastrointestinal tract. It is a true intestinal diverticulum, containing all normal layers of the intestinal wall and is located on the antimesenteric border of the small bowel.

The fetal midgut is attached to the yolk sac via the vitellointestinal duct, also known as the omphalomesenteric duct or yolk stalk. This duct normally obliterates between 5 and 8 weeks' gestation. Meckel's diverticulum results from failure of the proximal duct to obliterate.

Clinical features

Meckel's diverticulum has been called the 'great imitator' because of its varied manifestations. It accounts for nearly 50% of all instances of lower gastrointestinal bleeding in children, usually occurring in infants and toddlers. The common presenting problems of a Meckel's diverticulum are bleeding, obstruction and inflammation. The bleeding is due to ulcer formation from the acid secreted from the ectopic gastric mucosa and can be severe. Meckel's diverticulum can cause intestinal obstruction by one of the several mechanisms:

- Meckel's band
- Intussusception
- Volvulus
- Internal herniation
- Prolapse through a patent vitellointestinal duct

Meckel's diverticulum can mimic appendicitis very closely. Primary gastrointestinal neoplasias, such as carcinoid, sarcoma, lymphoma, adenocarcinoma and leiomyoma, are rarely reported in patients with Meckel's diverticulum.

Investigations

Blood investigations in bleeding child

- Full blood count
- Coagulation profile

Radiological investigations

Technetium-99m pertechnetate scintigraphy (Meckel's scan) is the investigation of choice. It is used to detect heterotopic gastric mucosa. Pentagastrin, histamine blockers and glucagon may enhance the accuracy of diagnosis. Fasting, nasogastric suction and bladder catheterisation may increase the yield of scanning.

However, if the diagnosis is still strongly suspected after negative scintigraphy, alternative investigations which may be considered are:

- Ultrasonography
- Colonoscopy
- Angiography in patients with severe active bleeding
- Laparoscopy

Differential diagnosis

- Malrotation
- Acute appendicitis
- Gastroenteritis
- Peptic ulcer disease
- Intestinal duplication
- Cow's milk protein intolerance/allergy

Treatment

The bleeding child should be placed nil by mouth and appropriately resuscitated. Elective resection of incidentally discovered diverticulum is indicated in uncomplicated patients with palpable thickening suggestive of heterotopic mucosa and in those with peritoneal band attachments. In immune-compromised patients, in patients undergoing insertion of prosthetic material and in babies with gastroschisis, elective resection of an incidental diverticulum is generally not recommended.

In symptomatic patients, the diverticulum is removed using a laparoscopic, laparoscopic-assisted or open technique. The technique comprises either a simple resection of the diverticulum and transverse closure across the base or resection of a short segment of ileum, containing the diverticulum, followed by end-to-end ileal anastomosis. The latter technique is recommended in bleeding patients because it deals with any ulcer which may be present in the adjoining 5 cm of distal ileum. The feeding diverticular artery on the surface of the ileum should be clearly identified and ligated. Concomitant incidental appendicectomy is often performed.

Further reading

Chatterjee CR. Sarcomas of Meckel's diverticulum. Can J Surg 1970; 13:163–165.

Meckel J. Uber die divertikel am darmkanal. Arch Physiol 1809; 9:439–453.

Moyana TN. Carcinoid tumors arising from Meckel's diverticulum: a clinical, morphologic, and immunohistochemical study. Am J Clin Pathol 1989; 91:52–56.

Snyder CL Meckel's diverticulum. In: Grosfield L, et al (eds). Paediatric surgery, 6th en. Mosby, 2006.

Related topics of interest

Meconium ileus

Learning outcomes

- To be able to recognise meconium ileus
- To understand the underlying aetiology
- To be aware of the medical and surgical management options

Overview

Meconium ileus (MI) is intestinal obstruction in the newborn, secondary to inspissation of abnormally viscid meconium in the terminal ileum; it is usually associated with cystic fibrosis (CF).

Epidemiology and aetiology

- Male to female incidence is approximately equal
- About 9–33% of neonatal intestinal obstruction is caused by MI
- About 90% of patients presenting with MI will have CF
- About 16–20% of CF patients will present with MI

CF is the most common potentially lethal genetic defect affecting Caucasians (1 in 25 have carrier status), with an incidence of 1 in 3000 live births per year.

The most common mutation is F508del (~70%), previously called ΔF508, but there are over 1000 mutations known. F508del, a three-base pair deletion, produces an autosomal recessive mutation in the CF transmembrane-conductance regulator (*CFTR*) gene on chromosome 7 (q31.2).

The *CFTR* gene codes for a cell membrane chloride channel which also regulates the flow of bicarbonate. The abnormal electrolyte content in the environment around the cell results in desiccation, and with the defective secretion of bicarbonate it produces a hyperviscous mucus. This results in a thickened meconium that accumulates and eventually obstructs the intestine lumen, leading to the presentation of MI. The role of pancreatic insufficiency is now believed to be minimal.

Clinical features

This can present in two forms:
1. Simple (66%) – abdominal distension, failure to pass meconium and visible bowel loops that feel 'doughy' on palpation
2. Complicated (33%) – secondary to local volvulus leading to antenatal perforation, with the development of a meconium pseudocyst and intestinal atresia

Investigations

In simple MI, a plain X-ray will demonstrate dilated loops of bowel with a 'soap bubble' appearance (Neuhauser's sign), representing swallowed air mixing with thick meconium and an absence of air-fluid levels.

Additionally in complicated MI, calcification may be seen, consequent to an antenatal perforation, and USS may be used to delineate a palpable mass suggestive of a meconium pseudocyst. Contrast enema (**Figure 42**) may be used where diagnostic doubt occurs and can be both diagnostic and therapeutic.

Differential diagnosis

- Meconium plug syndrome
- Ileal or colonic atresia
- Hirschsprung's disease
- Small left colon syndrome
- Imperforate anus

Treatment
Medical

The basis of non-operative management is clearance of the inspissated meconium by hypertonic water-soluble contrast enema performed under careful fluoroscopic control. The following criteria are required:
- Simple MI
- Intravenous antibiotic cover
- Fluid and electrolyte resuscitation with the procedure

Most commonly used is a 25–50% solution of meglumine diatrizoate (Gastrografin),

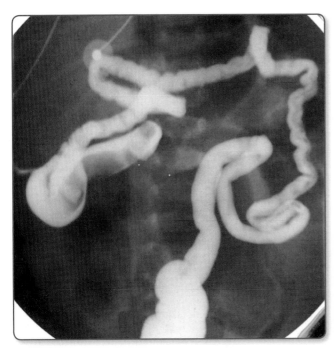

Figure 42 Lower gastrointestinal contrast showing the characteristic collapsed microcolon with filling defects proximally representing inspissated meconium. Courtesy of Dr N Broderick.

a hyperosmolar (1900 mOsm/L), water-soluble radiopaque solution, containing 0.1% polysorbate 80 (a solubilising or wetting agent).

Reflux of this enema into the inspissated meconium in the terminal ileum is critical for the obstruction to be relieved. Plain abdominal films can be taken as clinically indicated to confirm evacuation of obstruction and exclude late perforation. If evacuation of obstruction is incomplete, repeat enemas can be performed as long as no signs of peritonitis or clinical deterioration are evident.

Following a successful enema, up to 10 mL of 5–10% solution of N-acetylcysteine may be given via a nasogastric tube 6 hourly to maintain gut clearance. Contemporary studies report successful evacuation being achieved in 36–39% which is significantly lower than historically reported (63–83%).

Surgical

Surgical management is required if medical management fails or if there is evidence of perforation.

- **Simple:** Laparotomy via a supraumbilical transverse incision is performed with an enterotomy in the small bowel above the inspissated meconium. Irrigation with 25–50% Gastrografin clears the obstructing inspissated meconium and either a double-barrelled ileostomy is fashioned or the enterostomy is closed after clearance of the obstructing meconium.
Historically, resection with a distal chimney enterostomy, such as the Bishop-Koop or Santulli enterostomy, was performed. These enabled ongoing distal obstruction to be irrigated later, whilst achieving decompression of the proximal loop; these have fallen out of fashion
- **Complicated:** This can be a much more difficult procedure with multiple dense vascular adhesions and an associated pseudocyst with a thick fibrous wall. A conservative approach with a proximal ileostomy, followed by definitive surgery after 6 weeks is recommended

Postoperative management includes
- Antibiotics
- Total parenteral nutrition

- Enteral N-acetylcysteine via the nasogastric tube or ileostomy if ongoing obstruction
- Pancreatic enzymes once half feeds are established
- Early closure of stoma between 4 and 6 weeks
- The diagnosis of CF should be confirmed via
  - Sweat test (pilocarpine iontophoresis) (performed at > 1 month of age) – 100 mg of sweat required. A chloride of < 40 mEq/L is normal, > 60 mEq/L is diagnostic
  - *CFTR* gene mutation analysis – common mutations screened for detecting 98% of CF in Caucasian populations, but rarer forms are missed especially in non-Caucasian populations
  - Immunoreactive trypsinogen – raised in CF
  - Stool sample for trypsin (< 80 mg/g in CF), chymotrypsin and albumin (normally < 5 mg/g)
- Involvement of CF team for long-term management

Survival rates approach 100%. Long-term health of patients with CF and MI is as good as those with only CF.

MI equivalent or distal intestinal obstruction syndrome

In older children or adolescents with CF, the most common gastrointestinal problem is that of MI equivalent or distal intestinal obstruction syndrome. Patients present with symptoms and signs suggestive of bowel obstruction. These include, but are not restricted to, crampy abdominal pain, abdominal distension, constipation and vomiting. A plain abdominal film can be used to aid assessment. Partial bowel obstruction occurs in these children due to steatorrhoea or patients' non-compliance with supplementary pancreatic enzymes, causing thickened intraluminal bowel contents. The preferred treatment, once the diagnosis is made, is with solubilising agents, such as acetylcysteine and Gastrografin, given orally and per rectum. Operative management is rarely necessary.

Further reading

Carlyle BE, Borowitz DS, Glick PL. A review of pathophysiology and management of fetuses and neonates with meconium ileus for the pediatric surgeon. J Pediatr Surg 2012; 47:772–781.

Coran A, Adzick NS, Krummel TM, et al; Meconium Ileus. Pediatric surgery, 7th edn. Philadelphia, PA: Elsevier Saunders, 2012:1073–1083.
Docherty JG, et al. Meconium ileus: a review 1972–1990. Br J Surg 1992; 79:571–573.

Related topics of interest

Minimal access surgery in neonates

Learning outcomes

- To understand the basic principles of minimal access surgery (MAS)
- To develop an awareness of the indications for and the advantages of MAS
- To be familiar with the basic operating room set-up
- To understand the techniques for some index neonatal procedures

Overview

The advent of MAS has been one of the most important and dramatic surgical developments of the last century since the introduction of a cystoscope in the peritoneum of a dog by Kelling in 1901. Landmark innovations which enabled this progress were the introduction of cold light by Forestier in 1952, fibreoptic technology by Hopkins in 1953, thereby doubling the light-carrying capacity of the laparoscope, the automated insufflation device in the 1970s and invention of the charged couple device in 1985. MAS allows the surgeon to perform major intracavitary procedures with significantly less pain and morbidity compared with traditional open surgery. While MAS techniques have been embraced by adult surgeons over the last two decades, its utilisation in the paediatric community has progressed very slowly due to poorly adaptable equipment for use in small children in earlier years combined with the technical challenge of operating in small spaces in this population. In addition, it has been difficult to prove whether neonates and infants undergoing MAS have less postoperative discomfort and stress than those undergoing conventional surgical procedures because such patients are unable to articulate their distress. Over the last decade, many obstacles have been overcome with increasing surgical expertise, a marked improvement in video equipment and instrumentation and advances in anaesthetic techniques. Neonatal procedures that can now be performed safely and with good outcomes using MAS include:

- Pyloromyotomy
- Duodenal atresia repair
- Ladd's procedure for malrotation
- Intestinal atresia repair
- Diagnostic laparoscopy for necrotising enterocolitis
- Fundoplication
- Gastrostomy
- Colonic pull-through for Hirschsprung's disease or anorectal malformation
- Choledochal cyst excision
- Hepatic cyst excision
- Repair of congenital diaphragmatic hernia
- Repair of tracheo-oesophageal fistula and other thoracoscopic procedures, such as pulmonary lobectomy, lung biopsy and ligation of patent ductus arteriosus
- Resection of thoracic and abdominal teratoma
- Excision of retroperitoneal lymphatic malformations
- Salpingo-ophorectomy for ovarian torsion

There are no absolute contraindications for performing laparoscopic or thoracoscopic procedures in neonates. However, when the patient is haemodynamically unstable, is not on conventional ventilation, cannot be safely transported to the operating suite or is of extremely low birth weight, the pros and cons of a MAS approach must be considered. Laparoscopic procedures in neonates are not only safe and effective but have advantages such as:

- Significantly decreased morbidity
- Reduced physiologic stress
- Reduced postoperative pain leading to fewer pulmonary complications. Pulmonary benefits afforded by minimal access approach play a significantly greater role in neonates with congenital cardiac disease where the ability to avoid respiratory complications has a dramatic benefit
- Improved rates of extubation

- Shortened postoperative intensive care stay
- Reduced hospital stay
- Fewer days of supplemental oxygen
- Decreased postoperative pneumonias
- Earlier return of gastrointestinal function
- Improved cosmesis
- For some procedures, operative times are shorter due to improved operative visibility
- Multiple procedures can be performed simultaneously with minimal additional morbidity
- Long-term benefits of decreased adhesion and scar tissue formation may be the strongest argument for pursuing this approach in neonates
- Reduced overall hospital costs

Average complication rates vary based on the experience of the operating surgeon and have been between 1 and 3% in our experience. Complications unique to a MAS approach include trocar-related vascular and visceral injuries, trocar site bleeding or hernia and wound infection, but these are extremely rare. Most of the intra-operative complications can be managed laparoscopically, depending on the technical expertise and comfort level of the operating surgeon. There is a steep learning curve for MAS in neonates, and surgeons should be prepared to convert to an open procedure when needed. Conversion rate to open at our institution is <2%, but conversion to open to complete a procedure safely should not be considered to be a complication. Problems with overinflation and associated haemodynamic consequences have been minimised by optimal anaesthetic management and availability of modern CO_2 insufflators.

Basic technique

The importance of ergonomics in the setting of MAS cannot be overemphasised. Ergonomic integration and suitable laparoscopic operating room environment are essential to improve efficiency, safety and comfort for the operating team. A few of the challenges faced by trainee surgeons are absence of direct three-dimensional vision, loss of depth perception, loss of peripheral vision, loss of tactile feedback, fulcrum effect with tremor enhancement and decoupling of the visual and motor axes. Furthermore, it has been observed that the operating surgeon assumes a more static posture during MAS compared with the traditional open approach, potentially causing disabling and harmful effects. To overcome these factors, it is advisable to follow a few basic rules of laparoscopy:

- Choose an ergonomically convenient operating position
- Adjust the operating table height to keep instruments at elbow level
- Adjust the monitor image at or within 25° below the horizontal plane of the eye to avoid neck strain
- Additional monitors should be used as necessary for assistants
- Port positioning is dictated by the individual surgeon but should follow the rule of triangulation (**Figure 43**) to allow the instruments to work at a 60–90° angle with the target tissue without interference with each other and the abdominal wall
- Adjust the manipulation angle, ranging from 45 to 75°, with equal azimuth angles when possible
- The arms should be slightly abducted, retroverted and with inward rotation at shoulder level. The elbows should be bent at about 90–120°
- Try to use the best technology available, if feasible, while performing MAS in neonates in confined spaces, including high-resolution cameras, × 10–15

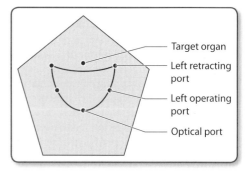

Figure 43 Ergonomics – principle of triangulation in laparoscopy.

magnification on the optical system to reduce the visual challenges, instruments with higher degree of freedom, articulating and flexible instruments and use of modern CO_2 insufflators

- Convert to open procedure when needed

Operative procedure

MAS in neonates is performed using specially designed 3 mm (2.7–3.4 mm) instrumentation of shorter length and 4.0, 2.7 and 1.6 mm diameter telescopes, with high-resolution digital cameras. Carbon dioxide insufflation is used with pressures, ranging between 8–15 mmHg and flow rates of 1–3 L/min, based on patient weight and physiology. All patients are monitored intraoperatively by electrocardiography, pulse oximetry and end-tidal CO_2 monitor.

Congenital diaphragmatic hernia

The repair is performed either with three or four trocars placed in the upper abdomen or with three trocars thoracoscopically, with reduction of contents and repair of the defect using single interrupted non-absorbable sutures. On occasion, a patch closure is necessary for large defects.

Malrotation

Surgery is performed with the child in the supine position, with the aid of three trocars. The vitality and the rotational status of the intestines are assessed. Dissection is started at the proximal duodenum and an extensive Kocher manoeuvre is performed. The bowel is then run from proximal to distal. Ladd's bands are divided as they are encountered, and the bowel is derotated as the bowel is run. Occasionally this approach is not possible because of the complex nature of the defect. In these cases, the bowel can be run retrogradely from the ileocaecal valve. Because the intestines are gently rotated counterclockwise, Ladd's bands are divided and the base of the mesentery is widened. The final result is the small bowel is positioned on the right of the abdomen and the colon on the left. Concurrent volvulus can be managed laparoscopically if there is no bowel compromise.

There is emerging literature to support the use of laparoscopy in the elective management of malrotation in children, demonstrating comparatively decreased time to oral intake, decreased narcotic use and shorter hospital stay. The areas of controversy are the safety and efficacy of laparoscopy in effectively opening the anterior leaf of the mesentery, delineating the proper alignment of the SMA and its failure to incite adhesion formation, potentially increasing the risk of recurrent volvulus. However, we have not seen this in our series. Laparoscopy is not recommended in the setting of midgut volvulus with compromised bowel.

Congenital lung lesions

For all thoracoscopic lobectomies for congenital pulmonary airway malformation or pulmonary sequestration, patients undergo either mainstem or selective intubation on the opposite side, and a low-flow low-pressure CO_2 insufflation is used to assist with collapse of the involved lung. Operating room set-up is as shown in **Figure 44**. The patient is placed in lateral decubitus position. Three to four valved ports are used. The exact procedure varies depending on the lobe resected and the pathology encountered. Dissection is done following the same principles as open procedure, and vessel ligation is achieved with Ligasure or bipolar sealing device. The specimen is taken out via a slightly enlarged trocar site, and a chest drain is placed in all cases.

Duodenal atresia

Operating room set-up is as shown in **Figure 45**. Atresia repair is performed with the patient in the supine position with three ports: one at the umbilicus, one in the right lower quadrant and one in the left upper quadrant. With the surgeon standing at the patient's feet, the duodenum is kocherised, and the dilated proximal and distal segments are identified. Transabdominal retraction sutures can be used to retract the gallbladder and liver out of the way

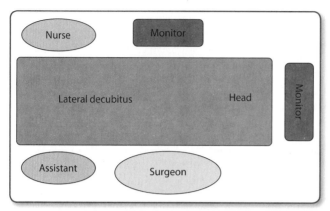

Figure 44 Operating room set-up for thoracoscopic lung resection.

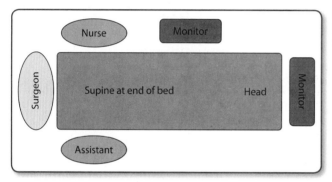

Figure 45 Operating room set-up for laparoscopic duodenal atresia repair.

as necessary. A proximal transverse and a distal longitudinal duodenotomy is then made. A stitch is placed transabdominally through the apex of the anastomosis and then back out through the abdominal wall. This stitch aligns the anastomosis and aids exposure. A diamond-shaped anastomosis is performed with either a running or interrupted absorbable suture. Intracorporeal knot tying is used. The distal bowel is examined in all cases to ensure that there are no obvious secondary atresias.

Further reading

Ponsky TA, Rothenberg SS. Minimally invasive surgery in infants less than 5 kg: experience of 649 cases. Surg Endosc 2008; 22:2214–2219.

Rothenberg SS. Thoracoscopic repair of esophageal atresia and tracheo-esophageal fistula in neonates: evolution of a technique. J Laparoendosc Adv Surg Tech A 2012; 22:195–199.

Rothenberg SS, Kuenzler KA, Middlesworth W, et al. Thoracoscopic lobectomy in infants less than 10 kg with prenatally diagnosed cystic lung disease. J Laparoendosc Adv Surg Tech 2011; 21:181–184.

Related topics of interest

Necrotising enterocolitis

Learning outcomes

- To be able to recognise the typical features of necrotising enterocolitis (NEC) and isolated small bowel perforations
- To be aware of the components of conservative management
- To outline the indications for surgery
- To be familiar with surgical management options

Overview

NEC is the commonest acquired cause of gastrointestinal problems in the premature infant. Mortality rates are high with severe disease and there is significant morbidity including short bowel syndrome, strictures and adhesional obstruction.

For the majority of babies with mild NEC, conservative management is successful. Surgery is performed in infants with ischaemic and/or perforated bowel, or disease refractory to conservative treatment. The aims of surgery are to preserve as much viable bowel as possible, remove the source of life-threatening sepsis and treat intestinal obstruction, when present.

Epidemiology/Aetiology

NEC occurs in 0.3–0.9% of live births and 2–5% of premature infants. Of all infants developing NEC, > 90% are premature and 80% are < 2 kg. Overall mortality ranges from 10–50% and approaches 100% in those with severe disease. NEC accounts for 6% of all neonatal deaths.

NEC is characterised by intestinal inflammation with disruption of the epithelial barrier, bacterial overgrowth and submucosal invasion, and in its most severe form by extensive disease and full thickness perforation.

Major risk factors are:
- Prematurity
- Hypoxic events
- Formula feeds, in premature infants

Minor risk factors include: blood transfusion, antenatal absent or reversed umbilical artery end diastolic flow, umbilical artery catheters, patent ductus arteriosus, congenital cardiac disease, pregnancy-induced hypertension, intrauterine growth retardation, chorioamonitis and gastroschisis.

Factors implicated in the pathophysiology of NEC in the premature infant are:
- Immature intestinal barrier: the epithelial barrier fails to protect the host due to immaturity of:
  - non-immunological factors (inefficient peristalsis, high gastric pH, higher mucosal permeability)
  - immunological factors (reduced number and function of B and T lymphocytes, impaired polymorphonuclear leukocyte function)
- Bacterial colonisation: a variety of bacterial and viral pathogens have been implicated, but no single organism appears to be responsible. NEC does not develop in animal models kept in sterile environments and the human intestine is devoid of bacterial flora at birth, but is rapidly colonised by maternal commensal and environmental organisms. Abnormal bowel colonisation may increase susceptibility to NEC and this may be compounded by antimicrobial treatments which alter gut flora.
- Enteral feeding: breast milk (BM) protects against NEC. Lucas et al. showed a 6–10 fold increase of NEC in formula fed infants compared to those fed BM. Beneficial effects are likely to be due to normal bowel colonisation and anti-microbial products including immunoglobulins, oligosaccharides, lactoferrin and cytokines within BM.

Studies investigating inflammatory cytokines have shown promise, but no conclusive role in pathogenesis or outcome.

Pathologically, NEC is a patchy mucosal disease with a predilection for the terminal ileum. The ascending and transverse colon are the second most commonly affected, followed by the jejunum and, rarely, the foregut or hindgut.

Occlusion of the microvascular bed by platelet aggregation in the submucosal capillaries causes oedema, patchy haemorrhage and ulceration, followed by inflammatory infiltration and bacterial invasion.

A pathognomic feature is pneumatosis intestinalis, characterised by air in the intestinal wall. It is thought to occur due to bacterial invasion, fermentation and production of hydrogen gas.

The intestinal microcirculation is more sensitive to stress than other vascular beds and the mucosa is easily injured. The processes following mucosal injury can be self-perpetuating.

Clinical features

There is a range of presenting symptoms and signs of NEC. The modified Bell's criteria (**Box 1**) attempt to standardise the diagnostic features with disease severity.

A neonate with mild disease may have light green gastric aspirates and mild abdominal distension. Although this type of NEC may progress to moderate or severe disease, it usually resolves with a brief period of gut rest with or without antibiotic cover.

Neonates with mild to moderate disease have feed intolerance, dark green bilious aspirates, some abdominal distension and macroscopic blood in the stool. This type of NEC may be reversible with conservative management, but can progress to extensive disease, perforation or a walled-off mass.

Neonates with advanced disease present with all the features of moderate NEC and can have abdominal wall cellulitis and/ or peritonitis reflecting the severity of their intra-abdominal disease. They are often grossly septic and frequently need high level respiratory and inotropic support.

Counter-intuitively, the severity of the clinical features does not always correlate with the length of bowel involved.

A premature baby with a spontaneous isolated terminal ileal perforation may present in a similar fashion to a baby with NEC, but aside from pneumoperitoneum, the abdominal X-ray (AXR) shows an unremarkable intestinal gas pattern. These infants generally have a less severe systemic and inflammatory response. They can occasionally be managed with needle decompression and subsequent laparotomy or primary laparotomy with anastomosis or stoma formation.

Box 1 Modified Bell's Staging criteria for NEC					
Stage			Systemic signs	Intestinal signs	Abdominal X-ray signs
I – Suspected disease	IA		Apnoea, bradycardia, temperature instability	Mild abdominal distension, high gastric residual volumes, microscopic blood in stool	Normal or mild ileus
	IB		Same as IA	Same as IA, macroscopic blood in stool	Same as IA
II – Definite disease	IIA – Mildly ill		Same as IA with metabolic acidosis, thrombocytopenia	Same as IB with absent bowel sounds, abdominal tenderness	Ileus, pneumatosis
	IIB – Moderately ill		Same as IIA	Same as IIA plus mass	As IIA with portal venous gas +/– ascites
III – Advanced disease	IIIA – Severely ill, bowel intact		As IIA with hypotension and shock. Metabolic acidosis, disseminated intravascular coagulopathy	Gross abdominal distension, abdominal wall discoloration, peritonitis	Definite ascites
	IIIB – Severely ill, bowel perforated		Same as IIIA	Same as IIIA with intestinal perforation	Definite ascites and pneumoperitoneum

Investigations

Blood tests:
- Complete blood count
- Urea and electrolytes
- Serum lactate
- C-reactive protein
- Blood gas
- Coagulation profile
- Blood cultures

These may show raised inflammatory markers, thrombocytopenia and a metabolic acidosis with raised lactate. Thrombocytopenia reflects consumption coagulopathy and bone marrow depression that occurs during severe sepsis. Metabolic acidosis occurs due to ischaemic tissue switching from aerobic to anaerobic respiration.

AXR – supine and/or lateral decubitus films may show:
- Pneumatosis intestinalis
- Portal venous gas
- Dilated intestinal loops or features of ascites
- Serial films may show gas pattern changes with a healthy bowel or static patterns with aperistaltic bowel
- Air/fluid levels in obstruction
- Pneumoperitoneum:
  - Sub-diaphragmatic free air
  - Air on either side of the falciform ligament or either side of the bowel wall (Rigler's sign). On a supine film, a central gas shadow is easily missed
  - Air taking the form of polygonal shapes, as opposed to circular or oval, is highly suspicious for pneumoperitoneum

Ultrasound (US) – vascular Doppler imaging can be useful in assessing the splanchnic circulation, and to evaluate for intestinal arterial or portal venous obstruction in recurrent cases.

Differential diagnosis

The main differential diagnosis is extra-abdominal sepsis with ileus.

Pneumatosis can also occur following a viral illness or repair of small bowel atresia in gastroschisis and, rarely, in malrotation.

A pneumoperitoneum can also arise following a perforation in untreated appendicitis, Hirschsprung's disease, intestinal atresia or anorectal malformations. Idiopathic perforations also occur. Translocated gas following mediastinal injury or pneumothorax can also cause a pneumoperitoneum.

Occasionally localised volvulus or vascular thrombosis may be found intraoperatively.

Treatment

In mild NEC, initial management is conservative. This comprises intestinal decompression with a nasogastric tube, broad spectrum antibiotics, gut rest, intravenous nutrition and circulatory support. It resolves the disease in the majority.

Decision-making regarding surgery and its timing can be challenging. Regular clinical assessment, review of recent observations, laboratory results and imaging informs surgical decision making.

Surgical intervention should be considered in:
- Pneumoperitoneum
- Those requiring increasing cardiorespiratory support
- Disease which is refractory to medical management; severe or rapidly progressive

The aims of surgery are to save life, remove septic foci and preserve as much viable intestine as possible to maximise the chance of enteral autonomy.

Surgical options should be tailored to the clinical status of the baby and the intraoperative findings.

The transverse laparotomy incision should be sited to avoid intraoperative injury to the liver which is extremely friable in these babies and if damaged can lead to uncontrollable, life-threatening haemorrhage.

In a critically unstable baby with severe disease, minimising the duration of anaesthesia is prudent and options include one or more of the following:
- A high jejunal or other small intestinal diverting stoma
- Clip and drop-back technique to resect gangrenous bowel
- Laparostomy to address potential abdominal compartment syndrome

These options are temporising measures to improve the acute situation and allow for a second look procedure on a more stable baby at 24–72 hours. During this second look, more definitive procedures can be undertaken and a further assessment made of the remaining bowel length.

In the stable baby with minimal to moderate bowel lengths affected options include resection and stoma or resection and primary anastomosis in selected cases.

A temporising peritoneal drain may stabilise cardiorespiratory physiology prior to transfer to a surgical centre in those < 1.5 kg. It may be applicable as a primary treatment in those < 600 g.

Lessin et al. reported a tube technique in babies with extensive NEC requiring multiple resections. Following a diverting jejunostomy, a feeding tube was passed through the remaining segments and the ends brought out through the abdominal wall. The segments spontaneously autoanastomosed and the tube subsequently removed. This technique maximised bowel length and avoided multiple stomata and subsequent anastomoses.

Diagnostic laparoscopy has been utilised in a few centres for equivocal cases.

In extensive disease with little or no viable small intestine, palliative care is justified with the alternative being evisceration, total parenteral nutrition and referral for small bowel transplantation with all the attendant problems which that entails. It is important to involve the family in the decision-making process.

Postoperatively, care is supportive until gut function returns. The re-establishment of feeds and management of adaptation can be a complex, long and difficult process. Multidisciplinary care including gastroenterologists and a specialised nutrition team is needed for those at risk of short bowel syndrome.

Complications

Affected intestine can stricture in 25–33% with symptoms characteristically developing 6–8 weeks following the acute episode of NEC. Adhesional obstruction is most common in the first year after surgery. Short bowel syndrome occurs in about 23% following intestinal resection.

Further reading

Bell MJ, et al. Neonatal necrotizing enterocolitis. Therapeutic decisions based upon clinical staging. Ann Surg 1978;187(1):1–7.

Lessin MS, et al. Multiple spontaneous small bowel anastomosis in premature infants with multisegmental necrotizing enterocolitis. J Pediatr Surg 2000;35(2):170–172.

Lucas A, Cole TJ. Breast milk and neonatal necrotising enterocolitis. Lancet 1990;336:1519–1523.

Vaughan WG, et al. Avoidance of stomas and delayed anastomosis for bowel necrosis: the 'clip and drop-back' technique. J Pediatr Surg 1996;31(4):542–545.

Related topics of interest

Neuroblastoma

Learning outcomes

- To be able to provide a simple description of the origin and pathology of the neuroblastoma cell line
- To be aware of anatomical sites of origin
- To recognise the typical clinical presentation
- To be able to instigate appropriate investigations
- To be able to formulate a management plan in conjunction with the multidisciplinary team (MDT)
- To be aware of the available surgical management options

Overview

Neuroblastomas (NBLs) are tumours of the autonomic nervous system that can develop anywhere along the sympathetic chain, although the majority arise in the adrenal gland. The characteristic histological appearance is a small, round blue cell with little cytoplasm. The neuroblast cells arise from the embryonic neural crest and display a range of behaviours from spontaneous regression to developing into a highly differentiated benign ganglioneuroma, to unremitting metastatic progression.

There are four major features that need to be assessed to diagnose and risk-stratify a NBL:

1. **Anatomical location:** Abdominal primaries are generally more aggressive than tumours arising from the pelvis, thorax or neck (**Table 8**)
2. **Age:** This is an important independent variable. Tumours arising below the age of 1 year have a much less aggressive course. There is debate about the true age cut-off, with some suggestion that 18 months is a better discriminator of behaviour
3. **Stage:** Traditionally, staging is based on the findings at surgery (**Table 9**). One disadvantage of this staging system is that it is dependent upon the degree of tumour clearance at surgery, which is in turn influenced by the skill and experience of the operating surgeon and cannot

be independently verified, hence the development of the image defined risk factors (**Table 10**). At present, this is being used solely as a research tool
4. **Biology:** Assessment of the tumour biology is an essential part of the risk stratification. Although numerous cytogenetic abnormalities have been identified, the only one used clinically is the presence

Table 8 Anatomical distribution of neuroblastoma primary lesion	
Abdomen	65% (35% adrenal, 30% extra-adrenal)
Thorax	20%
Neck	5%
Pelvis	5%
Other (or no primary identified)	< 5%

Table 9 International neuroblastoma staging system	
Stage 1	Localised tumours are confined to the organ of origin; complete resection with or without microscopic residual tumours; ipsilateral and contralateral lymph nodes are microscopically negative
Stage 2a	A localised tumour with incomplete gross resection; ipsilateral and contralateral lymph nodes are microscopically negative
Stage 2b	A unilateral tumour with incomplete or complete gross resection; ipsilateral lymph nodes are positive; contralateral lymph nodes are microscopically negative
Stage 3	The tumour crosses the midline with or without regional lymph node involvement; the unilateral tumour is associated with positive contralateral lymph nodes, or a midline tumour is found with positive bilateral lymph nodes
Stage 4	Distant metastases are present
Stage 4s	This occurs in infants with a localised tumour that does not cross the midline, with metastatic disease confined to the liver, skin and bone marrow (< 10% tumour cells in bone marrow)

Table 10 Image defined risk factors*		
Region	**Tumour appearance**	
Neck	Encases the vertebral or carotid artery	
	Encases brachial plexus roots	
	Crosses the midline	
Thorax	Encases the trachea or principal bronchus	
	Encases the origin and branches of the subclavian vessels	
	Thoracoabdominal tumour encases the thoracic aorta	
Abdomen	Infiltrates the porta hepatis	
	Encases branches of the superior mesenteric artery and/or coeliac artery at the root of the mesentery	
	Invades one or both renal pedicles	
	Encases the aorta or inferior vena cava	

*Data from Monclair et al (2009).

of N-Myc amplification, which confers a much higher risk

Management is broadly based on age, stage and biological activity (N-Myc status). Due to the complex nature of these tumours and the widely differing management plans, it is mandatory to involve the surgical oncology MDT prior to embarking upon major surgery.

Epidemiology and aetiology

NBL is the most common extracranial solid tumour of childhood and the most common malignancy diagnosed in infancy. The annual incidence of NBL in the UK was 9.2 per million children between 1991 and 2000. White children seem to have a slightly increased incidence compared with Blacks and Asians.

NBL is associated with measured Von Hippel–Lindau and Beckwith–Wiedemann syndromes. As one of the neurocristopathies, NBL has been described in association with neurofibromatosis (von Recklinghausen's disease), Hirschsprung's disease, central hypoventilation syndrome (Ondine's curse), hypomelanosis of Ito and multiple endocrine neoplasia type 2A.

During the 5th week of fetal life, neural crest cells migrate to populate, amongst other tissues, the sympathetic ganglia. Successful differentiation is dependent upon molecular signalling mechanisms thought to involve the gene products N-Myc and Sonic hedgehog (Shh). N-Myc is a transcription factor, high levels of which promote proliferation of neuroblasts, as well as causing their failure of terminal differentiation and exit from the cell cycle. These circumstances are thought to promote their transformation into NBL.

Clinical features

Presentation of the tumour can be very variable from an abdominal mass, general poor health, pyrexia and weight loss, to the paraneoplastic syndromes of dancing eyes or ataxia. Blueberry muffin lesions are classical of metastatic disease in the skin. Stage 1 or 2 tumours are often identified incidentally on imaging for other causes.

One unusual characteristic of NBL is its ability to spontaneously regress. This occurs up to 40 times more frequently than in clinically apparent NBL and is associated with age < 1 year.

Investigations

- **Tumour markers:** Urine catecholamines should be measured, even though these may not be raised. If they are raised, they serve as useful markers of recurrence and response to therapy
- **Radiological investigations:** Following initial imaging with ultrasound, the tumour should be formally investigated with cross-sectional imaging and a radioisotope metaiodobenzylguanidine scan. Typical features include calcification and a tumour that wraps around the great vessels
- **Bone marrow trephines and aspirates:**
- **Tumour biopsy:** Stage 1 or 2 tumours can often be diagnosed with imaging alone. Stage 3 and 4 tumours are usually diagnosed by a combination of imaging and biopsy. Sufficient tissue can be obtained with a Tru-cut needle inserted under ultrasound guidance by either a surgeon or an interventional radiologist. A coaxial needle and outer sheath that is

initially introduced into the tumour means that multiple biopsies can be taken with only a single puncture in the outer surface of the tumour. Staging investigations should be done at the same time with bilateral bone marrow trephines and aspirates

Differential diagnosis

- Rhabdomyosarcoma
- Desmoplastic small round cell tumour
- Wilms' tumour
- Lymphoma
- Hepatoblastoma
- Primitive neuroectodermal tumour (PNET)

Treatment

The treatment plan is typically formulated in an oncology MDT meeting.

Stage 1 and 2 tumours

Definitive treatment of stage 1 and 2 tumours requires complete surgical resection. As previously mentioned, these can occur anywhere in the body but are most frequently found in the adrenals or the sympathetic chain. If the surgeon is not familiar with the anatomical location, it is good practice to do the procedure jointly with a surgeon who is. For instance, a high cervical lesion can be resected jointly with an ear, nose and throat surgeon, hence combining expertise in NBL surgery with experience in operating around the skull base. Usually, these tumours are well encapsulated, and it is important to review the cross-sectional imaging with the radiologist preoperatively to get a good understanding of the local anatomy and the structures at risk. The tumour will usually push on the adjacent structures rather than invade them.

Because these are low-risk tumours, care should be taken to cause as little morbidity as possible. The principles of surgery involve good access and careful dissection by identifying and preserving the adjacent normal structures. Vascular control is always important, and consideration should be given preoperatively to the origin of the blood supply. For adrenal lesions, there will be three arteries, arising from the renal artery, the inferior phrenic artery and a branch directly from the aorta. The venous drainage is usually through one major vessel that drains directly into the inferior vena cava (IVC) on the right and into the renal vein on the left. There are often other multiple, small draining vessels which occasionally can be troublesome especially if the lesion is very large and metabolically active. The short venous drainage can be difficult to manage on the right, and care should be taken because it is easy to avulse this vessel. Small adrenal lesions can also be approached laparoscopically if the surgeon has the required expertise. Care should be taken to meticulously diathermy all the multiple small veins which otherwise cause a constant ooze which obscures the view.

Stage 3 and 4 tumours

High-risk tumours are treated with aggressive multimodal treatment, involving chemotherapy, surgery and radiotherapy. Surgery is usually performed at around day 100 of treatment. These tumours can be a surgical challenge. Evidence remains obscure regarding the degree of benefit from meticulous tumour clearance as by definition, even in the best hands, microscopic residual tumour will be left behind. Although it is clear that patients who have a complete macroscopic clearance will have a favourable outcome compared with those who have an incomplete resection, it is possible that this is a mere reflection of the biology and aggressiveness of the tumour. However, the considered opinion of both the UK's Neuroblastoma Working Group and the International Society of Paediatric Oncology is that if surgically feasible, this surgery should be attempted. The rationale for this is that despite the low mortality risk of surgery (much lower than the risk of chemotherapy), by debulking the tumours, radiotherapy and chemotherapy are more likely to be successful when used to treat the remaining microscopic disease.

Operative approach

The surgical approach is based on the fact that these tumours advance along the subadventitial plane of blood vessels and can therefore be dissected away from the vessel without vascular compromise. The surgical approach involves good access (rooftop incision for tumours around the coeliac axis), table-top retraction (Omnitract or Thompson retractor) and magnification. For thoracic tumours at the root of the neck, a trap-door incision (Dartevelle's approach) may be necessary. Because the anatomy may be confusing, it is important to start outside the area of the tumour, to sling the affected vessels and to follow these into the tumour following a subadventitial plane. Unlike most other oncological surgery, the tumour will be removed piecemeal and thus gradually exposing the involved vessels. A number of different approaches have been described for doing this dissection, including using scissors, diathermy, a knife or the cavitron ultrasonic surgical aspirator. There seems to be little difference in the efficacy of these techniques, but it is important that the surgeon develops experience with one piece of equipment rather than constantly changing.

Although the outcomes of surgery are somewhat unclear, it is important not to attempt overly radical or mutilating surgery, such as the radical resection of adjacent organs, even if macroscopic tumour is left behind. Any potentially controversial surgical decisions should previously have been discussed in the MDT meeting.

Complications of stage 4 NBL surgery

- Massive bleeding directly from the aorta or IVC
- Damage or ischaemia to adjacent organs, including liver, spleen, kidneys, bowel and pancreas
- Adhesive obstruction
- Chronic diarrhoea
- Chylous ascites
- Death, with a quoted mortality of 2%

In particular, care should be taken of the small bowel during dissection of the superior mesenteric artery and of the kidney during dissection of the renal vessels. Both structures can become ischaemic due to intimal damage caused by traction. During surgery of the retroperitoneum, chylous leaks are often noted and should be controlled at the time, with suture ligation with 6/0 prolene. If there is a general ooze of chyle or lymph noted at the end of surgery, then Tacosil is very effective at stopping the leak when placed on the retroperitoneum.

Further reading

Arul GS. Neuroblastoma. Surgery 2007 25;7:309–311.

Bolande, RP. The neurocristopathies: a unifying concept of disease arising in neural crest maldevelopment. Hum Pathol 1974; 5:409–429.

Carachi R, Azmy A, Grosfeld JL (eds) Neuroblastoma and other adrenal tumours. The surgery of childhood tumours, 2nd edn. Oxford, UK: Arnold Publishers, 2008.

Kiely EM. The surgical challenge of neuroblastoma. J Pediatr Surg 1994; 29:128–133.

Montclair T, Brodeur GM, Ambros PF, et al. The International Neuroblastoma Risk Group (INRG) Staging System: An INRG Task Force Report. J Clin Oncol 2009; 27:298–303.

Related topics of interest

- Haematological malignant disease (p. 146)
- Hepatoblastoma (p. 157)
- Soft tissue tumours (p. 326)

Oesophageal atresia and tracheo-oesophageal fistula

Learning outcomes

- To be able to make a clinical diagnosis of oesophageal atresia (OA)
- To understand the different anatomical types and how they can alter surgical management
- To be able to identify associated congenital abnormalities
- To understand the potential long-term complications faced by children born with OA

Overview

OA is the most common congenital anomaly of the oesophagus. There is interruption of the continuity of the oesophagus, with or without an abnormal communication with the trachea – a tracheo-oesophageal fistula (TOF). Once incompatible with life, it is now a congenital anomaly with overall survival rates > 90%. This reflects significant developments in surgical techniques and in neonatal care since the 1940s.

Epidemiology and aetiology

OA affects 1 in 4000 live births, with a slight male predominance. Associated chromosomal abnormalities are present in 10% of cases. Associated congenital anomalies are present in 50% of cases. The VACTERL association consists of vertebral, anorectal, cardiac, trachea-oesophageal, renal and radial limb abnormalities. Cardiac defects account for the majority of deaths. Five main anatomical subtypes were described by Gross, with 84% of affected infants having a distal TOF (**Figure 46**).

Type	Description	Frequency
A	OA alone	6%
B	OA with proximal TOF	5%
C	OA with distal TOF	84%
D	OA with proximal and distal TOF	1%
E	H-type fistula	4%

The motility of the oesophagus is always affected in OA, with the distal segment most commonly showing disordered peristalsis. The trachea is also abnormal, demonstrating varying degrees of tracheomalacia due to a deficiency of cartilage and an increase in length of the transverse muscle in the posterior tracheal wall.

The aetiology of OA remains largely unknown, but it is likely to be multifactorial, with a complex interplay of environmental and genetic factors, resulting in an embryological insult.

- **Embryogenesis:** This remains poorly understood. During the 4th week of embryonic life, the foregut divides into a ventral respiratory part and a dorsal oesophageal part. Animal models have shown that it is dependent on the temporospatial pattern of expression of foregut patterning genes (e.g. Sonic hedgehog and retinoic acid receptors). Disturbance of this pattern results in anomalies in trachea-oesophageal development
- **Environmental:** Various factors have been implicated, including maternal exposure to methimazole, alcohol, smoking and gestational diabetes. However, no strong evidence supports these environmental factors
- **Genetic:** The majority of cases are sporadic, but familial cases represent approximately 1%. The recurrence rate for siblings is 1% and for offspring is 2–4%. It is two to three times more common in twins. OA can occur as part of a genetic syndrome in up to 10% of cases. Associated chromosomal anomalies include trisomy 21, 18 and 13. OA is also a feature of autosomal dominant syndromes, such as CHARGE syndrome and Feingold's syndrome, and autosomal recessive syndromes, such as Fanconi's anaemia

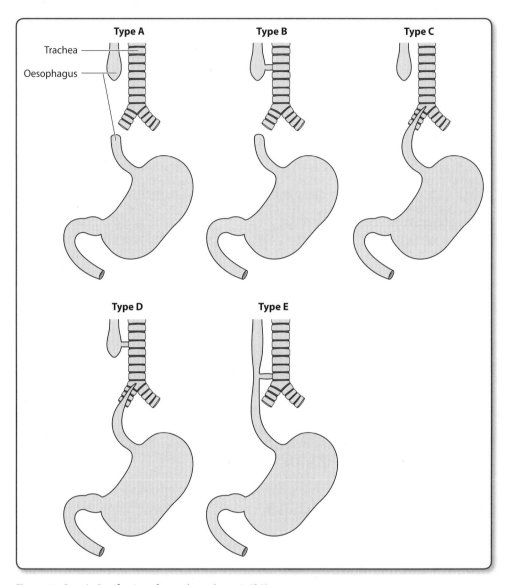

Figure 46 Gross's classification of oesophageal atresia (OA).

Clinical features

Antenatal

- Small or absent gastric bubble
- Polyhydramnios
- Distended oesophageal pouch
- Overall sensitivity of antenatal ultrasound is only 9–42% sensitivity

Postnatal

- Neonatal
  - Drooling/frothing of saliva
  - Respiratory distress
  - Cyanotic episodes
  - Choking on attempted feeds
  - Other VACTERL anomalies raising suspicion

- Passage of large-gauge nasogastric (NG) tube arrested about 10 cm from mouth
- Late diagnosis
  - Coughing with feeds
  - Abdominal distension
  - Recurrent pneumonia
  - Suggests isolated TOF

Investigations

The role of investigations is to confirm the diagnosis and assess for associated anomalies that may impact on operative management, including cardiac, renal and chromosomal abnormalities.

- **Chest and abdominal radiograph:** An NG tube arrested in the superior mediastinum confirms the diagnosis of OA. It is good practice for the operating surgeon to place gentle pressure on the tube whilst the X-ray is being taken to ensure it is maximally advanced and avoid an incorrect diagnosis. Presence of gas in the stomach indicates the presence of a distal TOF (**Figure 47**). Associated intestinal atresias, vertebral and rib abnormalities may be detected
- **Echocardiography:** Preoperative evaluation of significant cardiac anomalies, interruption of the inferior vena cava with azygos continuation and presence of a right-sided aortic arch that may alter operative timing and approach
- **Renal ultrasound:** Needed preoperatively if no urine output to rule out bilateral renal anomaly not compatible with survival
- **Chromosomal analysis and molecular genetic testing:** In presence of dysmorphic features or family history

Differential diagnosis

A differential diagnosis is unusual but may include:

- Laryngotracheoesophageal cleft – midline defect between posterior larynx, trachea and anterior wall of oesophagus
- Oesophageal web, ring or stricture – typically later presentation

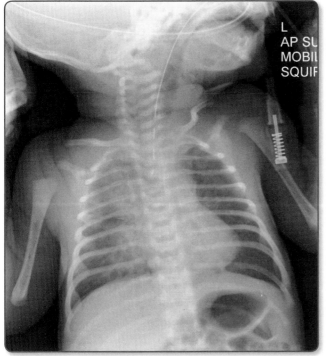

Figure 47 Anteroposterior chest X-ray of a neonate with oesophageal atresia (OA) and tracheo-oesophageal fistula (TOF).

- Tracheal atresia
- Oesophageal diverticulum

Treatment

Definitive treatment of OA is surgical. The timing of surgery is determined by the neonate's stability, but typically is not regarded as an emergency and is scheduled 12–24 hours after admission to a specialist paediatric surgical centre.

An exception to this is neonates, particularly those born prematurely, with respiratory distress requiring assisted ventilation. In such cases, urgent ligation of the TOF is necessary. Neonates with bilateral renal agenesis, trisomy 18 and non-correctable major cardiac defects should be considered for non-operative management.

Preoperative management

- Aim is to minimise risk of aspiration pneumonia
- The upper pouch is continuously aspirated using a Replogle tube attached to low-pressure suction

Operative management

- Aim:
  - Ligate the TOF
  - Restore oesophageal continuity
- Approach (thoracotomy versus thoracoscopy):
  - Traditionally surgery has been performed through a posterolateral extrapleural right-sided thoracotomy. The increased use of minimally invasive techniques in neonates resulted in the first thoracoscopic repair in 1999, and this is being increasingly adopted in specialist centres. Comparative studies are awaited
- Operative steps:
  - Some surgeons will perform an intraoperative bronchoscopy or rigid endoscopy. This aids identification of tracheomalacia, an upper pouch fistula and the length of the upper pouch, and also can identify the point where the distal fistula enters the airway.
  - The chest is opened through the fourth or fifth intercostal space. The azygos vein is exposed and ligated as this guides the surgeon to the oesophageal segments. The proximal pouch is exposed and the TOF is identified and divided close to the trachea. The proximal pouch is mobilised and a proximal fistula is excluded. The proximal and distal oesophageal segments are then anastomosed over a transanastomotic tube. A chest drain is seldom required
- Special considerations:
  - A delayed primary repair will be required in cases of long gap OA or extremely low-birth-weight neonates. In such cases, the fistula is ligated and a gastrostomy fashioned in order to allow feeding and growth until such time as a delayed anastomosis or oesophageal replacement can be performed.

Postoperative

Feeds are commenced via the transanastomotic tube on the second or third postoperative day. Oral feeds can commence once the neonate can swallow saliva. If the oesophageal anastomosis is performed under tension, elective paralysis and ventilation, with the neck flexed, is recommended for 5 postoperative days.

Complications

- Early:
  - Anastomotic leak 15%
  - Oesophageal stricture 30%
  - Recurrent TOF 10%
- Late:
  - Gastro-oesophageal reflux 40%, half of whom require antireflux surgery
  - Tracheomalacia 10%, half of whom require aortopexy
  - Long-term oesophageal dysmotility – improves with age
  - Respiratory disorders – improves with age

Further reading

De Jong EM, et al. Etiology of esophageal atresia and tracheoesophageal fistula: 'mind the gap'. Curr Gastroenterol Rep 2010; 12:215–222.

Rothenberg SS. Thoracoscopic repair of esophageal atresia and trachea-oesophageal fistula in neonates: evolution of a technique. J Laparoendoscopic Adv Surg Tech 2012; 22:195–199.

Spitz L. Oesophageal atresia. Orphanet J Rare Dis 2007;2:24.

Related topics of interest

- Long gap oesophageal atresia (p. 185)

Osteosarcoma

Learning outcomes

- To understand the role of paediatric surgeons in this condition
- To understand the rationale for surgical intervention
- To understand the mode of intervention

Overview

Osteosarcoma is a rare tumour although it is the most common malignant bone tumour in the paediatric age group. It has an association with hereditary retinoblastoma amongst others. Most arise in an area of normal bone and there are a number of different types. Treatment includes preoperative chemotherapy and surgical excision. Paediatric surgeons are involved in performing pulmonary metastasectomies.

Epidemiology and pathology

The annual incidence in the UK is 8.7 per million. It is slightly more frequent in males with a peak at 15–17 years of age; in females it is 13 years. Risk factors include radiation and exposure to alkylating agents.

A genetic predisposition is present in those patients with

- **Hereditary retinoblastoma:** These patients are at increased risk for secondary non-ocular tumours of which osteosarcoma makes up 44%
- **Li–Fraumeni:** This is a rare autosomal dominant syndrome with a germline TP53 mutation in which patients are predisposed to cancer
- **Rothmund–Thomson:** An autosomal recessive association of congenital bone defects, hair and skin dysplasias, hypogonadism and cataracts

Most tumours arise spontaneously in area of bone without any abnormality in contrast to adults in whom 25% arise in pre-existing pathologic osseous conditions. Biologically, most tumours have some type of combined inactivation of the retinoblastoma gene (*RB1*)

and p53 pathways, with alterations affecting *RB1* in up to 80%. There are structural alterations in the TP53 tumour-suppressor gene locus and within the *MDM-2* gene whose product is important in regulating p53 function.

Allelic loss at other loci is also recognised (3q; 13q; 18q) in up to 75%, with alterations in insulin growth factor-1 and 1R, playing a role. P-glycoprotein, a drug-resistance protein, also plays a role and its levels can predict outcomes.

Pathologically, an osteosarcoma is a sarcoma with the production of osteoid directly from the sarcomatous stroma. There are three major groups, depending on the predominant cell type.

1. 50% osteoblastic (predominantly osteoid)
2. 25% chondroblastic (predominantly malignant cartilaginous)
3. 25% 'herringbone pattern' similar to fibrosarcomas and are termed fibroblastic

There is no difference in outcome although the fibroblastic type may have a better histological response.

A small proportion present with clinical subtypes that are characterised by distinct clinical, radiological and histological characteristics:

- **Telangiectatic:** These are blood-filled spaces divided by septae and represent < 4% of total cases. On X-ray, it has an onion skin appearance and is purely lytic. Outcome is similar to conventional osteosarcoma
- **Low-grade intramedullary osteosarcoma:** These are found in < 1% of cases, mostly in 3rd decade of life with a predilection for distal femur and proximal tibia, lytic foci and dense areas, poorly demarcated. Incomplete resection results in local recurrence
- **Surface osteosarcoma:** These originate and grow on surface of bone
  - Low grade: paraosteal and periosteal
  - High grade: high-grade surface osteosarcoma

Clinical features

- Pain and swelling
- Pathological fractures
- Palpable swelling
- Painful limp that increases with with weight bearing
- Uncommon features are fever and weight loss

It has a predilection for the long bones mostly around the knee. Distal femur and proximal tibia are the most common sites and then proximal humerus. In children, < 10% present with tumours in the axial skeleton. 20% develop metastases and in 5% the disease is multifocal. This is more aggressive, has a higher incidence of lung metastases and a very poor prognosis.

Staging depends on:

- Grade: low (G1) or high (G2)
- Local extent of the primary: intracompartmental (T1) or extracompartmental (T2)
- Metastases: no spread (M0) or spread (M1)
  Stage 1: G1;T1/2;M0
  Stage 2: G2;T1/2;M0
  Stage 3: all M1 tumours regardless of grade or extent

Investigations

- Raised lactate dehydrogenase and alkaline phosphatase (ALP) which is also useful in monitoring
- A radiological assessment of the primary and a search for distant metastases
- X-ray features include
  - Metaphyseal lesion with periosteal new bone formation, destruction of pre-existing cortex
  - Soft tissue mass in > 90%
  - Codman's triangle (a triangular area visible radiographically where the periosteum, elevated by a bone tumour, rejoins the cortex of normal bone)
- A chest CT should always be performed to identify lung metastases, which are non-calcified in 75%. However, it can miss 40–50% of metastases.

Treatment

At diagnosis, metastases are missed in 75–85% of patients, and without adequate treatment, most patients with localised disease will develop secondary metastases within 1 year. Of those with localised disease, 60–70% can be cured with an appropriate multidisciplinary approach.

Chemotherapy options include a mixture of doxorubicin, cisplatin, high-dose methotrexate, ifosfamide, etoposide and liposome-encapsulated muramyl tripeptide (L-MTP-PE)

The goals of surgery are to safely remove the tumour and preserve as much extremity function as possible. This involves a wide resection margin with amputation being reserved for those that are unresectable. Criteria for performing limb sparing surgery include

- Absence of major neurovascular involvement
- Feasible wide local excision (WLE) to include normal muscle in all directions and en bloc removal of all biopsy sites
- Resection of adjacent joint and capsule
- Adequate motor reconstruction using regional muscle transfers
- Adequate soft tissue coverage

The surgical technique is beyond the scope of this book.

Paediatric surgeons become involved when pulmonary metastases are present as complete resection improves prognosis and survival. The procedure should take place by thoracotomy because some of the metastases cannot be seen and are appreciable on palpation only.

The question of whether to explore both sides at a single sitting is a matter for debate because the majority of those patients with unilateral disease on imaging will actually have bilateral disease. In addition, in relapsed patients, those with a second remission had 2- and 5-year survival of 60% and 38%, respectively. Survival in those with no second remission was 4% and 0%.

Most would advocate unilateral thoracotomy, with a staged contralateral exploration, due to the debilitating effects of bilateral thoracotomies. A median sternotomy gives poor access to the posterior chest and left lower lobe. Recurrent metastases occur in 40–75%, with 60–70% occurring within 12 months.

Surgical techniques are as follows:

- Lateral thoracotomy through the appropriate rib space
- Palpate metastases
- Wedge resection with a good margin. This is best accomplished with a stapling device
- Test for air leak: fill cavity with saline and over-sew any leak
- Chest drain is a matter of preference. Air can be drained in theatre by a nasogastric (NG) tube attached to an underwater seal. This passes through the space into the hemithorax, and then hand ventilation of the lung by the anaesthetist is performed as the NG tube is slowly withdrawn
- Closure in layers

The best prognostic factor is the percentage of tumour necrosis following chemotherapy, with >90% necrosis giving an excellent overall survival. The presence of metastases is the most adverse factor, with axial primaries also conferring poor prognosis. In localised disease, high tumour burden, high ALP and LDH, poor response to chemotherapy, hyperdiploidy and increased expression of p-glycoprotein are adverse factors.

Paediatric anaesthesia

Learning outcomes

- To understand the concepts of balanced anaesthesia
- Understand the role of preoperative assessment
- Understand postoperative implications including pain and fluids

Overview

Classically anaesthesia has been described as the triad of hypnosis, analgesia and muscle relaxation. Whilst these remain the underlying concepts, with more modern drugs the margins are more blurred with a number of drugs having analgesic and muscle-relaxant properties or analgesic and hypnotic effects.

In terms of divisions between local, regional and general, in the whole these are often not succinct categories as they are in adults, but instead most surgeries involve at least two if not three of these modalities in the paediatric population. It is very rare to see an entire procedure carried out under a regional block in children but very common to see this as part of the anaesthetic in combination with a general anaesthetic.

Anaesthetic assessment

The purpose of the preoperative visit can be broken down into three areas – patient factors, condition factors and surgical factors.

- Patient factors
  - Gaining rapport with the child
  - Discussion of anaesthetic induction type (gas versus intravenous)
  - Anaesthetic history
- Condition factors
  - Further information about the disease process
  - Relevant investigations
  - Previous related illnesses or specific conditions pertinent to anaesthesia (e.g. malignant hyperpyrexia and muscular dystrophies)
- Surgical factors

  - Actual operation to be performed
  - Requirement for regional block
  - Positioning issues
  - Requirement for intensive or high-dependency care postoperatively

Factors indicating that elective surgery should be postponed in a child presenting with an upper respiratory tract infection are as follows:

- Systemically unwell
- Fever > 38°C
- Mucopurulent nasal secretions
- Lower respiratory symptoms or signs
- There is a lower threshold for postponing surgery if the patient is younger than 12 months or if surgery requires tracheal intubation

American Society of Anesthesiologists' classification of physical status is as follows:

I   Normally healthy patient
II Patient with mild systemic disease
III Patient with severe systemic disease that is not incapacitating
IV Patient with incapacitating systemic disease that is a constant threat to life
V   Moribund patient who is not expected to survive 24 hours with or without an operation

Emergency cases are designated by the addition of 'E' to the classification number.

Preoperative investigations

The ability to obtain a full set of investigations, particularly in small children, can be limited by difficulties with intravenous access and potential distress to the child. Some investigations are easy to undertake and others less so with potential pitfalls therein. In general, long procedures and those mandating overnight stay will require more intense work-up. In children requiring blood tests it should be borne in mind that, if these are needed preoperatively, sitting a cannula at the same time will cause the child less distress later on and enable an intravenous route to be used for anaesthesia. If the investigation results are not required before anaesthesia, these may be taken at the time of surgery immediately after induction of anaesthesia.

Certain conditions will require particular investigation but would not be considered routine. For example, a chest radiograph is indicated in thoracic or cardiac surgery, but probably not necessary in all cases. Children with underlying cardiac disease or with a newly discovered murmur should have echocardiography and cardiac review if they have not had one previously or within the last few months. In a child with a soft early systolic murmur and no other symptoms or signs and a normal electrocardiogram (ECG), surgery could proceed.

Analgesic modalities

Anaesthesia in children quite often involves a dedicated technique for analgesia whether this is a local, regional or central neuraxial block. This commonly involves the use of a long-acting local anaesthetic, such as bupivacaine, with many centres favouring the L-isomer for cardiac safety. This can be used in combination with adjuncts, such as opioids, clonidine and ketamine.
Examples include

- Local – direct nerve block such as ring block for digital surgery, infraorbital nerve block for cleft lip and penile block for circumcision and hypospadias repair
- Regional – nerve block involving more than one nerve such as inguinal field block for inguinal hernia, transversus abdominis plane (TAP) block for abdominal wall surgery and lumbar plexus block in hip and femur surgery
- Central block – epidural commonly used in abdominal and thoracic surgery, caudal block in perineal surgery and more rarely spinal block classically used in ex-premature babies for inguinal hernia repair
- Paravertebral block – whilst not truly a central block, used more commonly now in renal and thoracic surgery both for good efficacy and for when an epidural might be contraindicated (e.g. coagulopathy and sepsis)

Anaesthesia

Discussion of a detailed anaesthetic plan is beyond the scope of this Topic; however, consideration is given to the following:
- Induction of anaesthesia
  - Inhalational: sevoflurane, with or without N_2O
  - Intravenous: propofol, ketamine, thiopentone
- Neuromuscular blockade
  - rocuronium, atracurium (suxamethonium)
- Airway management
  - Face mask with or without oropharyngeal airway
  - Laryngeal mask airway
  - Tracheal intubation: cuffed or uncuffed endo- or nasotracheal tube
- Maintenance of anaesthesia depends on the surgery, underlying and current conditions of the patient
  - Inhalational: isoflurane, sevoflurane, desflurane, with or without N_2O
  - Total intravenous anaesthesia involving
    - a sedative hypnotic: commonly propofol
    - analgesia: commonly remifentanil or fentanyl
    - others: ketamine, midazolam
  - Ventilation: spontaneous, assisted or controlled
- Other factors include
  - Fluid management
  - Thermoregulation and maintenance of body temperature
  - Prevention of hypoglycaemia

Postoperative considerations

Anaesthetic involvement does not cease when the patient is awake but continues into the postoperative period. Careful monitoring of analgesic infusions, whether they are in the form of an epidural, local anaesthetic or opioid patient-controlled analgesia infusions, requires anaesthetic and pain team support. Fluid therapy is best tailored to the age of the child and the type of surgery performed. Whilst Hartman's solution is very suitable in most cases, small babies will need a glucose-based solution and care must be taken with sodium levels in premature and term neonates.

Close collaboration between surgical, anaesthetic and nursing staff is essential to ensure high-quality postoperative care in terms of analgesia, fluid management and general well-being.

Further reading

Bingham R, Thomas AL, Sury M. Hatch and Sumner's textbook of paediatric anaesthesia, 3rd edn. Hodder Arnold, 2007.

Motoyama EK, Davis PJ. Smith's anaesthesia for infants and children, 7th edn. Mosby: Elsevier, 2006.

Rusy L, Usaleva E. Pediatric anesthesia review. Update Anesthesia 1998; 8:2–14.

Paediatric bariatric surgery

Learning outcomes

- To be able to identify morbid obesity
- To be aware of the indications for bariatric surgery in adolescence
- To be familiar with the principles of obesity management

Overview

Obesity is an increasing problem in children. Overweight and obesity are defined by the World Health Organization as 'abnormal or excessive fat accumulation that may impair health'. Body Mass Index (BMI) is a weight-for-height index that is commonly used to classify overweight and obesity:

$$BMI = \frac{weight\ (kg)}{height\ (m)^2}$$

A definition of paediatric obesity categories is as follows:

	BMI	BMI centile comparison
Overweight	25–29	85th–95th
Obese	>30	>95th
Morbidly obese	>40	>99th

BMI adjusted for age and gender is recommended as a measure of overweight in children. The UK 1990 BMI charts should be used to provide age- and gender-specific information.

Although diet and exercise remain the mainstay of obesity management, bariatric surgery in the adolescent population leads to more sustained weight loss, offering longer durable improvements in comorbidities and quality of life.

Epidemiology and aetiology

National statistics from the Health and Social Care Information Centre in 2010 indicated that 17% of boys and 15% of girls aged 2–15 years were obese, and it has been predicted that if current trends persist, 25% of children in the UK will be obese.

There are many causes of obesity, but the principal causes are prolonged periods of increased intake of energy-dense foods combined with decreased physical activity due to a sedentary lifestyle, with changing modes of transportation, increasing urbanization and prolonged use of television and computers.

Conditions predisposing to obesity

- Genetic conditions:
  - Prader–Willi syndrome
  - Melanocortin-4 receptor mutations
- Metabolic conditions:
  - Cushing's disease
  - Polycystic ovary syndrome
- Drugs:
  - Corticosteroids
  - Antidepressants, antipsychotics and mood stabilisers

Clinical features

Obesity is identified by increasing fat deposition and weight and is measured by calculation of the BMI. It may lead to various comorbid conditions, if not controlled, which are:

- Type 2 diabetes mellitus
- Obstructive sleep apnoea
- Non-alcoholic fatty liver disease
- Non-alcoholic steatohepatitis
- Pseudotumor cerebri
- Cardiovascular risk
- Quality of life
- Depression
- Metabolic syndrome
- Decreased exercise tolerance
- Polycystic ovary syndrome

Most children are referred by paediatricians or dieticians when an initial weight management programme has failed. Assessment should focus on identifying the cause of the obesity and should involve taking a detailed history, including dietary habits, and performing a physical examination and investigations for comorbidities.

Investigations

Investigations include:
- Height, weight, blood pressure and BMI calculations
- Anthropological measurements such as waist circumference and hip circumference
- Genetic studies to identify genetic defects and obesity syndromes such as melanocortin-4 receptor abnormalities and Prader–Willi syndrome
- Blood tests – fasting and postprandial blood glucose, liver function tests, renal function test, serum cholesterol and triglycerides
- Glucose tolerance test
- Ultrasound scan of the liver to look for fatty liver and pelvis to look for polycystic ovaries in girls
- Sleep study to investigate sleep apnoea
- Psychological assessment of:
  - The possible causes of obesity
  - Maturity to understand the consequences of surgery
  - Motivation for weight loss

Treatment

Prevention and medical management

- Dietary measures include the introduction of healthy foods (five portions of fruits and vegetables per day), decreased calorie intake and monitoring of meal portion sizes
- Exercise (at least 60 minutes of physical activity per day)
- Behavioural intervention by a trained specialist
- Drug treatment is not recommended in children younger than 12 years. In those aged 12 or more, orlistat, which inhibits pancreatic lipase, is the only drug which is recommended but only if physical or severe psychological comorbidities are present. It acts by preventing the absorption of fat, thereby reducing caloric intake
- Metformin has recently been used. It decreases gluconeogenesis by the liver and increases muscle consumption of glucose

- Obese or overweight children with complex needs, such as learning difficulties or significant comorbidity, should be referred to an appropriate specialist

Surgery

Surgery is considered a last resort for the treatment of adolescent obesity after appropriate conservative measures have been tried and shown to have failed.

Adolescent patients should also meet criteria recommended by the National Institute for Health and Clinical Excellence. All the following criteria should be met before bariatric surgery is recommended:
- BMI ≥ 40 kg/m^2 or > 35 kg/m^2 in presence of other significant disease that could be improved if the patient lost weight
- All non-surgical measures have been tried but have failed to achieve or maintain weight loss for at least 6 months
- Receiving or will receive intensive management in a specialist obesity service
- Commitment to long-term follow-up

It should be noted that bariatric surgery in children and young people should only be recommended under exceptional circumstances and only in patients who have achieved or nearly achieved physiological maturity.

Bariatric operative techniques

There are three main types of operations:
1. Restrictive procedures:
   I. Laparoscopic adjustable gastric banding (LAGB)
   II. Sleeve gastrectomy
   III. Vertical banded gastroplasty (not commonly used)
2. Malabsorptive procedures:
   I. Biliary pancreatic diversion
3. Mixed procedures:
   I. Roux-en-Y gastric bypass

Procedures most commonly performed in the adolescent population are LAGB, sleeve gastrectomy and Roux-en-Y Gastric bypass. All adolescent bariatric surgery can be performed laparoscopically. Preoperative preparation must take into account thromboprophylaxis.

LAGB

A Silastic band with an inflatable balloon is placed around the proximal part of the stomach to create a small pouch of about 30–50 mL capacity (**Figure 48**). The balloon is connected to a port placed in the abdominal wall through which the balloon size can be adjusted, thereby controlling the aperture of the outlet from the pouch to the rest of stomach. This technique works by slowing and limiting the amount of food which can be consumed at any one time and also leads to early satiety through the release of peptide YY by L cells in the mucosa.

The advantages of LAGB are that it is a simple and quick procedure to perform and is associated with a short hospital stay. However, frequent hospital visits are required to adjust band fill, and the procedure is not as effective as other procedures in achieving weight reduction. It is expected to achieve a weight loss of 20 kg in 1 year.

Sleeve gastrectomy

A gastric tube is formed along the lesser curvature of the stomach and more than 85–90% of the stomach is removed (**Figure 49**). This procedure is more effective than LAGB, requires less follow-up hospital visits and is associated with less metabolic changes than gastric bypass. Disadvantages are the invasiveness and irreversibility of the procedure, a long suture line, with more potential for postoperative complications and a lack of long-term outcome data in children.

Roux-en-Y gastric bypass

The stomach is divided transversely, creating a small proximal gastric pouch (**Figure 50**). The jejunum is divided about 50 cm from the duodenojejunal flexure, and a 75–150 cm jejunal Roux loop is anastomosed to the gastric pouch. This procedure achieves good weight loss of approximately 45–50 kg in 1 year, and there is significant improvement in comorbidities. However, there is a relatively high perioperative complication rate, with a 10% readmission rate and long-term nutritional deficiencies of iron, vitamin B_{12}, vitamin D and rarely vitamin B_1 have been reported, requiring lifelong supplementation.

Bariatric surgery is slowly being accepted as a safe and reliable procedure in the adolescent age group as long as a strict protocol is followed. It is effective in treating comorbidities but requires lifelong commitment and long-term follow-up.

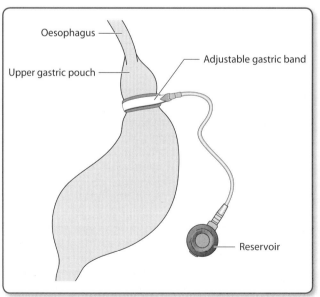

Figure 48 Laparoscopic adjustable gastric banding

Oesophagus

Upper gastric pouch

Adjustable gastric band

Reservoir

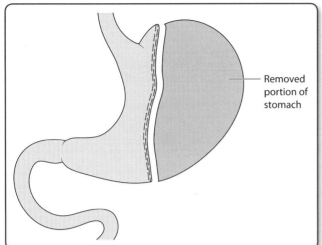

Figure 49 Sleeve gastrectomy

Removed portion of stomach

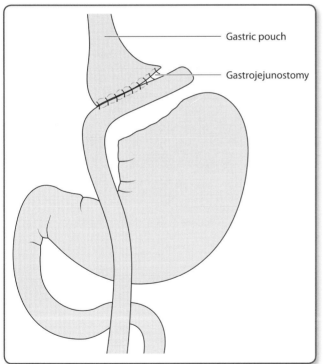

Figure 50 Roux-en-Y gastric bypass

Gastric pouch

Gastrojejunostomy

Further reading

Aikenhead A, Knai C, Lobstein T. Effectiveness and cost-effectiveness of paediatric bariatric surgery: a systematic review. Clin Obes 2011; 1:12–25.

Messiah SE, Lopen-Mitnik G, Winegar D, et al. Changes in weight and comorbidities among adolescents undergoing bariatric surgery: 1-year results from the bariatric outcomes longitudinal database. Surg Obes Relat Dis 2012.

National Institute for Health and Clinical Excellence. Obesity: guidance on the prevention, identification, assessment and management of overweight and obesity in adults and children. London: NICE, 2006.

Related topics of interest

- Endocrine conditions presenting to paediatric surgery (p. 99)
- Growth disorder (p. 143)

Paediatric breast disease

Learning outcomes

- To understand the range of breast disease presenting to paediatric surgery
- To define disease-specific aetiology
- To be able to form a management plan

Overview

Breast disease presents infrequently to paediatric surgeons and the majority of pathology is gynaecomastia. True breast absence occurs in Poland's syndrome, which is associated with absent or diminished underlying chest wall structures, including pectoralis muscles and ribs. The ipsilateral upper limb may also be affected.

Benign premature thelarche is isolated breast development in females aged 6 months to 9 years. Physical examination should seek out other signs of puberty, such as pubic hair, thickening of the vaginal mucosa or accelerated bone growth. If no other signs of puberty are present, reassure the patient and family that it is a benign finding. Examine the child every 6–12 months. If other signs of puberty are evident, precocious puberty should be entertained as a diagnosis.

Breast pain

Epidemiology and pathology

Breast pain accounts for 25% of visits to adult breast clinics and is the presenting feature of breast cancer in 15% of cases.

Clinical features

Initial evaluation to exclude localised lesions and inflammatory conditions. Pain is categorised into non-cyclical and cyclical, usually occurring in the fourth and third decades of life respectively.

Treatment

This includes removal of methylxanthines from the diet and reassurance. Evening primrose oil, danazol and bromocriptine can be effective as adjuncts.

Breast lumps

Epidemiology and pathology

Cysts occur throughout childhood and are most common at the onset of breast development. Juvenile fibroadenomas occur in young adolescents and are often single. The adult variant is multiple in 10–15% and confers a relative risk of 1.3–1.9 for cancer development. There is considerable overlap of the adult form with phyllodes tumours, and these may be part of a spectrum.

Phyllodes tumours occur at a mean age of 44 years and are exceedingly rare in paediatric practice. They have minute projections from the surface that are invisible to the naked eye. Fibrous areas are interspersed with soft, fleshy areas and cysts are filled with clear or semisolid bloody fluid. On microscopy epithelial and stromal elements show hyperplasia and may have areas of atypia, metaplasia and malignancy.

Breast cancer in children can be a primary or secondary malignancy or part of a metastatic tumour. Only 0.2% of primaries occur before 25 years, and > 90% are first seen as a breast lump.

Aetiology

- Physiological
  - Normal breast bud or premature puberty
- Pathological
  - Inflammatory
    - Mastitis, breast abscess, fibrosis, fat necrosis
    - Benign neoplasm
    - Children – haemangioma, cyst, lipoma, papilloma
    - Adolescents – fibroadenoma, phyllodes tumour, cyst, fibrocystic disease, neurofibroma
  - Malignant neoplasm
    - Metastatic, secretory
    - Primary – rhabdomyosarcoma, lymphoblastic non-Hodgkin's lymphoma

- Secondary – retinoblastoma, osteosarcoma, neuroblastoma, leukaemia, lymphoma, rhabdomyosarcoma
  - Others
    - Lymph or haemangioma

Clinical features

Simple cysts occur with the onset of breast development and are soft, painless and mobile. Adult fibroadenomas occur in the older adolescent and juvenile fibroadenomas in peripubertal adolescents. The adult variant is 1–2 cm in diameter. They are well circumscribed, rubbery and mobile. The juvenile form is often larger and may cause significant asymmetry. Phyllodes tumours are well circumscribed range in size from 1 to 40 cm.

Investigations

- Ultrasound
- Fine-needle aspiration (FNA)
- Biopsy

Treatment

FNA commonly results in complete resolution of cysts, with persistence an indication for biopsy. Excisional biopsy should be undertaken in a solitary breast lump which is present for several months in an adolescent girl.

Fibroadenomas and phyllodes tumours are difficult to differentiate preoperatively. FNA may not yield a definitive diagnosis. When known to be a fibroadenoma, they can be safely followed up if 1–2 cm, solitary, firm, rubbery, non-tender and well circumscribed. Those enlarging should be excised to avoid further deformity. Development is usually normal as tissue compressed prior to excision fills the defect over time.

A 2 cm excision margin is recommended for a phyllodes tumour; 20% will recur if resected without adequate margins. Recurrence rate of benign tumours > 5 cm diameter is 39% and smaller ones 10%. One-fifth of recurrences show malignant transformation.

Breast abscess or mastitis

Epidemiology and pathology

Primarily it affects the neonatal breast. About 84% cases occur in the first 3 weeks of life. There is a male–female ratio of 1.0:1.8

Aetiology

Primary organisms are *Staphylococcus* in 90%, but *Streptococcus*, *Salmonella* and *Escherichia coli* contribute.

Clinical features

The skin and nipple are red with occasional induration due to swelling and oedema. Fluctuance indicates an abscess. The majority do not develop pyrexia, irritability or feeding difficulty.

Treatment

Appropriate intravenous antibiotics resolve the infection in the majority. If fluctuant, an FNA may be the first line to avoid breast deformity in later life. In a confirmed abscess or recurrence post-FNA, incision and drainage is required.

Gynaecomastia

Epidemiology and pathology

Gynaecomastia is defined as benign proliferation of glandular tissue of the male breast great enough to be seen or felt as an enlarged breast. About 30–60% of boys have gynaecomastia. It first appears between 10 and 12 years of age, but the highest prevalence is between 13 and 14 years of age. Involution is generally complete at 16 or 17 years of age.

Aetiology

Imbalance between oestrogen and androgen may contribute to its pubertal development. Testicular or adrenal tumours cause overproduction of oestrogen, or peripheral conversion of androgens to oestrogen may increase their levels (excessive extraglandular aromatase activity). Decreased androgen levels or effects can be due to primary testicular defects, loss of pituitary gonadotropin stimulation or increased androgen binding to sex hormone-binding globulin.

Many drugs cause displacement of androgens from their receptors and result in unopposed oestrogen effects, e.g. spironolactone. Other aetiologies include

- Ectopic production of human chorionic gonadotropin (β-hcg)
- Primary or secondary hypogonadism
- Androgen insensitivity, Kleinfelter's syndrome
- Liver disease
- Starvation
- Renal disease and dialysis
- Idiopathic
- Physiological – neonatal, pubertal, involutional

Pseudogynaecomastia is due to increased amounts of adipose tissue beneath the breast.

Clinical features

Adolescent boys commonly present with a tender and painful breast. They often describe some minor trauma and the injury is usually incidental. True gynaecomastia can be felt as a disk of rubbery tissue, arising concentrically from beneath and around the nipple and areola. Tanner testicular staging should be formally undertaken.

Investigations

Oestradiol, testosterone, β-hcg levels

Treatment

Initial treatment of the underlying cause is recommended if one is found. The majority resolve spontaneously. Tamoxifen and anastrozole have been tried. Studies showed anastrozole had no benefit over placebo. Tamoxifen reduced pain and breast size. Surgery should be reserved for those with the persistent, severe form.

Options are as follows:

- Subcutaneous mastectomy using an inferior partial circumareolar extendable incision can result in poor cosmesis
- Reduction mammoplasty using the nipple–areolar complex and an anchor

or keyhole incision as the site of removal of breast tissue. This gives good cosmesis and allows removal of lateral, medial and superior sited breast tissue, with preservation of the nipple blood supply
- Mastectomy or subtotal mastectomy

Nipple discharge

Aetiology

Inappropriate lactation not related to pregnancy or which continues postpartum without breast feeding is called galactorrhoea. There are five pathophysiological groups:

1. Neurogenic: local breast and nipple irritation and stimulation
2. Hypothalamic: prolactinoma (rare in children and adolescents, but often accompanied by delayed puberty), most common cause in boys
3. Endocrine: cessation of oral contraceptive, polycystic ovary, adrenal and gonadal tumours, hypothyroidism
4. Pharmacological: neuroleptics, oestrogens and opiates all described in adults
5. Idiopathic

Purulent discharge indicates an abscess. Serous drainage may indicate the presence of a communicating breast cyst. Bloody discharge (a sign of tumour in adults) is generally drainage from an intraductal papilloma or duct ectasia in children.

Clinical features

The type of discharge indicates the underlying problem.

Investigations

- Prolactin, oestradiol, and thyrotropin levels with an MRI sella turcica in galactorrhoea

Treatment

- Galactorrhoea: treatment aimed at the underlying cause
- Purulent: culture, antibiotics then incision and drainage if fluctuant
- Bloody: generally self-limiting

Further reading

Laituri CA, Garey CL, Ostlie DJ, et al. Treatment of adolescent gynaecomastia. J Ped Surg 2010; 45:650–654.

Related topics of interest

- Paediatric gynaecology (p. 242)

Paediatric cardiac surgery

Learning outcomes

- To be aware of different types of congenital heart defects
- To understand how cardiac surgery may be undertaken
- To be aware of the presentation and management of two commonly occurring conditions

Overview

The heart is the most common organ system to be affected by congenital abnormalities, with an incidence of 0.8% live births. The signs and symptoms relate to the type and severity of the defect, with many conditions not requiring surgery.

Traditionally defects have been considered as 'simple' and 'complex' and subdivided into

- Obstructive lesions, e.g. aortic stenosis, coarctation and interrupted aortic arch
- Left to right shunts – 'pink' or acyanotic conditions, e.g. atrial septal defect (ASD), ventricular septal defect (VSD), patent ductus arteriosus (PDA) and atrioventricular septal defect (AVSD)
- Right to left shunts – 'blue' or cyanotic conditions, e.g. tetralogy of Fallot, pulmonary atresia
- Complex mixing defects, e.g. transposition of great arteries, truncus arteriosus, total anomalous pulmonary venous drainage and hypoplastic left heart syndrome

With this classification in place, it is possible to approach each surgical operation with the object of relieving obstruction which may occur at the inflow as well as the outflow to a heart chamber, correcting, if possible, shunts and balancing pulmonary blood flow against an adequate systemic blood flow.

The natural history of defects is important with respect to the timing of repair. There has been a move away from early palliation and later repair to single-stage repair, often in the early neonatal period.

Surgical approach via a median sternotomy is the most common access to the heart, with partial or complete removal of the thymus gland. For some procedures a thoracotomy is used, e.g. aortic coarctation repair or PDA ligation. Currently thoracoscopic techniques have a limited role used in some centres for clipping a PDA or creation of a pericardial window.

The next consideration is whether the surgery will require the use of cardiopulmonary bypass (CPB). Simple lesions, not requiring work within the heart, such as pulmonary artery banding and PDA ligation, can usually be performed without CPB. As the surgical complexity increases, CPB is required to give the surgeon maximum control of the operative field without compromising systemic perfusion and oxygenation, control temperature and acid, base and electrolyte balance whilst allowing the heart to beat empty. CPB requires complete systemic anticoagulation that is later reversed with protamine sulphate.

Intracardiac repair or surgery requiring a still heart and bloodless field necessitates cross-clamping the aorta and diastolic cardiac arrest using crystalloid or blood cardioplegia, containing high concentrations of potassium. In some complex cases (e.g. aortic arch repair and complex intracardiac neonatal repair), the circulation may be stopped entirely using deep hypothermic circulatory arrest. This requires systemic cooling to temperatures of 15–18°C and is tolerated for periods up to 45 minutes in children.

Surgical repair frequently requires the placement of patches, valves and conduits made from autologous tissue (e.g. the patient's own pericardium), homografts, heterografts (bovine pericardium, porcine or bovine valves or conduits) or synthetic material (e.g. Dacron or Gortex). The child may be treated with an antiplatelet drug, such as aspirin or dipyridamole, to prolong the life of the tissue patches or prevent thrombus formation. Similarly children with mechanical prosthetic valves will be taking warfarin to prevent thrombus formation. This should not be stopped or omitted without consultation with the child's cardiac centre. In addition, such foreign tissue may become infected and advice should be sought regarding antibiotic prophylaxis at times of invasive procedures or surgery.

Tetralogy of Fallot and transposition of the great arteries are two commonly occurring conditions that demonstrate many of the principles of paediatric cardiac surgery.

Tetralogy of Fallot

Epidemiology and pathology

Tetralogy of Fallot is the most common cyanotic heart condition and accounts for 5–10% of all congenital heart diseases. The condition is characterised by a large VSD, an overriding aorta, right ventricular outflow tract obstruction (RVOTO) and secondary right ventricular hypertrophy.

Clinical features

The heterogeneity of this condition is such that it may present in the neonatal period due to severe RVOTO, with limited pulmonary blood flow being dependent upon ductal blood flow. More commonly children present within the first year of life, with cyanosis due to right to left shunting via the VSD, as the RVOTO worsens. Classically the children may have episodes of acute desaturation, with cyanotic 'spells' secondary to muscular spasm of the RVOTO.

Investigations

The diagnosis is made using echocardiography. If there are concerns about the size of the branch pulmonary arteries or coronary artery pattern, then angiography or MRI may be undertaken.

Treatment

Historically, the condition was palliated with a systemic–pulmonary artery shunt (the Blalock–Taussig shunt) to provide additional pulmonary blood flow until the child was considered old enough for definite repair. This is now much less commonly performed, and usually reserved for small neonates where complete repair may be difficult. Currently, surgical repair is generally performed at 4–5 months of age when the child is around 6–7 kg in weight. The operation is performed via a median sternotomy on CPB. The VSD is closed using a prosthetic patch, working through the tricuspid valve via the right atrium. The right outflow tract is enlarged by dividing and resecting muscle bundles, but usually also requires the placement of a patch across the small pulmonary artery to establish an adequate size outflow tract from the right ventricle.

The procedure restores normal anatomy and physiology and is associated with 98–99% survival. However, children need regular follow-up because they tend to develop increasing pulmonary regurgitation across the reconstructed outflow tract, with consequent dilatation of the right heart. This is well tolerated and produces minimal symptoms, but most patients eventually require a pulmonary valve replacement in early adulthood to restore pulmonary competence. This is a good example of the need for specialist follow-up and life-long surveillance in congenital heart disease.

Transposition of the great arteries

Epidemiology and pathology

The defect consists of transposed great vessels, with the aorta arising from the right ventricle and the pulmonary artery from the left ventricle, creating two parallel circulations. Adequate mixing of right and left circulations is required for survival, and this can occur via an ASD, VSD or PDA.

Clinical features

Increasingly this condition is detected antenatally, and the child is commenced on a prostaglandin infusion (Prostin) at birth to maintain the PDA to ensure adequate mixing between circulations. The baby will be cyanosed and, if undetected, their condition may worsen when the duct closes spontaneously, especially if an adequate ASD or VSD to enable mixing is not present.

Investigations

Echocardiography is the investigation of choice.

Treatment

Without intervention the condition is fatal. Mixing of the circulations is promoted by maintaining the PDA using a prostaglandin infusion, and a balloon atrial septostomy may be required to stretch or create an ASD to stabilise the circulation. Surgical repair is planned within the first 2 weeks of life before the left ventricle looses muscle mass and 'involutes' due to pumping against the lower pressure pulmonary circulation.

Surgery is performed on CPB and involves dividing and mobilising the great arteries, swapping them around and reanastomosing them to achieve anatomical correction. In addition, the coronary arteries, which arise from the native aorta from the right ventricle, have to be excised from the aorta, mobilised and then reimplanted into the root of the pulmonary artery which will become the neoaorta, thereby restoring them to the systemic circulation. This is the arterial switch procedure, which has an operative mortality < 1% and restores normal physiology. These children will continue to need surveillance because some may develop valvular regurgitation or arterial narrowing at the site of the original surgery. However, such problems are very rare, and current outcomes suggest that > 95% of these children would now be expected to reach adulthood without requiring any further intervention, with entirely normal physiology and quality of life.

Further reading

Stark JF, De Leval MR, Tsang VT (eds). Surgery for congenital heart defects, 3rd ed. Oxford: Wiley, 2006

Paediatric gynaecology

Learning outcomes

- To understand the range of gynaecology presenting to paediatric surgery
- To define disease-specific aetiology
- To be able to form a management plan

Labial adhesions

Epidemiology and pathology

Labial adhesions should be considered an acquired rather than a congenital condition, as they were not identified in 9000 female neonates – most often found between 6 months and 6 years, with peak around 2 years. It is thought to develop as oestrogen levels fall and irritation occurs.

Clinical features

Generally it is asymptomatic but found on routine assessment or at catheter insertion for another purpose. Careful assessment is needed to ensure that the 'dark line' of a patent vagina can be seen behind the adhesions.

Treatment

If left alone, the adhesions will separate as oestrogens rise at puberty. Various creams (oestrogen, Vaseline) can be used, but the main benefit is from the pressure of the finger which applies the cream, causing physical separation. The adhesions will recur (even after separation under general anaesthetic) if the area is allowed to become soggy, so waterproofing with Vaseline should continue after separation.

Vaginal foreign bodies

Epidemiology and pathology

Vaginal foreign bodies are most common in the toddler age group where foreign bodies range from plugs of tissue to crayons and small toys. Non-accidental injury should always be considered.

Aetiology

The presence of the foreign body leads to irritation and possible secondary bacterial infection.

Clinical features

Most common symptom is discharge though this can take some time to be recognised. The younger the child, the more likely that a foreign body is implicated.

Investigations

Gentle clinical examination, if irritation is a marked feature, may be better conducted under anaesthesia.

Treatment

Examination is carried out under anaesthetic, with endoscopic inspection of the vagina and removal of the foreign body. Microbiological swabs should be taken before endoscopic irrigation begins.

Ovarian or fimbrial cysts

The objective should be to preserve as much ovarian tissue as possible.

Epidemiology and pathology

Ovarian cysts can arise from all three ovarian cell lines:

- Mesenchyme of the urogenital ridge
- Germinal epithelium that covers that mesenchyme
- Germ cells

These are the same cell lines that are needed to form the follicles (16–20 weeks' gestation) which persist into adult life stimulated by oestrogens. In utero stimulation results from maternal oestrogens, placental human chorionic gonadotropin (HCG) and fetal gonadotropins. After birth, the stimulation can be the result of normal oestrogen activation in menarche, or oestrogens, arising from an abnormal source. Ultrasound is the most useful investigation, with MRI rarely performed.

Aetiology

Variable oestrogen levels cause the follicular cells to secrete fluid which accumulates and is identified as a 'cyst'.
It is best regarded in three phases – fetal, premenarchal and postpubertal.

- Fetal

- Clinical features: This is usually picked up coincidentally at booking scan or late scanning for other reasons
- Treatment: This depends on size, with 4–5 cm usually being taken as the point above which spontaneous resolution is unlikely. Postnatal intervention depends on diagnostic confidence and/or failure of resolution. Intervention is influenced by the presence of a solid component, giving rise to the suspicion of cystic teratoma. Arguments are made to operate to prevent the heavy cyst from causing torsion of the ovary and tube, leading to loss. Even when torsion of the ovary is presumed to have happened prenatally, there can be confusion between torsion and bleeding into an ovarian cyst, which will resolve. Surgeons who have taken the decision to keep the asymptomatic patient under ultrasound review have been pleased to see the resolution of the cystic lesion and clear evidence of two ovaries. Surgery (whether open or laparoscopic) almost invariably leads to ipsilateral oophorectomy

- Premenarchal: Malignant ovarian lesions in this age group are rarely cystic
  - Clinical features: Of girls younger than 8 years having pelvic ultrasound examination for another reason, 2–3% will have cysts identified. If these are < 1 cm, they should be considered normal. If precocious puberty is what has brought the child to attention, then the ovarian cyst may well be significant
  - Treatment: Cysts which are hormonally active, do not resolve on serial ultrasound, are complex in nature or are symptomatic require excision. At the time of surgery, simple cysts, or hormonally active cysts with normal alpha-fetoprotein (α-FP) and β-HCG, may be considered suitable for deroofing or excision with ovarian sparing

- Postpubertal: in this group, follicles develop up to 2–3 cm in the first half of the cycle and subside in the second half. If ovulation does not occur, the cyst may persist and continue to expand in each succeeding cycle. The corpus luteum (which results when the follicle ruptures mid cycle) can also persist and continue to expand (though usually not to such large dimensions – 6 cm) and can then rupture and bleed significantly
  - Clinical features: It is usually pain that brings girls to seek help, though irregular periods and a palpable mass may feature. In a large series in 1995, > 90% of even the large cysts resolved spontaneously
  - Treatment: In the first instance, they should be observed for resolution. Hormonal suppression (with oral contraceptives) has nothing to contribute. The debate regarding torsion, if the cyst is large, continues. If the cyst is complex, the question of dermoid cyst arises and α-FP and β-HCG should be measured. The distinction between a solid lesion and a bleed into a cyst takes two to three cycles to determine, as the clot lyses and a fluid level develops. Taken with a normal α-FP and β-HCG, then dermoid is most unlikely and ovarian sparing surgery should be attempted

Hydrocolpos and imperforate hymen

Epidemiology and pathology

Incidence is between 1:1000 and 1:10,000. It results from a failure of canalisation of the tissue, marking the junction of the upper and lower vagina.

Aetiology

- 5th embryonic week: Wolffian ducts connect mesonephros to cloaca
- 6th embryonic week: Müllerian ducts develop lateral to Wolffian and move into midline caudal to the mesonephros
- 7th embryonic week: Urorectal septum separates rectum from urogenital sinus
- 9th embryonic week: Müllerian ducts continue caudally and merge into urogenital sinus
- 12th embryonic week: Müllerian ducts fuse to form primitive uterovaginal canal

– proximal portion becomes fimbria and Fallopian tubes, and distal portion forms uterus and upper vagina. This must connect with an indentation (the vaginal plate) which canalises from caudal to cranial by the 5th embryonic month to form the distal vagina. The point of contact represents the hymen which canalises just before or shortly after birth

Clinical features

Hydrocolpos and imperforate hymen depend on when the problem is identified; they are occasionally found antenatally, with distension of the vagina on ultrasound. Because the vagina above the hymen fills with secretions, it can be seen as a bulge at the introitus. If this compresses the bladder or rectum, urinary or bowel symptoms can develop. The most common presentation is with delayed menarche, cyclical lower abdominal pain as the vagina fills with the fluids which cannot escape, and eventually a lower abdominal mass.

Investigations

Usually it is obvious on clinical examination which can be supplemented with ultrasound scanning and MRI.

Treatment

If picked up coincidentally before puberty, surgery should be planned after its onset because the rise in oestrogens will prevent closure. If identified due to symptoms, it will require early intervention with the possible need for further surgery at a later stage.

Further reading

Brandt ML,Helmrath MA. Ovarian cysts in infants and children. Semin Pediatr Surg 2005; 15:78–85.

Kanizsai B, Orley J, Szigetvari I, et al. Ovarian cysts in children and adolescents: their occurrence, behaviour and management. J Pediatric Adolesc Gynecol 1998; 11:85–88.

Leung AK, Robson WL, Tay-Uyboco J. The incidence of labial fusion in children. J Paediatr Child Health 1993; 29:235–236.

Paediatric neurosurgery

Learning outcomes

- To be aware of the range of conditions presenting to paediatric neurosurgery
- To understand the pathophysiology, classification and management of hydrocephalus
- To understand the embryology and management of myelomeningocele

Overview of the specialty

Paediatric neurosurgery is a specialist discipline dealing with the central nervous system. Conditions presenting include tumours, hydrocephalus and epilepsy. Amongst other things paediatric neurosurgeons can undertake procedures for epilepsy, place shunts to drain cerebrospinal fluid (CSF) and insert baclofen pumps for children with spastic conditions.

Two conditions common to the speciality are described below.

Hydrocephalus

Overview

Hydrocephalus is the abnormal accumulation of CSF within the ventricle and subarachnoid spaces, which is often associated with dilatation of ventricles, causing pressure on the adjacent cerebral tissue. It mostly occurs as a result of interruption of CSF flow but rarely can also be due to increased production.

Hydrocephalus is classified as follows:

- **Non-communicating:** In this case, the flow of CSF from the ventricles to subarachnoid space is obstructed. Thus, there is no communication between the ventricular system and the subarachnoid space. The most common cause of this is aqueduct of Sylvian blockage
- **Communicating:** In this case, the flow is not obstructed, but CSF is inadequately reabsorbed in the subarachnoid space. Thus, there is communication between the ventricular system and the subarachnoid space. The most common

cause of this group is postinfective and posthaemorrhagic hydrocephalus

Epidemiology

The exact incidence is unknown, but the incidence of isolated congenital hydrocephalus is 1–3 in 1000 live births.

Clinical features

Patient presentation varies depending on age.

- Premature infants: accelerated head circumference, tense fontanelle, widened sutures, distended scalp veins, apnoeic episodes and bradycardia, 'Sun setting' sign
- Infants: accelerated head circumference, irritability, vomiting, drowsiness, distended scalp veins, 'Sun setting' sign
- Toddlers and older children: Headache, vomiting, lethargy, diplopia, papilloedema, lateral rectus palsy

Investigations

- MRI brain scan is the investigation of choice.
- CT head scan is more commonly used because of easy availability and access
- Cranial ultrasound can be used in infants with open fontanelles

Differential diagnosis

- Ex vacuo dilatation of ventricles
- Arrested hydrocephalus

Treatment

- Non-surgical
  - Serial lumbar punctures or ventricular puncture can be used to temporise the progressive ventriculomegaly in premature infants with intraventricular bleed
- Surgical
  - Non-shunting options
    - Third ventriculostomy
    - Excision of the obstructing lesion
  - Shunting options
    - Ventriculoperitoneal
    - Ventriculoatrial
    - Ventriculopleural (now very rarely used)

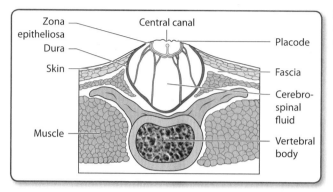

Figure 51 Cross-sectional view of an open meningomyelocoele showing the anatomy.

Myelomeningocoele

Overview

Myelomeningocoele is the most common significant birth defect involving the spine (**Figure 51**). Its aetiology remains unknown, but there is evidence to suggest that both genetics and environment do play a role. Evidence suggests that periconceptional folic acid intake by mothers decreases the incidence of spina bifida.

Embryology

This defect manifests between 3 and 4 weeks of gestation. The neural plate folds into the neural tube (neurulation) which begins in the dorsal midline and proceeds both cephalad and caudal simultaneously. The last portion of tube to close is the posterior end (neuropore) at 28 days, and failure of the closure or reopening due to distension with cerebrospinal fluid, causes myelomeningocoele.

Management

1. Assessment and management
   I. Measure the defect and assess whether it is ruptured or unruptured
   II. If ruptured, commence broad-spectrum antibiotics
   III. Cover the lesion with sponges or gauze soaked in normal saline and then cover with a non-adhesive plastic cover (such as cling film)
   IV. Nurse the baby prone on the stomach in Trendelenburg position
   V. Consider closing the defect within 36–72 hours
2. Neurological assessment
   I. Watch for spontaneous movement in the lower limbs and perform a neurological examination by checking the pain response in the lower limbs
   II. Measure head circumference daily
   III. Check external genitalia and if the anus is patulous. Also see if there is urinary dribbling which can indicate the status of the bladder sphincter
   IV. Babies need to be to be started on regular clean intermittent catheterisation, and an ultrasound of the renal tract and bladder along with a urological consultation should be obtained once the lesion is repaired
   V. Orthopaedic consultation is to be obtained because these babies can have associated hip, knee and foot deformities
   VI. Cranial or spinal imaging should be arranged (non-emergent)

Further reading

Dias MS, McLone DG. Myelomeningocele. In: Leland Albright A, Pollack IF, David Adelson P (eds) Principles and practice of pediatric neurosurgery, 2nd edn. New York: Thieme Medical Publishers, 2007:338–366.

Sutton L. Spinal dysraphism. In: Rengachary SS, Ellenbogen RG (eds), Principles of neurosurgery, 2nd Edn. Philadelphia: Elsevier Publishers, 2005:99–115.

Wang PP, Avellino AM. Hydrocephalus in children. In: Rengachary SS, Ellenbogen RG (eds), Principles of neurosurgery, 2nd edn. Philadelphia: Elsevier Publishers, 2005:117–135.

Related topics of interest

- Bladder dysfunction (p. 31)

Paediatric ophthalmology

Learning objectives

- To know the initial evaluation of the eye
- To appreciate the range of conditions
- To be aware of the conditions requiring ophthalmological input

Overview

The eye is a complex sensory organ and is affected in several developmental brain disorders. The development of the eye is complete at 7 months of gestation. The first few years of life are crucial for visual development. Adequate stimulation of both eyes in the first 6–8 years of life is essential to achieve normal visual acuity as adults.

Examination and assessment of visual acuity

Visual acuity tests for children must be age appropriate, and include preferential looking tests (e.g. teller cards) or picture and letter recognition charts. Other useful observational clues to vision include interest in human faces, social smile, stranger anxiety and navigation around obstacles.

- External examination – for dysmorphic features like low set or slanted eyelids and palpebral fissures, wide set eyes (telecanthus), lid colobomas, squint, ptosis (droopy eyelids) or abnormal eye size, e.g. microphthalmos
- Direct ophthalmoscopy – a very useful screening tool to detect cataracts as well as tumours (retinoblastoma)
- Eye movement testing – assess the centration and symmetry of the light reflex (Hirschberg corneal reflex test) to screen for squint. Eye movements can be tested with a toy or light
- Refraction and fundus examination – usually performed by the ophthalmologist

Common conditions

Squint

The term 'squint' (or strabismus) refers to misalignment of the eyes, and may be horizontal, vertical or both. An inward turn of the eye is a convergent squint (esotropia), while an outward turn is a divergent squint (exotropia). The eyes can deviate for the first 2–3 months while the fixation system is still developing (neonatal ocular misalignment), and these can be observed unless there are concerns about the child's vision. Persistence beyond 3 months warrants referral to the ophthalmologist. Neurogenic causes include nerve palsy (IIIrd, IVth or VIth) or skew deviation following intracranial pathology, such as tumours or trauma.

Treatment of squint

- Correct refractive error with spectacles or contact lenses
- Treatment of amblyopia with occlusion (patching) of the better seeing eye
- Surgery if spectacles do not correct the squint, to preserve or restore binocular vision, and to improve cosmesis

Abnormal eye movements

Abnormal eye movements may be rhythmic, to and fro (nystagmus) or random (nystagmoid). Nystagmoid movements indicate extremely poor visual function. All such cases should be referred to an ophthalmologist to look for a cause. Acquired nystagmus merits urgent referral and a head CT scan.

Refractive errors in childhood

Refractive errors are common in childhood (up to 5%). These include hypermetropia (long-sighted), myopia (short-sighted) and astigmatism. Significant errors should be corrected with glasses (or contact lenses where appropriate) to provide clear vision, and prevent amblyopia (lazy eye).

Retinopathy of prematurity

Premature birth interferes with normal retinal vascularisation, with risk of abnormal retinal vascular proliferation that can cause retinal scarring and/or detachment – retinopathy of prematurity (ROP).

Babies < 32 weeks' gestation or birth weight ≤ 1500 g are at risk of ROP, and fortnightly screening examinations are recommended (UK ROP Guidelines May 2008, Royal College of Ophthalmologists and RCPCH). Most cases do not require treatment, but ROP beyond a certain threshold will require prompt laser treatment of the avascular retina to reduce risk of visual loss.

Delayed visual maturation

The visual pathways can take a few months to mature in some cases, and more so with coexistent developmental delay. Most cases improve spontaneously by 6 months of age. If there is no improvement, or if there are abnormal eye movements, brain scan and electrodiagnostic testing electroretinography and visual evoked potentials are indicated.

Cataracts in childhood

Congenital (present at birth) or developmental (occur later) cataracts can be unilateral or bilateral. There may be a metabolic or systemic cause in bilateral cases (and must be investigated), although most are genetic or unexplained. If visually significant, early surgery within weeks can maximise vision. Considerable aftercare is needed, including spectacles, or contact lenses, with lifelong follow-up.

Glaucoma in childhood

Childhood glaucoma is a blinding illness, and can present with watering, enlargement of the eye and photophobia. The treatment is primarily surgical, with additional medical treatment as needed. Lifelong follow-up is required and multiple operations are common.

Ocular trauma – accidental and non-accidental

Accidental ocular trauma is rare in young children. Accidental chemical injuries and burns can occur in toddlers, but one must rule out non-accidental causes or neglect. The eyelids usually protect the ocular surface, and corneal burns are very rare. Chemical injuries need urgent prolonged washout with water and saline, followed by steroid and antibiotic eyedrops. Thermal burns need specialist care because eyelid contracture can result in ectropion and corneal exposure.

Non-accidental injury (NAI) or abusive head injury are terms commonly used to describe physical abuse, often involving shaking injury, with or without impact. Children with suspected NAI should receive eye examination by an experienced ophthalmologist looking for external evidence of trauma, and dilated fundoscopy for retinal haemorrhages. Accurate documentation, with retinal photography where available, is essential.

Eyelid disorders

Colobomas (partial absence of eyelid) can be isolated or occur as part of facial clefting disorders or syndromes. Surgical repair is necessary but rarely urgent. Dermoid cysts are commonly seen at the medial or lateral orbital rim. Surgical excision is indicated for large or growing dermoid cysts. Chalazia (meibomian cysts) are common in children, often presenting with localised swelling and inflammation of the eyelid margin. Treatment is usually conservative, with surgery needed in resistant cases.

Orbital cellulitis

Orbital cellulitis is common in children because the thin bone between the paranasal sinuses (ethmoid or maxillary) and the orbit permits easy passage of infective organisms. Preseptal (anterior) cellulitis responds well to intravenous antibiotics, but orbital (posterior) cellulitis needs close monitoring (CT scan if there is proptosis) and surgical drainage of abscess where indicated. Orbital rhabdomyosarcoma can present with inflammatory signs, and orbital cellulitis unresponsive to medical management needs imaging.

Congenital globe malformations – anophthalmia and microphthalmia

The choroidal fissure closes at 7 weeks, and incomplete closure can result in chorioretinal and/or optic nerve colobomas. They may be unilateral or bilateral, incomplete or complete, and affect the iris (keyhole pupils) or retina and choroid (producing a white reflex on fundus photographs) which can also affect the vision.

Acute red eye

Acute red eye in a child warrants urgent assessment. Trauma (often chemical) and foreign bodies (corneal or subtarsal) must be considered in the differential diagnosis, as should infective conjunctivitis. Inflammation and glaucoma are rare causes.

Painful eye

Accompanying photophobia (light aversion) and redness indicates an ocular surface problem (corneal foreign body, abrasion or ulcer) or subtarsal foreign body. Inflamed meibomian cysts or stye (hordeolum externum or infected eyelash follicle) can also cause periocular pain.

Paediatric orthopaedic surgery

Learning outcomes

- To be able to recognise the most common paediatric orthopaedic conditions that may cause a limp in a child
- To be aware of the management options available and indications for surgery
- To be able to provide first aid care prior to referral to the orthopaedic service

Overview

The clinician providing musculoskeletal care must be able to decipher sinister or joint threatening causes from the more stable, sometimes self-limiting cause of a limp in a child. Traumatic causes are beyond the scope of this Topic. We discuss some of the most common differentials of an atraumatic limp in a child.

Bone and joint infections

Bone and joint infections are common and are associated with significant morbidity and mortality. Early diagnosis and timely treatment is essential to prevent chronic illness and irreversible joint destruction.

Epidemiology and aetiology

Septic arthritis (SA) is an infection of the synovium and joint space. In children the incidence ranges from 2 to 12 per 100,000. Most cases occur in the first and second years of life, and the male–female ratio is 2:1. Osteomyelitis is a bone infection and has a similar prevalence.

Bacteria enter the bone or joint by direct inoculation or haematogenous spread. SA can develop from osteomyelitis especially in neonates where infection spreads from the metaphysis through transepiphyseal blood vessels. The hip joint is one of the most frequently affected joints, with its deep anatomical location, making joint swelling impossible to identify. The femoral head has a precarious blood supply, and the results of infections can potentially be disastrous.

The causative organism depends on patient age. *Staphylococcus aureus* is the most commonly implicated organism for both septic arthritis and osteomyelitis across all age groups. *Streptococcus* sp. is the second most frequent, with *Haemophilus influenzae* playing a prominent role prior to immunization. There is a small but steady incidence of methicillin-resistant *S. aureus* and an increasing trend for Panton–Valentine leukocidin *Staphylococcus* and Gram-negatives, including *Kingella kingae*.

Clinical features

Symptoms often develop over several hours.
- A history lasting several days is unusual unless patients have been partially treated with oral antibiotics
- Fever, pain, swelling, limited movements of the affected joints and often inability to weight bear
- Blood inflammatory markers may also be deranged

The main differential diagnosis is transient synovitis: a reactive arthritis often secondary to upper respiratory tract infection (URTI), ear infection or urinary tract infection. It is self-limiting.

Investigations

- X-rays:
  - SA: normal or osteopenia
  - Osteomyelitis: periosteal reaction or lytic lesions (may take several days to appear)
- Ultrasound scans (USS):
  - Detect fluid effusions (although cannot differentiate between purulent or reactive effusion) with a positive result an indication for surgery
- Magnetic resonance imaging (MRI):
  - 100% sensitive, 75% specific for joint effusions, soft tissue changes and bone infection
  - If USS rules out joint effusion, MRI is indicated to rule out osteomyelitis, Legg-Calve–Perthes (LCP) disease and psoas abscess

Treatment

The standard of care is expedient surgical drainage of any collection followed by antibiotics. Blood cultures and joint samples should be obtained before commencing antibiotic treatment to maximise the possibility of isolating the causative bacteria. In confirmed cases of septic arthritis, the joint fluid white cell count is usually > 50,000 mm^3.

Traditionally, antibiotics were given for several weeks or months. Recent studies suggest that a 3 days' course of intravenous antibiotics, followed by a 3 weeks' course of oral, is sufficient in two-thirds of uncomplicated acute SA and osteomyelitis.

Antibiotic treatment is based on clinical presentation, likely organisms and the results of microbiological investigations. Empirical treatment is started with high-dose intravenous flucloxacillin and can be adjusted based on microbial tests. The mainstay of treatment of acute osteomyelitis is antibiotic therapy and surgical drainage of collections.

If treated promptly the majority make a full recovery. Diagnostic delay leads to irreversible hip avascular necrosis (AVN), resulting in stiffness, leg length discrepancy and joint replacement in early adult life.

Developmental dysplasia of the hip

Dysplasia of the hip (DDH) refers to a spectrum of disorders of the growing hip, ranging from a subtle hip or acetabular dysplasia with an enlocated hip through to more severe forms of dysplasia associated with frank dislocation.

Epidemiology and aetiology

The incidence is variable due to inconsistencies in definition, screening tools used and study populations. Estimated prevalence rates range from 1.3 in 1000 in unscreened populations to 34 in 1000 in populations screened by both clinical and ultrasonographic examinations.

The precise aetiology is unknown, but mechanical, hormonal and genetic factors are implicated. Breech presentation, positive family history, female sex, first-born status and oligohydramnios are all recognised risk factors. Eighty percent are girls, with the left hip more commonly affected.

Clinical features

In neonates, the Ortolani and Barlow tests are screening tools to assess hip stability clinically, but even in expert hands, they may fail to identify 50% of cases and will miss potentially stable dysplastic hips. Both tests will miss a dislocated irreducible hip or a stable but shallow hip (acetabular dysplasia). In the older child
- Limited hip abduction in 90° of flexion is the most sensitive indicator
- Limp and leg length discrepancy in the second year of life

The condition is not associated with pain until arthritis develops in adolescence or early adult life.

Investigations

Femoral head ossification occurs at 4–6 months so neonatal X-rays are of limited use. USS makes an accurate assessment of the cartilaginous static anatomy of the femoral head and acetabulum as well as dynamic hip stability. It is 100% sensitive and specific. In the UK, only babies at risk (breech, family history) have routine scans although in certain parts of Europe all babies are scanned at birth.

Treatment

Treatment is easier and more effective the earlier it starts. Non-operative treatment – abduction brace or harness (Pavlik) – is successful in > 90% if diagnosed in the first 3 months of life.

In a clinically dislocated hip confirmed by ultrasound, treatment is commenced immediately. Dysplastic, enlocated hips can be observed with USS until 6 weeks because many resolve spontaneously.

Surgery is indicated if non-operative treatment fails or in children diagnosed late. Closed reduction under anaesthetic confirmed with an arthrogram may be possible up to about 1 year age. The reduction has to be maintained in a cast (hip spica) for 3–4 months. If this is not possible, open reduction is performed involving
- Release of tight adductors, psoas tendon, capsule, ligamentum teres and transverse ligament

- Postoperative immobilisation in hip spica

In children older than 18 months, the shallow acetabulum (dysplastic) will often not resolve even once the femoral head is enlocated. A pelvic osteotomy is then indicated either at the primary surgery or later. In children presenting at > 30 months, a femoral shortening osteotomy is also needed to allow reduction of the femoral head without pressure.

Slipped capital femoral epiphysis

Slipped capital femoral epiphysis (SCFE) refers to a separation of the femoral capital epiphysis and the metaphysis of the femoral neck through the intervening physis (growth plate). It has been postulated that the growth plate widens and the femoral head displaces posteriorly and inferiorly in the vast majority of cases.

Epidemiology and aetiology

The incidence varies according to sex, race and geographic location. Reported prevalence rates vary from 0.2 in 100,000 to 10 in 100,000, depending on the study population. It is more common in males than females and in blacks than Caucasians. The average age at diagnosis tends to coincide with the period of maximal skeletal growth (14 years for boys and 12 years for girls).

The cause is unknown in the vast majority, but several factors are implicated. Mechanical factors (obesity, relative or absolute femoral retroversion, increased obliquity of the growth plate relative to the femoral neck and shaft) combine with biological factors (endocrine) to create a weakened growth plate which predisposes it to failure.

Clinical assessment

- Limp and groin, hip, thigh or knee pain
- Acute or chronic (months) onset

Acute slips may be associated with damage to the vascular supply to the head of the femur

(AVN). Unstable slips (defined by inability to weight bear due to pain) are associated with 50% incidence of AVN.

Investigations

- Anteroposterior and frog-leg lateral X-rays of both hips demonstrate posterior inferior displacement of the epiphysis relative to the metaphysis. A subtle, early slip can easily be missed if lateral views are not taken
- Computed tomography can identify significant risk factors, e.g. femoral neck retroversion
- MRI is needed if concerns about the state of health (AVN) of the femoral epiphysis preoperatively

Management

The primary aim of first aid for SCFE patients is to prevent further progression of the slip and minimise the risk of complications. Patients should be provided with non-weight-bearing crutches or a wheelchair, pending access to an orthopaedic surgeon. Surgery is required on the next available operating list. Definitive surgical intervention depends on slip severity:

- Mild or moderate slips – single screw in situ fixation with the advantages of percutaneous pin placement and low incidence of further slippage, AVN and chondrolysis
- Severe SCFE management is more controversial
  - In situ fixation will improve pain in the short term, but risks of osteoarthritis due to impingement are high
  - As a result, surgical correction of the deformity by an osteotomy through the femoral neck has become popular. This surgery carries a risk of inducing AVN of about 10%

In patients presenting later with pain following previous SCFE, intertrochanteric osteotomies will reliably restore leg length and range of internal rotation. Such surgery is often worthwhile up to age 20 years, but many patients will require joint replacement in middle age.

Legg–Calvé–Perthes (LCP) disease

Epidemiology and aetiology

LCP disease is relatively common, with reported prevalence rates ranging from 5 in 100,000 to 17 in 100,000 children, depending on geographical location. It can affect a wide age range of children, but is most common between 4 and 8 years, with a male:female ratio of 4:1. It is bilateral in 10–15% of affected patients.

Aetiology is unknown although vascular insufficiency, repetitive microtrauma and skeletal retardation have been proposed. The outcome is AVN of the femoral head. The blood supply recovers over a period of 2–4 years, but during this period the femoral head becomes soft and deformable and the long-term prognosis is directly related to its residual deformity.

Clinical assessment

- A limp with groin, thigh or knee pain that may be related to physical activity
- Symptoms usually slowly evolve over several weeks
- Isolated knee pain without groin pain may occur, leading to a delay in diagnosis

Careful examination of the hip is required in all limping children regardless of the suspected aetiology. Physical examination may show

- Antalgic or Trendelenburg gait
- Limited abduction and internal rotation of the hip
- If chronic, wasting of the thigh and calf muscles
- Leg length discrepancy

Radiological assessment

X-rays are generally diagnostic although they may be normal for the first few weeks. LCP passes through stages of sclerosis, fragmentation, reossification and remodelling which can be seen radiographically. Disease severity can be graded by the degree of collapse.

Treatment

Main objectives are to

- Obtain and maintain containment of the femoral head within the acetabulum
- Maintain a good range of motion

Since the acetabulum is not primarily affected, it acts as a mould maintaining a spherical femoral head. Surgical intervention in children younger than 7 years has no long-term benefit over conservative treatment. Older children with grade B disease have been shown to have superior results, with containment surgery either by femoral varus osteotomy or Salter pelvic osteotomy.

Differential diagnosis of the limping child (atraumatic)

The conditions above are not exhaustive, and there is a wider differential diagnosis in the limping child. For example, intra-abdominal pathology (psoas abscess) and testicular torsion may present as a limp.

- Infective or Inflammatory
  - Transient synovitis
  - SA
  - Osteomyelitis
  - Juvenile idiopathic arthritis
  - Psoas abscess
  - Discitis
- Neurological
  - Cerebral palsy
  - Muscular dystrophy
- Anatomical
  - DDH
  - LCP
  - SCFE
  - Limb length discrepancy
- Neoplasms
  - Osteoid osteoma
  - Leukaemia

Further reading

Aronsson DD, et al. Slipped capital femoral epiphysis: current concepts. J Am Acad Orthop Surg 2006; 14:666–679.

Dezateux C, Rosendahl K. Developmental dysplasia of the hip. Lancet 2007; 369:1541–1552.

Kim HK. Pathophysiology and new strategies for the treatment of Legg–Calvé–Perthes disease. J Bone Joint Surg Am 2012; 94:659–669.

Paediatric otorhinolaryngology

Learning outcomes

- To have an overview of the breadth of paediatric ear, nose and throat (ENT) surgery
- To understand the details of two conditions within the speciality

Overview

Paediatric ENT surgeons, in addition to managing conditions involving the ears, nose and throat, undertake assessment and management of congenital and acquired conditions affecting the airway, breathing, swallowing, skull base and head and neck. Although a detailed history and examination remains vital, improvement in microscopic and endoscopic techniques has revolutionised clinical assessment and management of many conditions. The introduction of implantable devices has transformed the lives of deaf children.

Children with syndromes, such as CHARGE (coloboma, heart defects, atresia choanae, growth and/or developmental retardation, genitourinary abnormalities, ear abnormalities and deafness), craniofacial and Down syndrome, require ENT input as part of their multidisciplinary management.

ENT procedures account for 40% of all surgery on children and range from simple procedures, such as adenotonsillectomy, to complex endoscopic nasal tumour surgery, implantable hearing devices and ear surgery, laryngotracheal surgery and head and neck surgery on branchial and lymphovascular malformations. In some centres this includes cleft palate repair.

Two conditions with particular relevance to paediatric surgery are discussed here.

Laryngomalacia

Anatomically the larynx is divided into the supraglottis (epiglottis, aryepiglottic folds, false cords and laryngeal ventricles), glottis (vocal cords) and subglottis (from the undersurface of the vocal cords to the inferior border of the cricoid cartilage).

Laryngomalacia predisposes to partial or complete collapse of the supraglottic structures during inspiration, causing airway obstruction.

Epidemiology and pathology

Congenital abnormalities of the airway occur in 1 in 10,000 to 1 in 50,000 births, and 20% have a second airway anomaly. Laryngomalacia is the most common cause of congenital stridor. The pathophysiology remains unclear, but the following anatomical abnormalities of the supraglottis are common:

- A long, curled (omega-shaped) epiglottis which may be soft
- Tall, bulky, floppy arytenoid tissue
- Short aryepiglottic folds

These features result in a tall, narrow supraglottis. The negative pressure generated during inspiration causes the epiglottis and the redundant arytenoid mucosa to collapse into the airway, obstructing it. Neuromuscular discoordination may also contribute.

Clinical features

A characteristic high-pitched, fluttering inspiratory stridor is usually present at, or shortly after, birth. It is exacerbated when the infant is active, upset or feeding and may reduce with rest or during sleep.

Increased work of breathing (tracheal tug, intercostal, costal and subcostal recession) may be evident. This may cause or exacerbate gastro-oesophageal reflux (GOR) which in turn compounds supraglottic oedema and alters laryngeal sensation. Desaturation and cyanosis is not unusual. The airway obstruction, altered laryngeal sensation and increased work of breathing impacts on the infant's ability to coordinate breathing with swallowing, leading to feeding difficulties, failure to thrive (FTT) and/or aspiration.

Comorbidities, such as a syndromic or congenital cardiac, respiratory or neurological disease, compound the symptoms and may lead to cor pulmonale.

Prolonged sternal and costal recession increases the risk of permanent chest deformity (pectus excavatum).

Investigations

- Outpatient transnasal or transoral flexible fibreoptic laryngoscopy demonstrates supraglottic collapse during inspiration
- Laryngotracheobronchoscopy (LTB) under general anaesthesia if the diagnosis is in doubt or a second anomaly is suspected
- Other indications for LTB include
  - Stridor that is severe enough to cause cyanosis
  - Biphasic or expiratory component to the stridor
  - Aspiration or FTT
- During LTB the larynx, trachea, carina and main bronchi are examined for a concurrent pathology. Then, under light anaesthesia, with the beak of the laryngoscope in the vallecula, the collapse of supraglottic structures on inspiration is witnessed

Treatment

In 90%, the condition is mild and self-limiting although their symptoms may worsen as the child becomes more active in the first 3–12 months of life. Symptoms diminish and usually disappear by 2 years of age. Very rarely it may persist until later in childhood.

The child is given antireflux medication until weaned onto solids or the reflux settles. Surgery is required for severe laryngomalacia – where there is significant respiratory distress, feeding difficulty with FTT or recurrent aspiration.

Surgery

Restoration of an adequate airway can be achieved by performing an endoscopic aryepiglottoplasty.
- The procedure begins with an LTB
- Once the diagnosis is confirmed and other airway pathology is excluded, a nasotracheal tube is passed. This maintains the airway and protects the interarytenoid mucosa from trauma, reducing the risk of posterior glottic web formation

- With the aid of suspension laryngoscopy and the operating microscope the larynx is visualised
- Using a cup forceps and scissors, each aryepiglottic fold is divided, releasing it from the edge of the epiglottis, allowing the epiglottis to relax anteriorly, increasing the calibre of the supraglottic airway. Redundant tissue is then resected from over the arytenoids, with reduction or resection of the cuneiform cartilages where necessary. Haemostasis is achieved by the application of topical 1:10,000 epinephrine on neurosurgical patties

Stridor usually improves immediately postoperatively, although oedema may make it worse for a day or two prior to improvement. This is usually managed with a couple of doses of steroids.

Where significant stridor and feeding difficulties persist following aryepiglottoplasty, the possibility of an underlying hypotonic state or other neurological disorders must be considered. Aggressive GOR management is essential as GOR may cause recurrent oedema and stridor, if left untreated.

Choanal atresia

Choanal atresia occurs when the posterior nasal choana is obliterated, interrupting continuity between the nasal passage and the nasopharynx.

Epidemiology and pathology

Choanal atresia has an incidence of 1:7000 live births and a female–male ratio of 2:1. It is unilateral in 70%. The most popular theory is failed rupture of the oronasal membrane around the 38th day of development. However, 70% of cases are complex, involving the choanae and the bone of the medial wall (vomer), lateral wall and the floor of the nasal cavity – suggesting a more complex aetiology.

Clinical features

Nasal obstruction identified in the
- Newborn, by the absence of misting on a metal spatula placed below the anterior nares, or by the failure to pass a nasal catheter into the oropharynx

- Older child, by unilateral nasal discharge or a sensation of nasal obstruction

Bilateral choanal atresia often features as part of a polymalformation syndrome, such as CHARGE, and presents with signs of severe airway obstruction and cyclical cyanosis (as an obligate nasal breather the neonate experiences periods of cyanosis that are relieved by crying) at birth.

Investigation

- CT scan to delineate the nature (bony, membranous or both), degree and site of the obstruction

Treatment

In bilateral choanal atresia, the airway is secured by means of endotracheal intubation or an adapted nipple from a feeding bottle. Comorbidities permitting, definitive surgery should take place within the first week of life, with an aim to establish adequate and stable choanal patency.

Surgery

In the majority, unilateral atresia is well tolerated and surgery can be deferred until 1–5 years of age. Surgery is rarely required in the first months of life (where there is obstructive sleep apnoea).
Bilateral atresia necessitates urgent surgery.

- Intranasal approach
  - After decongestion the atretic area is visualised with a nasal endoscope
  - Simple membranous atresia can be perforated with a metal probe (e.g. urethral sound), carbon dioxide (CO_2) or potassium titanyl phosphate laser
  - However, for compound atresia (70% of cases), the choanae need to be drilled under direct vision (through the nasopharynx using a mirror or a 120° endoscope)
  - The use of choanal stents is controversial
- Transpalatine approach
  - This is a viable alternative, but does not afford a direct view of the choana and requires the detaching and cutting of healthy palatine mucosa
- Complications
  - The main risk of both techniques is restenosis, especially in the neonate. To maintain an adequate airway, repeated dilatation under anaesthesia may therefore be required (on average 1.5–3.0 surgical procedures). More predictable long-term results are obtainable with revision surgery when the child is older (access is easier), but there is no consensus as to the optimal timing

Further reading

Bailey M. Congenital disorders of the larynx, trachea and bronchi. In: Gleeson M, Browning GG, Burton MJ, et al. (eds), Scott Brown's otorhinolaryngology, head and neck surgery, vol. 1, 7th edn. London: Hodder Arnold, 2008:1135–1136.

Bailey M. Congenital disorders of the larynx, trachea and bronchi. In: Graham JM, Scadding GK, Bull PD (eds), Pediatric ENT. Heidelberg: Springer-Verlag, 2007:190.

Froehlich P, Ayari-Khalfallah S. Management of choanal atresia. In: Graham JM, Scadding GK, Bull PD (eds), Pediatric ENT. Heidelberg: Springer-Verlag, 2007:291–294.

Paediatric plastic surgery

Learning outcomes

- To understand extravasation injuries as emergencies
- To understand how agents affect tissue and be able to administer 'first aid'
- To understand treatment options and be able to administer those
- To understand the difference between normal, hypertrophic and keloid scars
- To understand the basic principles of scar treatment
- To understand basic principles of initial treatment in burn and scald injuries

Overview

Plastic surgery consists of two components: reconstructive and aesthetic surgery. Reconstructive surgery aims at restoring appearance and function after illness, accident or congenital deficiencies, whereas aesthetic surgery is performed to change the appearance by choice. In children it is paediatric plastic surgery and comprises burns, craniofacial, cleft and hand surgery, vascular anomalies, reconstruction of facial and trunk anomalies, obstetric brachial plexus palsy, skin and soft tissue anomalies and other problems.

Paediatric plastic surgeons are frequently part of multidisciplinary teams, such as for epidermolysis bullosa, liver and small bowel transplant and others. Three conditions are discussed here.

Extravasation injury

Extravasation injury is the leakage of an intravenously administered drug into the perivascular space. An extravasation is considered an emergency and should be treated immediately by medical personal experienced in treating extravasations.

Epidemiology and pathology

The risk of causing lasting skin and tissue damage depends on drug characteristics, such as osmolarity, pH, cytotoxicity and vasoactivity. Drugs can be classified into vesicants, exfoliants and irritants.

- Vesicants are drugs potentially causing tissue necrosis, with skin loss and damage to underlying structures, resulting in permanent damage
- Exfoliant drugs cause inflammation and skin shedding, less likely to cause tissue death
- Irritant drugs cause an inflammatory reaction. Symptoms are usually transient and do not have a long-lasting effect

Clinical features

- Vesicant drugs: skin blanching, blistering, if untreated, demarcation and tissue necrosis
- Exfoliant drugs: inflammation and skin shedding
- Irritant drugs: aching, burning, tightness, pain, warmth, erythema and tenderness (irritant drugs can cause lasting damage if the extravasated quantity causes a compartment syndrome)

Treatment

A variety of treatment options are advocated: application of ice, injection of hyaluronidase, local injection of steroid to combat inflammation, injection of saline to dilute the toxic agent and injection of specific antidotes, such as phentolamine, in the case of extravasation of vasopressor agents, but no consensus has been reached so far on an optimal algorithm.

- Check your local institutional policy and get the extravasation kit
- Assessment – what drug type, how much infused and when infusion was stopped – choose appropriate treatment
- Leave a cannula in situ and mark area of extravasation with a pen
- Aspirate as much of extravasated fluid through the cannula as possible; the cannula can also be used to flush
- If neutralisation is needed
  - Several stab incisions, infiltration of 1500 units of diluted hyaluronidase and flush, ideally stab wounds are for exiting fluid

- Topical steroids can be used, elevate, thermal compress
- Antidotes should be administered as soon as possible. Phentolamine may be given in cases of vasopressor extravasation (e.g. dopamine, norepinephrine and epinephrine)

Scars

Scars are a common outcome after surgical intervention, and although expected, they are not always welcome because they can cast a negative light on an otherwise good surgical result.

Scars are collagenous areas replacing normal skin after injury. The specific unidirectional alignment of this collagen leaves scar tissue less resistant and of inferior quality than skin.

Epidemiology and pathology

The word 'scar' derives from the old French 'escharre', which is derived from the late Latin 'eschara', which is the Latinisation of the Greek ἐσχάρα (eskhara), meaning 'hearth, fireplace', but in medicine 'scab, eschar on a wound caused by burning or otherwise'. Only humans are affected by keloid scars. Dark-skinned people and patients in their second decade have a greater risk of developing keloids.

Aetiology

In hypertrophic and keloid scars, the balance between collagen synthesis and collagen lysis is never achieved. Collagen synthesis and deposition persists; collagen lysis is decreased for an indefinite period.

Clinical features

- A keloid scar is scar tissue that progressively invades surrounding normal tissue ('tumorous' growth)
- A hypertrophic scar is scar tissue that remains confined to the area of tissue damaged by the initial injury
- Both can be bulky, reddish discoloured, itchy and sometimes even painful

Treatment

Multiple topical treatments have been trialled and described, but as the reasons for keloid formation are unknown, specific targeted treatment strategies are not available. Treatment strategies described include surgical intralesional excision, pressure garments, silicon cream and sheets, local tissue hypoxia, cryotherapy and laser therapy. Pharmacological treatment modalities include penicillamine, vitamin E, colchicine, retinoids, dextran sulphate and systemic chemotherapy like methotrexate.

Only intralesional steroid therapy, specifically triamcinolone, has proven to consistently effectively reduce keloid scars. This must be administered strictly intralesionally because it may cause irreversible atrophy in the surrounding tissue. Injections can be repeated three to four times every 4–6 weeks, until an effect is seen. In older children, this can be done with local anaesthetic cream, and in younger non-cooperative children general anaesthesia may be required. Intralesional injections can progress to intralesional surgical excision (especially earlobe keloids), but the risk of recurrence is high.

Any postoperative scar suspected to be prone to develop a hypertrophic or keloid scar (e.g. postinfection or prolonged secondary healing) should be treated immediately with silicon cream or gel sheeting for several months.

Initial treatment of burns and scalds

Despite constant efforts to prevent burns and scalds in children, these injuries remain very common in emergency departments where the situation can be governed by crying children, frightened parents and an unsure physician. Primary treatment in every emergency department should be directed at pain relief, fluid resuscitation, wound management and basic life-support measures. The child may then be treated on site or transferred to a specialised burns unit.

Epidemiology

The annual incidence of severe burns in Europe is stated to have been 0.2–2.9 in 10,000 inhabitants, with a decreasing trend in time. About half of those are below 16. In children the main causes are hot liquids.

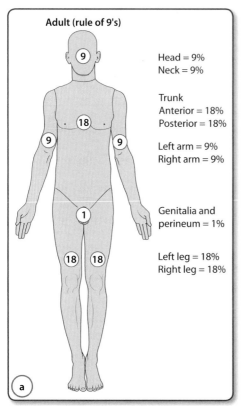

Figure 52 (a) Rule of 9's, (b) Lund and Browder chart.

Adult (rule of 9's)

Head = 9%
Neck = 9%

Trunk
Anterior = 18%
Posterior = 18%

Left arm = 9%
Right arm = 9%

Genitalia and
perineum = 1%

Left leg = 18%
Right leg = 18%

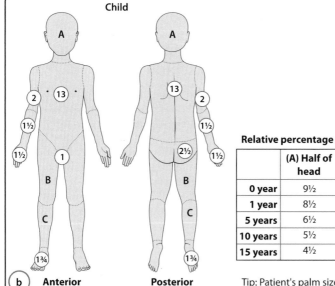

Child

Anterior   Posterior

Relative percentage of body surface area (BSA%)

	(A) Half of head	**(B) Half of one thigh**	**(C) Half of one lower leg**
0 year	9½	2¾	2½
1 year	8½	3¼	2½
5 years	6½	4	2¾
10 years	5½	4¼	3
15 years	4½	4½	3¼

Tip: Patient's palm size is approximately 1% BSA

Treatment

- **Surface estimation:** Whenever a child is seen in the emergency department, the burn distribution should be plotted exactly and the total area involved added up and expressed as a percentage. Lund and Browder charts (**Figure 52**) for estimating the severity of burn wound are used and intravenous fluid resuscitation is started if the surface is estimated at being ≥ 10% total body surface area (TBSA)
- **Resuscitation fluids:** All children with burns ≥ 10% TBSA will receive fluid according to the Parkland formula: 4 mL/kg/% burn over 24 hours from the time of injury given 1/2 in the first 8 hours and 1/2 in the second 16 hours as Hartmann's fluid (compound sodium lactate solution). If presentation is delayed then the delay in fluid resuscitation must be kept in mind

Referral criteria for specialised burn service

Consider if > 2% TBSA partial thickness burn, all deep dermal and full thickness, circumferential burns and burns involving the face, hands, soles of feet or perineum. All burns associated with smoke inhalation, electrical shock or trauma, severe metabolic disturbance.

Children with burn wound infection, all children 'unwell' with a burn, unhealed burns after 2 weeks, neonatal burns of any size, all children with burns and child protection concerns, progressive non-burn skin loss condition (toxic shock syndrome, staphylococcal scalded skin syndrome).

Differential diagnosis

- Toxic shock syndrome
- Staphylococcal scalded skin syndrome

Further reading

Devika R, Arockiamary SN. Aetiology of keloids – an overview. Res Biotechnol 2011; 2:37–43.
Gault DT. Extravasation injuries. 1993; Br J Plast Surg; 46:91–96.

O'Sullivan ST, O'Shaughnessy M, O'Connor TPF. Aetiology and management of hypertrophic scars and keloids. Ann R Coll Surg Engl 1996; 78:168–175.

Paediatric transplantation

Learning outcomes

- To understand the history of clinical transplantation
- To understand the principles of transplant immunology and immunosuppression
- To understand the principles of graft procurement, preservation, engraftment and postoperative management
- To know the expected long-term outcomes

Overview

Organ transplantation has been one of the great success stories of modern surgery. Notable successful firsts were kidney (1954), pancreas (1966), liver (1967), heart (1967), heart and lung (1981), intestine (1988) and single lung (1983).

Over the subsequent decades, most of the technical issues were solved and the following principles were established:

- All vascular and anatomical connections are restored without flow compromise
- There is adequate space in the recipient for the graft to be accommodated without increasing the surrounding pressure

Early advances were the legal acceptance of brain death for deceased donors and the preservation of the organ for retrieval and storage before reimplantation.

The first and remaining challenge to long-term graft survival is rejection. Recognition of rejection processes, the discovery of tissue HLA and DR immune recognition sites and that foreign tissue would be aggressively attacked and destroyed was initially managed from the stance that if the recipient was sufficiently immunosuppressed the graft would survive. Whilst largely true, the recipient often succumbed to infections or drug side effects.

There are at least seven genes in the major histocompatibility complex on chromosome 6, which code for HLA antigens. Each of these genes is polymorphic, and each of these variants codes for different HLA antigens. Since HLA antigens are genetically determined, HLA identical individuals can be found within a family, but rarely the general population. The HLA antigens that receive the most attention are HLA-A, HLA-B and HLA-DR. Since each person carries a chromosome 6 of maternal and paternal origin, there are two copies of each HLA gene, all of which are expressed codominantly. Therefore, a 'perfect' match is a six-antigen match (2 HLA-A, 2 HLA-B and 2 HLA-DR) although there are other minor histocompatibility antigens that may be important (HY-A1 and HA-1).

In the early 1980s, cyclosporine was introduced and was much more effective than steroids, azathioprine and antilymphocyte globulin, which although effective in immunosuppression, rendered the recipient immune incompetent with all its consequences, in addition to drug side effects.

In 1990, tacrolimus, a drug similar to cyclosporine in action but much more powerful, with a slightly different side effect profile, was introduced and has become the prime immunosuppression drug in most centres (**Table 11**).

Rejection

Medawar with skin transplant experiments demonstrated that

- Graft rejection is donor specific
- Rejection possesses memory and responds to a second graft from the same donor in an accelerated manner
- First-set rejection is cell mediated
- Second-set rejection is largely antibody mediated

Thus, hyperacute rejection (minutes to hours post-transplant) is caused by preformed cytotoxic antibodies in the recipient's serum. Acute rejection (most commonly 3–14 days' post-transplant but may occur years later) is cell mediated and equivalent to Medawar's first-set rejection response. In renal transplants, the timing of the first rejection in a second graft may be accelerated if the graft shares antigens with the first graft. Chronic rejection is multifactorial, but the result is microvascular endothelial damage and ischaemia-induced organ pathology.

Table 11	Immunosuppressants: mechanism of action and common side effects	
Agent	Mechanism of action	Side effects
Antibody therapy	Targets multiple antigens on lymphocytes	Serum sickness
Anti-thymocyte globulin (ATG) and anti-lymphcyte globulin (ALG)	Modification of cell surface and cell lysis	Cytokine release Prolonged leucopoenia Viral infections Increased post-transplantation lymphoproliferative disease (PTLD)
OKT3	Binds to T-lymphocyte surface antigen CD3	Same as ATG/ALG
IL-2 receptor antibody		
Basiliximab	Binds to T-cell surface IL-2 receptor CD25	Minimal complications
Daclizumab		
Calcineurin inhibitors		
Cyclosporine	Inhibits calcineurin, decreased IL-2 production	Hypertension Nephrotoxicity Neurotoxicity Hirsutism Gingival hyperplasia
Tacrolimus	Inhibits calcineurin, decreased IL-2 production	Hypertension Nephrotoxicity Neurotoxicity Glucose Intolerance
Sirolimus	Inhibits IL-2 cell-cycle process	Inhibits wound healing Hyperlipidemia
Antimetabolite		
Mycophenolate mofetil	Inhibits purine synthesis	Gastrointestinal discomfort Diarrhoea Bone marrow suppression
Azathioprine	Inhibits purine synthesis	Bone marrow suppression Drug-induced hepatitis
Corticosteroids	Blocks cytokine production	Glucose intolerance Hypertension Growth delay Osteopenia Dermatological complications

Organ preservation and procurement

The next challenge was procuring the organ in an intact state and preserving it during transportation, preparation of the recipient and engraftment. Various preservation solutions that stabilize cell membranes along with storage at 4°C to inhibit metabolism have resulted in reliable reperfusion function, in some organs up to 24–48 hours. However, short cold preservation times still equate with less organ damage, better function after reperfusion, a reduced incidence of rejection and better long-term graft survival.

The current major challenge is the shortage of organs, and need or demand now far outstrips the supply. This has led to a great drive for cadaveric organs within all countries that culturally accept deceased donation. In the others, living donor transplantation has been favoured. In a commercial world where demand exceeds supply there will inevitably be tension. The ethics of transplantation medicine have been sorely tested with deceased donation from executed prisoners, rampant organ theft and organs for sale in a marketplace of desperate recipients who want to buy an extension of life at almost any cost and desperate donors who want to sell their organs, usually as a short-term solution out of poverty.

Indications

The essential indication is organ disease, leading to severe dysfunction or failure. Uniquely liver transplantation may be to correct an enzyme defect where the consequence is on another organ or system or in primary non-metastatic hepatic neoplasia. Contraindications are few and relate mainly to the overall fitness of the patient to tolerate an operation with subsequent immunosuppression.

- Absolute contraindications: metastatic neoplasia, uncontrolled infection, systemic disease in other organs, with limited life expectancy, major neurological deficit
- Relative contraindications: extensive vascular thrombosis, immune hypersensitivity or immune deficiency syndrome; mismatch of ABO blood type, tissue or viral serology (EBV/CMV); presence of resistant organisms (of particular relevance in lung transplantation)

Donor-recipient size matching must ensure an adequate domain for the new organ and generally a donor size < 20% of the recipient and an adequate size or volume to take up the functional work required of the graft are required. This is particularly relevant in liver (0.8% of recipient body weight is thought safe) and bowel transplantation.

Strategies to address the size mismatch problem and increase donor numbers include

- Preoperative recipient tissue expansion, graft size reduction and staged abdominal closure, with prosthetic patch replacement of the abdominal wall and skin graft onto exposed organs.
- Kidney: congenital structural abnormalities, nephritis, hereditary metabolic diseases, focal segmental glomerulosclerosis, nephronophthisis and associated ciliopathies, nephrotic syndromes, Wilms' tumour. Congenital and hereditary problems predominate, therefore the strategic integration of urological surgery and transplant surgery is crucial

- Liver: cholestatic disorders, metabolic disease, autoimmune disease, acute liver failure, graft failure, tumour
- Intestinal transplant: intestinal failure (short bowel, dysmotility and congenital diarrhoea), complications from parenteral nutrition (recurrent sepsis and loss of venous access)
- Lung: cystic fibrosis, pulmonary vascular disease, primary pulmonary hypertension and pulmonary hypertension, with congenital heart disease, Eisenmenger's syndrome, pulmonary fibrosis and diffuse pulmonary parenchymal disease, graft failure, congenital lung disease
- Heart: severe congenital heart disease, cardiomyopathy, acute myocarditis, graft failure

Transplant assessment

All children require diagnostic confirmation, intensive medical investigation (cardiovascular, respiratory, renal, gastrointestinal, neurodevelopmental) to assess residual function in the diseased organ and to assess suitability for transplant. Most will require intensive medical management prior to transplant, including nutritional resuscitation and specific interventions for systemic consequences of the failing organ. Viral serology and immunizations are checked. Disease assessment includes identification of risk factors and contraindications.

The family and social circumstances also need to be fully assessed. Living-related transplant requires extensive physical and psychological evaluation of the potential donor.

Immunosuppression strategies

These have become fairly standardised across all transplants (**Table 11**).

- An induction agent inhibiting T-cell function (monoclonal antibodies directed at IL-2 receptor): daclizumab and basiliximab
- 'Triple–drug' maintenance immunosuppression

- Calcineurin inhibitor: cyclosporine and tacrolimus
- Cell-cycle inhibitors: azathioprine and mycophenolate mofetil
- Prednisolone

Surgical options

A poor general condition prior to transplant, particularly nutritional deprivation, is associated with a poor outcome. Organ procurement is usually part of a multiorgan procedure from deceased donors with heart, lungs, liver, kidneys and sometimes pancreas and/or bowel procured at the same operation. The organs are flushed with preservation solution and stored at 4°C in plastic bags, containing the preservation solution and in slush ice cool boxes suitable for transport. Living donor transplants have the advantage of timing of the procedure, a healthy graft, short ischaemic times and a possible improved immune compatibility. The operations are in three stages:
1. Diseased organ explant (often not required in renal transplants)
2. Graft implantation
3. Reperfusion and wound closure

Postoperative care is according to intensive care and immunosuppression protocols, with bacterial, fungal and viral prophylaxis as required.

The graft is monitored for signs of acute rejection manifested by organ dysfunction and systemic response to the inflammatory process and confirmed by tissue biopsy. Rejection is treated according to severity, in most cases with a short course of increased immunosuppression supplemented with steroid bolus doses.

Liver transplant

Types of grafts used are
- Whole liver orthotopic
- Reduced size: the section not used is discarded
- Split liver: the donor organ is divided into two functioning units, usually Couinaud segments 2–3 to a child and segments 4–8 for an adult; a left and right split can be used for two equal sized small adult donors

- Living donor: left and right lobe, left lateral segment
- Auxiliary partial orthotopic transplant is occasionally used for acute liver failure as a bridge to recovery of the acute insult after which immunosuppression can be withdrawn, allowing the graft to resorb and the recovered native liver to function normally

Intestinal transplant

Graft types depend on the indication:
- If bowel only is affected then an isolated intestinal transplant is sufficient
- In established liver disease, a combined liver and intestine graft is used. Size mismatch may dictate that the donor liver and possibly bowel be reduced in size. The hepatoduodenal complex is usually left intact
- If dysmotility extends into the foregut, a multivisceral transplant of liver, stomach, duodenum, pancreas and intestine is indicated
- Occasionally in infants with short bowel syndrome and early-onset liver failure due to parenteral nutrition, an isolated liver transplant is undertaken, with the expectation of eventual gut adaptation

A distal stoma is created initially for close monitoring of effluent and as access for biopsy to monitor for rejection. Bowel transplants require more immunosuppression to prevent rejection than other organs.

Renal transplants

Most grafts are adult to children (cadaver and living donor) requiring special care to make space for the large kidney and to place the vascular anastomoses as proximal as possible on the common iliac vessels or in adult size kidneys into infants, the aorta and inferior vena cava.

All grafts may suffer from primary poor function due to preservation injury, technical complications with the tubular structures reanastomosed as well as the usual wound complications. All are particularly sensitive to increase in intracompartmental pressures which may require emergency decompressive laparostomy or thoracostomy.

Follow-up

All patients are closely followed up lifelong because complications in the long term relate to chronic rejection, infections (bacterial, viral, protozoan and fungal), drug toxicity (from immunosuppressive agents and those used to treat infective complications), post-transplant lymphoproliferative disorder and lymphoma, disease recurrence and malignancy in the long term.

The liver has the capacity to regenerate, and after the first year there is very little attrition of the graft with 5-, 10- and 15-year survivals only decreasing by a few percentage points per year. This is not true for other organs transplanted where graft function deteriorates with time such that at 10 years there is often a > 50% loss of graft function and at 20 years an 80% loss. This can be ameliorated to some extent if there is a good HLA cross-match and the patient has been well cared for.

Adherence with medication is crucial to a good long-term outcome, and the most difficult time is the transition from a paediatric environment to an adult follow-up programme during the teenage years. Great care should be taken to support children through this time to avoid the tragic consequences of non-adherence, with cycles of rejection, leading to graft loss and increased immunosuppression leading to infections, drug toxicity and neoplasia.

Further reading

Agarwal A, Pescovitz M. Liver, kidney, heart and lung and intestinal transplants and immunosuppression. Semin Pediatr Surg 2006; 15:142–152.

Millar AJ, Gupte G, Sharif K. Intestinal transplantation for motility disorders. Semin Pediatr Surg 2009; 18:258–262.

Related topics of interest

Pancreatitis

Learning outcomes

- To understand the aetiology of pancreatitis in children
- To understand the management of pancreatitis and place of surgery within it

Overview

Acute pancreatitis is an inflammatory condition resulting from intrapancreatic activation, secretion and digestion of the pancreas by its own enzymes. It is rare in childhood.

Acute pancreatitis accounts for 75% of cases and is abrupt in onset, but usually self-limiting. Recurrent acute pancreatitis, characterised by repeated acute episodes, is associated with obstructive disease, such as pancreatic ductal abnormalities, biliary tract obstruction, duplication cysts and biliary lithiasis.

In chronic pancreatitis, the pancreatic inflammation and gland destruction are progressive. There are a number of classifications, but the simplest is to divide it anatomically into calcifying or obstructive. This most common aetiology in children is familial or hereditary pancreatitis.

Surgery is rarely required, but includes necrosectomy, drainage of intra-abdominal collections, management of abdominal compartment syndrome and complications such as pseudocysts and management of specific aetiologies once the pancreatitis subsides.

Epidemiology

Drugs and toxins (12–18%) and systemic disease (12–35%) are major causes of acute pancreatitis. Abdominal trauma accounts for 14–29% and is related to blunt abdominal trauma, surgical trauma or child abuse. Up to 25% of cases are idiopathic.

Pancreas divisum is present in as many as 10–15% of patients undergoing magnetic resonance cholangiopancreatography (MRCP) and is associated with 2.5% of acute pancreatitis in children. Acute pancreatitis can occur within the first month of life, but most cases present around the age of 5 years and during adolescence.

The pathophysiology by which inappropriate activation of pancreatic enzyme occurs is unknown; possibilities include

- Reflux of duodenal enterokinase into the pancreas, activating trypsin that then inappropriately activates other proenzymes
- Ductal obstruction with extravasation of enzyme-rich ductal fluid into the pancreatic parenchyma
- Fusion of lysosomes with zymogen granules inside the acinar cells, allowing lysosomal enzyme activation of proenzymes

Once activated, elastase, phospholipase and superoxide free radicals are thought to be the principal mediators of tissue damage.

Aetiology

- Systemic disease
- Systemic lupus erythematosus (SLE), Reye syndrome, fulminant liver failure, Henoch–Schönlein vascultitis, Kawasaki disease, haemolytic–uremic syndrome, renal failure, hyperparathyroidism, Crohn's disease, hypertriglyceridemia, malnutrition, cystic fibrosis (CF), solid organ transplantation, hyperlipoproteinaemia (types 1 and 5), α1-antitrypsin deficiency
- Drugs and toxins
  - Sodium valproate, thiazides, furosemide, cimetidine, L-asparaginase, azathioprine, 6-mercaptopurine, cyclosporin A, tacrolimus, didanosine, corticosteroids, oestrogen, sulfonamides, tetracycline, erythromycin
- Infections
  - Mumps, Coxsackie B virus, Epstein–Barr virus, hepatitis A and B, measles, malaria, mycoplasma, rubella, influenzae A and B virus, varicella, HIV

- Obstructive disease
  - Pancreatic ductal abnormalities, biliary tract malformations, pancreas divisum, duplication cyst, pancreatic pseudocyst, biliary lithiasis, tumours, ascariasis
- Trauma
  - Blunt or penetrating abdominal injury, surgical trauma, child abuse
- Hereditary pancreatitis
  - Familial, e.g. cationic trypsinogen gene mutation (*PRSS1* gene)
  - SPINK 1 mutation: acute-phase protein-inhibiting trypsin activation, or CTFR (cystic fibrosis transmembrane conductance regulator)
- Idiopathic
- Endoscopic retrograde cholangiopancreatography (ERCP)
- Scorpion bites

Clinical features

Clinical features are sudden-onset midepigastric pain, radiating to the back or left upper quadrant, vomiting and low-grade pyrexia. Pain is not well localised in young children, and nausea and vomiting feature predominantly.

Abdomen is distended, diffusely tender with peritonism and paucity of bowel sounds. In severe necrotising or haemorrhagic pancreatitis, haemorrhage passes along tissue planes and appears as flank (Grey-Turner's sign) or umbilical (Cullen's sign) ecchymoses which characteristically take 1 or 2 days to develop.

Investigations

- Hyperamylasemia has a high specificity within the first 24 hours, but the degree of elevation does not correlate with disease severity. Salivary inflammation and trauma, intestinal disease, renal failure and macroamylasemia also elevate blood amylase levels
- Initial C-reactive protein level of > 150 mg/L has a positive predictive value of > 90% for severe acute pancreatitis. A level > 210 mg/L in the first 4 days or > 120 mg/L after 7 days suggests

severe disease. Trypsin, elastase and phospholipase A_2 are elevated, but these tests are expensive, uncommon and their prognostic value unknown. Lipase is not in common use in the UK
- Ranson's or Glasgow score can be used to grade severity although with low specificity and sensitivity for initial evaluation
- An abdominal X-ray to exclude differential diagnoses may show a paralytic ileus pattern with a sentinel loop, 'colonic cut-off' with local spasm of the transverse colon, with proximal dilatation or retroperitoneal gas. Pancreatic calcifications suggest chronic disease. Chest X-rays may show pleural effusions and pulmonary oedema
- Abdominal ultrasound scan can delineate pseudocysts, pancreatic ascites, vascular thrombosis and guides paracentesis in cases of proven pancreatitis. Endoscopic ultrasound provides detailed information on pancreatic parenchymal and ductal anatomy, biliary ducts and presence of cystic lesions
- Contrast-enhanced computerised tomography (CT) gives an accurate determination of the extent of necrosis and peripancreatic collections. CT signs of acute pancreatitis include marked glandular enlargement, reduced pancreatic density and extrapancreatic extension of inflammation. Specificity for acute pancreatitis approaches 100% and sensitivity 85%. It allows detection and assessment of intra- and extrapancreatic necrosis. A repeat examination (after 48 hours) may provide dynamic information and help differentiate between oedematous and necrotising pancreatitis
- ERCP can evaluate relapsing pancreatitis and demonstrate obstructing lesions, stones, ductal strictures, duplication cysts and other anatomic anomalies. This is contraindicated in the acute phase and has a 10% incidence of acute pancreatitis
- MRCP can demonstrate dilatation, stricture, pseudocysts and ductal filling defects, including calculi, mucinous plugs and sludge

Differential diagnosis

- Other causes of acute or chronic abdominal pain in children

Treatment

Medical management is to maintain normovolemia, normoglycemia, electrolyte and acid–base balance, identify and treat systemic and local complications. Early nutrition reduces the rate of septic complications. There is no consensus on antibiotic therapy and local practice varies. Cochrane review found a consistent beneficial trend when using imipenem, but with no significant data to support this. Octreotide or somatostatin reduces mortality without affecting complications. Insulin therapy to maintain blood glucose $\leq 110\,mg/dL$ reduces morbidity and mortality, but all this data comes from adult studies.

Aggressive intensive medical care is the mainstay of treatment, with specific criteria for operative intervention. One randomised study identified a better prognosis in adult patients undergoing delayed necrosectomy. Surgical or percutaneous drainage of intra-abdominal collections with large gauge drains is essential if sepsis is suspected. Early decompressive laparotomy is the treatment for acute compartment syndrome. Surgical treatment is delayed except in gallstone pancreatitis with cholangitis or progressive obstructive jaundice.

- Early complications
  - Capillary leak syndrome; systemic inflammatory response syndrome; circulatory, metabolic, respiratory, renal or cardiac failure; pancreatic necrosis; abdominal compartment syndrome; disseminated intravascular coagulopathy; encephalopathy
- Late complications (>2 weeks)
  - Infection of necrosis or pseudocyst; disruption of pancreatic duct (pancreatic ascites), pleural or pericardial fistula, pseudocyst; viscus perforation; pseudoaneurysm; splanchnic venous thrombosis; bowel infarction

Chronic pancreatitis can result in early complications of obstructive cholestasis and cholangitis, with late complications being pseudocyst, ascites and fistula; pancreatic fibrosis; abscess; pseudoaneurysm; splanchnic vein thrombosis; pancreatic exocrine and endocrine insufficiency.

Pseudocysts complicate acute pancreatitis in 10–23% of cases. Their incidence is >50% when associated with traumatic abdominal injury. They can be drained percutaneously or by endoscopic, open or laparoscopic cystogastrostomy or ERCP with transpapillary drainage where the cyst communicates with the pancreatic duct. ERCP can also be used to stent the pancreatic duct if transected or to manage a pancreatic fistula by internal drainage proximal to the fistula.

Further reading

UK Working party. UK guidelines for the treatment of acute pancreatitis. Gut 2005; 54:1–9.

Villatoro E, Mulla M, Larvin M. Antibiotic therapy for prophylaxis against infection of pancreatic necrosis in acute pancreatitis. Cochrane Database of Systematic Reviews 2010, Issue 5. Art. No.: CD002941. DOI:10.1002/14651858.CD002941.pub3

Wilson C, et al. C-reactive protein, antiproteases and complement factors as objective markers of severity in acute pancreatitis. Br J Surg 1989; 76:177–781.

Related topics of interest

Pelvi-ureteric junction obstruction

Learning outcomes

- To understand the aetiology and consequences of pelvi-ureteric junction obstruction (PUJO)
- To be able to assess a patient with hydronephrosis
- To understand treatment options and outcomes

Overview

Pelvi-ureteric junction (PUJ) obstruction causes reduced flow of urine from the kidney, resulting in pain or loss of renal function. It is not synonymous with hydronephrosis. Antenatal diagnosis of hydronephrosis has increased the early detection of PUJO but has also identified a large number of children without significant obstruction. The overall pyeloplasty is performed in about 1 in 1500 cases of hydronephrosis.

Epidemiology and aetiology

PUJO is twice as common in males as in females. The right and left kidneys are equally affected. There is an increased incidence in horseshoe kidneys, and in the lower moieties of duplex kidneys, both probably due to anatomical as well as vascular anomalies.

PUJO may have extrinsic or intrinsic causes. Extrinsic causes include aberrant lower pole vessels, crossing at the PUJ (found in about 30%), tumours and extrinsic scarring. Intrinsic causes include congenital strictures, folds within the upper ureter, polyps and stones.

Clinical features

The two main features of PUJO are hydronephrosis and/or pain. Hydronephrosis may be detected antenatally or incidentally during an ultrasound for other indications. Occasionally, haematuria or hypertension may be presenting features. A right-sided PUJO with hydronephrosis can give rise to vomiting because the large dilated renal pelvis compresses the second part of the duodenum. Vomiting may also occur in PUJO due to a vagal reflex triggered by renal capsular stretching and pain. Any child with hydronephrosis has to have the differential diagnoses fully considered and appropriate investigations carried out to determine the cause. Differential diagnoses for hydronephrosis include congenital self-limiting hydronephrosis, vesicoureteric reflux (VUR), vesicoureteric junction obstruction (VUJO), renal cystic disease and renal dysplasia. Clinical examination might demonstrate high blood pressure, an abdominal mass (if there is a very large hydronephrotic kidney), and abdominal or loin tenderness.

Investigations

A renal ultrasound scan (USS) will usually demonstrate hydronephrosis. The presence of a dilated ureter suggests VUJO or VUR, but these can coexist with PUJO. In the newborn, sequential ultrasound scans will help distinguish those likely to settle spontaneously (anteroposterior renal diameter of pelvis in the prone position of < 20 mm) and those likely to need surgery (increasing hydronephrosis over three successive measurements).

The key investigation to determine obstruction is a MAG3 renogram. MAG3 radiolabelled with 99-technetium is injected intravenously, and sequential scans of the kidney are taken between 1 and 30 minutes, with a late film at 60 minutes also being desirable. This will give an assessment of flow from the kidney as well as function of one kidney compared with the other. A number of different protocols have been established as to how best to carry out a MAG3 renogram to determine whether or not obstruction exists. Ideally, there should be the possibility of free flow of isotopes through the kidney and urinary tract, so some centres advocate a urethral catheter during the investigation.

If a catheter is not placed, a postmicturition image should be obtained. The timing of frusemide to obtain a maximum diuresis is also widely debated, either at the same time as injection of isotope or 15–20 minutes before or after.

A contrast CT or angiogram is occasionally performed to determine whether or not there is a lower pole and crossing blood vessels impinging on the PUJ. In the presence of a contralateral normal kidney, renal function is usually well preserved and so glomerular filtration rate (GFR), plasma urea and plasma creatinine will usually be normal. In bilateral cases, these parameters may be compromised.

Differential diagnosis

Other causes of hydronephrosis have already been mentioned. Other causes of abdominal pain, vomiting, haematuria and hypertension need to be considered in the absence of hydronephrosis.

Treatment

PUJO requires surgical treatment to relieve pain and to preserve renal function. The classical operation is the Hynes–Anderson dismembered pyeloplasty, originally carried out in 1949 because of obstruction at the PUJ due to a retrocaval ureter. A Culp pyeloplasty (rotated down flap) may have to be carried out in the presence of a mainly intrarenal pelvis where a dismembering procedure is difficult. Pyeloplasty may be carried out using open surgery or laparoscopic (robotic or not robotic) surgery. It may be carried out using a transperitoneal or extraperitoneal approach. Some centres have advocated endopyelotomy, but in children, the recurrence rate is high and this procedure is not widely adopted in this group of patients.

The success rate of a pyeloplasty is generally >95%, irrespective of which method is used. Complications include urinary leak, recurrent stricturing, complications of laparoscopy (if this is the method employed), and complications of any stents or drainage methods used. There is a wide variety in methods used to provide drainage of the affected kidney following a pyeloplasty, including a urinary catheter, a transanastomotic nephroureteric stent, a transanastomotic nephroureteric bladder stent, a simple wound drain or no drainage at all. The aim of utilising drainage for a variable period postoperatively (from days to weeks) is to reduce the risk of leakage and subsequent restricturing. Recurrence of PUJO due to scarring is most common in the first 12–18 months after surgery and usually occurs in <1% of cases.

Postoperative investigations usually include a follow-up USS to assess resolution of hydronephrosis and a MAG3 renogram. In very young children, early (within 3 months of surgery) postoperative USS may show little initial change from the preoperative scan.

Further reading

Cuckow P, Desai D. Upper urinary tract obstruction. In: Burge D, Griffiths DM, Steinbrecher HA, Wheeler RA (eds), Paediatric surgery, 2nd edon. Hodder Arnold, 2005.

Lee RS, et al. Antenatal hydronephrosis as a predictor of postnatal outcome: a meta-analysis. Pediatrics 2006; 118:586–593

Gordon I. Assessment of pediatric hydronephrosis using output efficiency. J Nucl Med 1997; 38:1487–1489.

Related topics of interest

Perianal disease

Learning outcomes

- To recognise and distinguish between perianal fissure and fistula
- To understand the management of these pathologies

Overview

The most common perianal pathologies in childhood are anal fissure and perianal fistula. If not treated actively, correctly and adequately, these benign conditions will recur or lead to chronic stool withholding and constipation, which can take years to resolve.

Epidemiology and aetiology

Perianal fissure occurs in infancy and early childhood, with equal frequency in males and females. Perianal abscess and fistula usually occur in early infancy. Almost all fistulae occur in males.

Anal fissures occur secondary to the passage of a hard stool in infancy, often at the time of weaning onto solid feed. Perianal fistula in infancy differs from that seen in adults in that the fistula is always low, its internal opening occurring at the level of the dentate line. A congenital aetiology has been postulated.

Clinical features

Parents of children with an anal fissure give a classical history. The child often has no symptoms or difficulty in stooling in early infancy. The problem commences with the passage of fresh blood preceding or on the surface of, but not mixed with, the stool. This is usually short lived, but following this, the child passes a hard stool with difficulty. This is associated with a lot of distress. The child will then pass a stool less frequently, and when doing so, will pass a large hard stool, an event that is accompanied by a lot of pain and screaming. If the fissure persists without treatment, then the child will try to avoid the pain of stooling by withholding. Parents will then describe the child hiding and straining.

The child may be reluctant to be examined. Abdominal examination may reveal palpable faecal loading. Inspection of the anal canal will demonstrate a fresh or healing fissure at the muco-cutaneous border of the anal margin, usually in an anterior position. With longstanding fissures, a sentinel skin tag may be visible adjacent to the fissure, which will persist after the fissure has healed – and it is often this skin tag that has prompted referral for advice. Rectal examination should not be performed with the child awake.

Perianal fistula usually presents with a perianal abscess in infancy. Parents may describe recurrent episodes of perianal infections or discharge. The fistula is almost always in a lateral position, extending radially from the anal crypt at the dentate line to a skin opening 1–2 cm from the anal margin.

Investigations

For most children with anal fissure, the diagnosis is made from the history and examination, and treatment may commence without further investigation. If a child has a longstanding or atypical history, then examination under anaesthesia and sigmoidoscopy are indicated.

For infants with recurrent perianal abscess or perianal fistula, examination under anaesthesia is indicated. In addition, older children should undergo endoscopy, serum erythrocyte sedimentation rate and albumin estimation to exclude Crohn's disease.

Differential diagnosis

In older children, anal fissure, abscess and fistula can be the presenting features of Crohn's disease. Chronic fissures can be secondary to lichen planus, and rarely non-accidental injury or sexual abuse. Multiple fissures can occur as a result of a group A streptococcal infection.

Treatment

Anal fissure is a self-limiting disease. The principle of treatment is to break the vicious cycle of stool withholding to enable the child to pass a soft stool past the fissure with the least discomfort. The mainstay of treatment is conservative with stool softening and bulking laxatives such as Movicol.

In the past, anal dilatation under anaesthetic was a standard treatment, but this has not been proven to be of any benefit. Topical glyceryl trinitrate paste and injection of Botox into the internal anal sphincter have been advocated for persistent fissure.

Perianal abscess should be treated by incision and drainage once pus has developed. The abscess will often be associated with a fistula – if this can be identified at the time of drainage, then this should be laid open. For male infants, if a fistula is not easily defined, the infant should undergo examination under general anaesthetic and laying open of the perianal fistula at a later date to prevent recurrent abscess. The tendency to treat with repeated courses of antibiotics should be resisted.

In this procedure, under general anaesthetic, the infant is placed in a lithotomy position with an assistant holding the legs. Gentle retraction at the anal margin will demonstrate the dentate line. Pressure on the perianal skin may extrude a bead of pus, helping identification of the internal opening. The fistula is defined with a blunt probe, which is passed toward the external opening of the fistula. This probe should be passed without force to prevent the formation of a false passage. The fistula is laid open by cutting down onto the probe with mono-polar diathermy. The exposed track is left to heal by secondary intention.

Further reading

Fitzgerald RJ, Harding B, Ryan W. Fistula-in-ano in childhood: a congenital etiology. J Pediatr Surg 1985; 20:80–81.

Novotny NM, Mann MJ, Rescorla FJ. Fistula in ano in infants: who recurs? Pediatr Surg Int 2008; 24:1197–1199.

Shafer AD, McGlone TP, Flanagan RA. Abnormal crypts of Morgagni; the cause of perianal abscess and fistula-in-ano. J Pediatr Surg 1987; 22:203–204.

Related topics of interest

- Crohn's disease (p. 74)
- Rectal prolapse (p. 296)

Perioperative care: surgical safety and human factors

Learning outcomes

- To develop awareness of patient safety and factors affecting it
- To understand the importance of non-technical skills for surgeons
- To understand the role of the surgeon in improving patient safety

Overview

The provision of healthcare is a hazardous activity; approximately 10% patients suffer adverse events during a hospital admission, of which at least half are potentially preventable. Each year in the UK alone, up to 7500 patients suffer serious harm and 3500 patients die as a result of adverse events, at an estimated cost of £2 billion.

Every healthcare professional has a duty of care to patients to try to reduce harm and maximise safety. To do this effectively, an understanding of why mistakes happen and how systems can be made as safe as possible is required.

Person approach versus systems approach

Reason's 'Swiss cheese model' suggests that organisational systems consist of layers of defence against harm; these layers can be likened to Swiss cheese because they contain many holes and are not infallible. These holes represent 'latent conditions' that are not errors themselves, but allow errors to pass undetected. Harm arises only when 'active failures' occur in conjunction with several latent conditions, aligning 'the holes' and allowing the error to reach the patient. Most large-scale disasters, such as the sinking of the Herald of Free Enterprise ferry (1987), can be attributed to the combination of active failures and latent conditions.

The person approach to error focuses on individuals and human errors, which can be divided into 'slips and lapses' (failures of execution) or 'mistakes' (failures of planning). A person approach attempts to eradicate these human errors by making people change their behaviour. By contrast, the systems approach acknowledges that humans are fallible and will make failures of both execution and planning. It seeks to eliminate system failures and emphasises the need to create systems that support and protect the individuals working within them by eliminating latent conditions that predispose to harm.

Non-technical skills

Surgical training traditionally focuses on knowledge and technical skills, but non-technical skills are just as important. Adverse events in surgery are usually the result of an accumulation of small non-technical errors. For example, poor communication is implicated in > 40% of errors during surgery.

Non-technical skills include cognitive and social skills. An understanding of these skills can be used to observe behaviour and aid training. The following are examples of some essential non-technical skills surgeons should develop:

- Situation awareness
- Gathering information – from the patient, operating theatre environment and other staff
- Understanding information – interpreting the findings based on knowledge and experience
- Projecting and anticipating future state, e.g. predicting which instrument will be needed next, planning operating lists
- Decision making
- Considering options – operative planning and intraoperative decision making
- Selecting and communicating options to other members of the team
- Implementing and reviewing decisions – including asking for help when required

- Communication and teamwork
- Exchanging information – intraoperative communication in a timely fashion
- Establishing a shared understanding – including team briefing and debriefing
- Coordinating team activities – including checking whether other members of the operating team have any concerns
- Leadership
- Setting and maintaining standards such as following theatre protocols
- Supporting others with positive feedback or constructive criticism
- Coping with pressure

Human factors

'Human factors' is the science of the inter-relationship between humans, their tools and the environment in which they work. It covers both the human-machine and human-human interfaces. Understanding human factors enables the design of a system that is as safe as possible, without trying to eliminate human error. The aim is to create a 'high reliability' environment free of latent errors in which to deliver patient care.

Human factors that can increase risk to patient safety include the following:

- High mental workload – stress and reliance on memory increase the risk of error, and cognitive bias leads to 'seeing what we want to see'
- Distractions – noise and interruption cause increased medication errors
- Adverse physical environment – including heat and lighting
- Extreme physical demands – staff who are tired make more mistakes

Factors that can reduce the risk to patient safety include the following:

- **Good product design:** Devices should be designed to make it easy to do the right thing and hard to do the wrong thing (e.g. ensuring that lumbar puncture needles have a different shape to intravenous needles so that intravenous drugs cannot be given intrathecally)
- **Teamwork:** Briefing and debriefing helps teams to develop and communicate a shared mental model so that risks can be predicted and mitigated in advance

- **Process design:** Simplification and standardisation of clinical processes reduces reliance on memory and improves safety.

Safety culture

Organisational culture is an elusive concept but, in essence, it relates to a shared set of values, norms and practices within a work place, it refers to 'the way things are done around here'. Culture is notoriously difficult to change but there are key elements to a safety-oriented culture that should be promoted by leaders:

- Open – staff can raise safety concerns
- Reporting – staff have the confidence to report any adverse event
- Learning – the organisation is committed to learning from incidents and preventing them from reoccurring
- Just – the organisation treats staff involved in incidents fairly
- Informed – learns from experience and implements best practice

Attempts to achieve these culture changes have been limited to date, with under-reporting of incidents and a lack of understanding of the nature of patient safety incidents, making a just culture an aspiration in most healthcare systems.

World Health Organization surgical safety checklist

In 2008, World Health Organization's (WHO) Patient Safety Program launched the second global patient safety challenge, Safe Surgery Saves Lives. The project's aim was to reduce the harm caused by unsafe surgery worldwide. Its centrepiece was the development and implementation of a checklist that covers the peri-operative period and helps ensure that essential, evidence-based steps are carried out for every patient undergoing surgery.

A large, multicentre evaluation of the checklist carried out in countries with varying levels of healthcare resource demonstrated a reduction in morbidity and mortality rates, following the introduction of the checklist.

Subsequent studies, using the WHO checklist and others, have confirmed a positive benefit from the use of checklists in the delivery of surgical care.

The precise reasons for improved outcomes using checklists are still unclear, but they do increase reliability and promote communication between professional groups. They also raise awareness of patient safety as an issue, and so promote safety-oriented cultural change. It seems likely that as the evidence base grows, their use will become increasingly widespread, in surgical practice and beyond.

Further reading

Catchpole K. Errors in the operating theatre – how to spot and stop them. J Health Serv Res Policy 2010; 151:48–51.

Haynes AB, et al. A surgical safety checklist to reduce morbidity and mortality in a global population. N Engl J Med 2009; 29(360):491–499.

Reason J. Human error: models and management. BMJ 2000; 320(7237):768–770.

Posterior urethral valves

Learning outcomes

- To understand the underlying pathophysiology of posterior urethral valves
- To recognise clinical presentations of this condition before birth, in infancy and in older children
- To be aware of the long-term problems and complex needs of patients with urethral valves

Overview

Posterior urethral valves (PUVs) cause outflow obstruction to the developing male bladder, resulting in abnormal development of the kidneys as well as the bladder. There is a wide spectrum of severity, but many will develop renal insufficiency and bladder dysfunction. Long-term follow-up is needed for all.

Epidemiology and aetiology

PUVs are the most common congenital cause of bladder outlet obstruction in boys, occurring in 1 in 4000–6000 male births.

Pathophysiology

- Valve membranes form at the level of the verumontanum as a result of an abnormality of migration of the junction between the cloaca and the Wolffian duct
- Early bladder outflow obstruction contributes to renal dysplasia. Tubular damage predominates, resulting in an increased loss of sodium and bicarbonate ions. Renal dysplasia may also be partly primary
- The bladder develops a higher ratio of collagen to muscle, causing reduced contractility and reduced compliance
- Dilatation of the bladder and kidneys may be detectable by 14 weeks' gestation
- Young defined three types of PUVs in 1919, but this description is generally losing favour. Most consist of obstructing membranes that radiate from the verumontanum towards the membranous urethra and fuse in the midline (Type I valves). Type III valves consist of a membrane distal to the verumontanum at the level of the membranous urethra. Type II valves are considered to be prominent non-obstructing urethral folds (plica colliculae)
- No identified causative factors have been found
- There is no established genetic predisposition, but many cases have been reported in first-degree relatives and also in identical twins

Clinical features

Antenatal

- Most will be detected antenatally with high-quality fetal ultrasonography
- Typical features are bilateral hydronephrosis, a distended bladder that cannot be seen to empty and a dilated posterior urethra (the 'keyhole' sign). Oligohydramnios suggests a poorer outcome because 90% amniotic fluid arises from fetal 'urine'

Presentation at/after birth

- May present at birth with delayed voiding, poor urine stream, distended abdomen (bladder and kidneys), failure to thrive, lethargy, poor feeding or urosepsis
- On examination may have palpable distended bladder and kidneys and/or urinary ascites
- May present later in infancy or childhood, with failure to thrive, urine infection or bladder function problems

Investigations

- **Ultrasound:** Assess bladder and kidneys
- **Micturating cystourethrogram (MCUG):** This shows a dilated posterior urethra, and a prominent bladder neck with a prominent posterior lip. The bladder is usually small and irregular following decompression. Valve leaflets may be seen. Reflux occurs in more than half. Some

have large para-ureteric diverticulae and reflux into the utriculus may also be seen (see **Figure 50**).

- **Assessment of renal function:** It is usually 5–7 days before the infant's urea and electrolytes reflect their own renal function, rather than their mother's, and enable assessment of prognosis
- **DMSA kidney scan:** This is usually done when a few months old to assess split renal function and to establish a baseline in case of later new renal scarring

Differential diagnosis

Urethral valves need to be considered in all boys presenting with urinary tract infection, urinary tract dilatation, high-grade vesicoureteric reflux (VUR), urethral or bladder outflow obstruction or bladder dysfunction

Treatment

The aims of treatment are to preserve renal and bladder function.

Prenatal

- Parental counselling

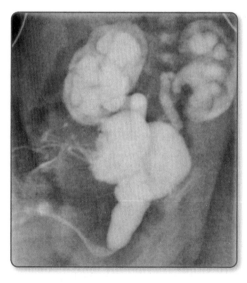

Figure 50 MCUG showing typical urethral configuration of PUV, irregular walled bladder, bilateral reflux and large para-ureteric diverticulae.

- Assess risk and prognosis. Poor prognostic features are early diagnosis (before 24 weeks), oligohydramnios, echogenic kidneys or cysts indicative of dysplasia, high fetal urinary electrolytes ($Na > 100$, $Cl > 90$ mmol/L and osmolality > 210 mmol/L) and raised β_2 microglobulin
- Termination of pregnancy can be considered in severe cases particularly if associated with chromosomal or other severe abnormalities
- Fetal shunting – to preserve renal function and reduce risk of pulmonary hypoplasia. This remains an area of debate with concern that the risks in terms of fetal loss and prematurity outweigh the potential benefits of limiting damage that has already been done
- Planned delivery in a centre with paediatric urology and nephrology facilities

At birth

- Supportive care as needed, including ventilation if there is pulmonary hypoplasia
- Confirm the diagnosis. Ultrasound if there is clinical doubt
- Decompress bladder using a 5–8 Fr tube. Insertion can be difficult because the tube tends to curl back in the dilated posterior urethra
- Start antibiotic prophylaxis
- Monitor urine output – likely to need fluid and electrolyte replacement particularly if diuresis > 5 mL/kg/min.
- MCUG when clinical condition stable
- Valve ablation. With a small urethroscope or resectoscope (8–9 Fr) the valve leaflets can be seen and incised at the 4, 8 and 12 o'clock positions, using a diathermy hook, bugbee electrode, cold knife or YAG laser. A catheter is usually left in situ for 2–5 days. Balloon disruption under radiological control can be considered in infants too small for safe urethroscopy. A check MCUG can be done at the time of removal of the catheter, and some centres carry out routine check cystoscopy at 4–6 weeks
- Urinary diversion is suitable for infants too small for instrumentation or who

fail to decompress after valve ablation, particularly with recurrent sepsis or deteriorating renal function. A Blocksom vesicostomy is the simplest procedure, but urine diversion above the level of the bladder (ureterostomy or nephrostomy) with or without ureteric stenting may be needed if there is ongoing obstruction or stasis at or above the ureterovesical junction

- Early circumcision has been recommended to reduce the risk of bacterial colonisation and infection of the dilated urinary tract
- Prenatal forniceal or renal parenchymal rupture can result in a perirenal urinoma or urinary ascites. If early drainage does not control or seal the leak, repair is needed or nephrectomy if there is no salvageable function in the affected kidney

Follow-up

All but the most mild cases need careful long-term review of renal and bladder function, growth and blood pressure. Many will benefit from a multidisciplinary clinic, including urologists, nephrologists, dietician and continence services.

VUR and bladder dysfunction

About one third will have unilateral reflux and one third bilateral reflux at presentation. High-grade reflux is associated with renal dysplasia, but some of this may also be due to abnormalities in nephrogenesis, arising from abnormal or ectopic insertion of the ureteric bud.

Pop-off mechanisms, which include unilateral reflux, large bladder diverticulae or urinary leak from the kidneys, may tend to protect the contralateral kidney by acting as a pressure reservoir but prognosis is still worse for those with unilateral reflux than those without reflux. This popular theory has been challenged.

VUR and bladder dysfunction are closely interrelated. About 75% will have persisting bladder dysfunction and more than half will have persistent upper tract dilatation after correction of obstruction.

Different patterns of urodynamic abnormality have been identified, including high voiding pressures as a result of sphincter dyssynergia or stricture, hyper-reflexia with poor bladder compliance, and many will develop myogenic failure and overflow incontinence. About half will have daytime incontinence well into late childhood.

The important principle is to optimise bladder function first because VUR improves after relief of obstruction and correction of bladder dysfunction. Surgical treatment may be needed if medical measures fail to halt recurrent infections or deteriorating renal function.

Active individualised treatment of bladder function is needed to develop continence and preserve renal function. Prophylactic antibiotics, anticholinergics for overactivity, alpha-blockers for sphincter dyssynergia and intermittent catherisation all have a role. Catheterisation can be very difficult in a distorted posterior urethra particularly with normal urethral sensation. Some will need an alternative catheterising channel (e.g. Mitrofanoff appendico-vesicostomy) with or without bladder reconstruction.

Prognosis

Approximately 20% will develop end-stage renal failure in childhood. PUV accounts for approximately 16% end-stage renal failure in children in the UK. Unfavourable prognostic factors are detectable dilatation on ultrasound at < 24 weeks' gestation, hyper-echogenic or dysplastic kidneys, lowest serum creatinine > 70 mmol/L, VUR and incontinence, bladder dysfunction and proteinuria. Polyuria may exacerbate damage associated with bladder dysfunction.

Sexual function and fertility may also be affected. Dry ejaculation can occur from pooling of semen in the dilated posterior urethra. Sperm may be extremely viscous, some may have recurrent epididymo-orchitis and there is a higher than normal incidence of testicular maldescent (12%). Poor renal function also contributes to infertility.

Further reading

Caione P, Nappo SG. Posterior urethral valves: long-term outcome. Paed Surg Int 2011; 27:1027–1035.

Morris RK, Kilby MD. An overview of the literature on congenital lower urinary tract obstruction to the PLUTO trial: percutaneous shunting in lower urinary tract obstruction. Aus N Zealand J Obster Gynecol 2009; 49:6–10.

Morris RK, Malin GL, Kilby MD, Collaborative Group PLUTO. The PLUTO trial: percutaneous shunting in lower urinary tract obstruction. Arch Dis Child Fetal Neonatal Ed 2011; 96:e-pub.

Related topics of interest

Postoperative care

Learning outcomes

- To understand the concept of homeostasis and its relevance to postoperative fluid and electrolyte management
- To be familiar with the principles of nutritional support
- To be aware of the range of options for pain management

Overview

Meticulous attention to fluid and electrolyte, nutritional and pain management is a prerequisite to achieving optimal outcomes following surgery in children. There is evidence that inappropriate fluid and electrolyte management is associated with considerable morbidity and mortality in children. According to the National Patient Safety Agency (NPSA) report, 80–90% of intravenous fluids are prescribed by doctors in training, and significant gaps in knowledge have been identified. Deaths and near misses have been reported as a result. It is therefore essential that this aspect of management receives due attention.

Careful management of the nutritional state of patients is required, with preoperative nutritional assessment and appropriate caloric support during both the pre- and postoperative phases. Management of the stress response and pain by a multimodal pain relief strategy is necessary. This service is provided by a dedicated pain team in many institutions.

Fluid and electrolyte management

The French physiologist Claude Bernard introduced the concept of homeostasis in the 19th century. He advocated that the constancy of the 'milieu intérieur' (internal environment) was a critical condition for maintaining health. Appropriate care of the postoperative child is not possible without having a good grasp of the concept of homeostasis.

During the postoperative phase, the constancy of the internal environment is challenged by:

- Fasting, which limits fluid, electrolyte and nutrient intake
- Normal fluid and electrolyte losses through insensible losses (sweat, respiratory tract), urine and stools
- Abnormal fluid and electrolyte losses through vomiting, loose stools, nasogastric tube, drain or stoma

The primary purpose of fluid and electrolyte management is to maintain homeostasis, by preserving the normal volume and composition of body fluids. This is achieved by replacing normal and abnormal losses through maintenance and replacement fluid therapy, respectively.

Maintenance fluid and electrolyte therapy

Maintenance fluid requirements for children are listed in **Table 12** noting that there is a reduction in requirements with increasing age and size. One reason for this is that normal fluid losses in the respiratory tract, urine and stool are higher in early life. In the first few days of life, fluid and electrolytes are restricted because of:

- A high level of antidiuretic hormone (ADH)
- A sodium (Na^+)-retentive state secondary to low mean arterial pressure, reduced glomerular filtration rate and high renin–angiotensin activity.

In contrast, premature neonates have excessive urinary sodium losses due to the immaturity of the proximal convoluted

Table 12 Paediatric fluid requirements*	
Weight	**Volume requirement**
< 2 kg	150 mL/kg/day
2–10 kg	100 mL/kg/day
10–20 kg	1000 mL + 50 mL/kg over 10 kg weight
> 20 kg	1500 mL + 20 mL/kg over 20 kg weight

*Volumes may need to be modified in the presence of pyrexia, hyperventilation, excessive sweating or renal disease.

tubules, which limit Na⁺ reabsorption. Na⁺ supplementation may be required (up to 6 mmol/kg/day). The two most important factors to consider are the volume and solute load to be administered, and therefore the appropriate choice of intravenous fluids is crucial. A selection of appropriate intravenous fluid preparations for use in children is listed in **Table 13**.

An understanding of osmolality and tonicity is essential for appropriate fluid management. Osmolality refers to the concentration of solutes in plasma (mOsm/kg), whereas tonicity refers to the osmotic pressure gradient across a (cell) membrane. As an illustration, both 0.9% saline and 0.18% saline with 4% dextrose have the same concentration of solutes as plasma and are therefore described as iso-osmolar. Approximately 0.9% saline has the same concentration of Na⁺ as the cell, does not cause an osmotic pressure gradient and is described as isotonic. In contrast, 0.18% saline with 4% dextrose has a lower concentration of Na⁺ than the cell. Its glucose content is actively transported into the cell in the non-diabetic child. This results in the fluid in the extracellular compartment becoming relatively dilute with respect to the solute Na⁺ (hypotonic) leading to an osmotic pressure gradient and water moves into cells, causing cellular oedema, injury and eventually death. The NPSA therefore recommends that 0.18% saline with 4% dextrose should be avoided in children.

It is important to be aware of the usefulness and limitations of serum electrolyte measurements in monitoring total body electrolyte status. Because the bulk of total body water is in the extracellular space, serum Na⁺ is a good marker of total body sodium. On the other hand, most of body's potassium (K⁺) is intracellular and serum K⁺ is therefore not a good marker of total body K⁺. Total body K⁺ may be severely depleted in spite of normal serum K⁺ and a normal serum K⁺ should not deter physicians from prescribing K⁺ in postoperative fluids. Omission of K⁺ from postoperative fluids in the patient with normal urine output is a common error. Standard teaching of fluid management readily addresses Na⁺ requirements for homeostasis (2–4 mmol/kg/day). The omission of K⁺ maintenance in fluid prescribing often leads to hypokalaemia. The administration of K⁺ should be considered in all postoperative fluid prescriptions (20–40 mmol KCl/L), except in the immediate postoperative oliguric phase.

Replacement fluid and electrolyte therapy

The aim of replacement fluid therapy is to prevent as well as to replace accumulated fluid deficits. The extent of the fluid deficit is gauged by the assessment of body fluid hydration (**Table 14**). Abnormal fluid losses from diarrhoea, vomiting, stoma and drains closely approximate plasma osmolality and should therefore be replaced millilitre for millilitre with isotonic fluids. Choice of fluids and rate of administration are both important. A commonly used fluid for this purpose is 0.9% saline with 20 mmol/L of KCl.

Management of postoperative oliguria

Anaesthesia and surgery results in a decrease in renal blood flow and an increase in ADH, plasma cortisol and aldosterone.

Table 13　Fluid solute concentrations							
Solution	Na⁺ (mmol/L)	Cl⁻ (mmol/L)	K⁺ (mmol/L)	Ca²⁺ (mmol/L)	Lactate (mmol/L)	Dextrose (%)	Osmolality (mOsm/L)
0.9% NaCl	154	154	0	0	0	0	308
0.45% NaCl 0.15% KCl 5% dextrose	75	95	20	0	0	5	445
Compound sodium lactate (Hartmann's)	131	111	5	2	29	0	279
Requirements mmol/kg/day	3–4	2–4	2–3	1–2	–	–	270–310

Table 14 Assessment of level of clinical dehydration			
Clinical Sign	Mild	Moderate	Severe
Degree of dehydration in: Infant	<5%	5–10%	>10%
Child and adult	<3%	3–6%	>6%
Skin turgor	Normal	Decreased	Markedly decreased
Mucous membranes	Thirsty	Dry	Parched
Skin colour	Normal	Pale	Mottled
Urine output	Decreased	Oliguria	Anuria
Blood pressure	Normal	Normal, ↓	↓↓
Heart rate	Normal, ↑	↑	↑↑
Capillary refill	Normal (<2 seconds)	Delayed (>2 seconds)	Very delayed (>3 seconds)
Fontanelle (<7 months)	Flat	Sunken	Very sunken
Mental status	Consolable	Irritable or lethargic	Limp, depressed consciousness

Urine output decreases and this oliguric phase lasts for 3–5 days. Management comprises postoperative fluid restriction and avoidance of KCl until urine output recovers. It is not uncommon for doctors in training to misinterpret the low urine output as a hypovolaemic state and to administer fluid boluses on this basis. It is important to be aware that urine output is not a good indicator of hydration status in the immediate postoperative phase and should not be used as the sole basis for assessing hydration status.

Nutrition

Assessment of nutritional state

The impact of nutritional state on tissue healing, repair and immune function and hence postoperative outcomes should not be underestimated. Clinical and biochemical markers can be used to estimate nutritional state.

- Clinical markers:
  - A loss of 10% of body mass has been shown to be clinically important and may lead to refeeding syndrome. It must be recognised that acute changes in nutritional state affect body weight quicker than length (asymmetric growth)
  - Other clinical markers used are anthropometric measures: triceps skin fold thickness, which assesses

subcutaneous fat reserves and mid-arm circumference, which assesses somatic muscle mass

- Biochemical markers:
  - Serum albumin, which has a half-life of 20 days but can be affected by hepatic function, hydration status and protein loss from the vascular compartment
  - Transferrin, which has a half-life of 8–9 days but can be inaccurate in the presence of iron-deficiency anaemia, liver failure or significant fluid shifts
  - Retinol binding protein, which has a half-life of 12 hours and which reflects most accurately the acute loss of protein but may be of limited use in renal failure when its excretion is reduced

Calorie requirements

It is useful to categorise calorie provision into protein and non-protein calories. The daily requirement for calories and protein is age-dependent and is as follows:

Age (years)	Calorie requirement	Protein requirement
<1	90–120 kcal/kg	2–3.5 g/kg/day
1–12	60–90 kcal/kg	2–2.5 g/kg/day
>12	30–60 kcal/kg	1.5 g/kg/day

Protein intake should provide 15% of caloric intake, the remainder being used for anabolic needs. It is not unusual to find postoperative patients being prescribed insufficient calories in the form of carbohydrate and lipids, which results in breakdown of body protein stores for calorie needs.

Introduction of postoperative feeding is important in infants and children. This should be as early as possible and the enteral route should be the preferred route. Many infant formula feeds only contain 65–70 kcal/mL. Higher energy feeds may contain 100 kcal/mL or more, with variable protein concentrations available. Specific energy (glucose and medium chain triglyceride) supplements are available but may significantly affect the osmolality of the feed and therefore the tolerance to the modification. Formulae for premature infants may have energy concentrations of 70–80 kcal/mL. The wide variation (in excess of 150 formulae) in feed constituents and requirements makes the role of the specialist paediatric dietitian essential in ensuring that the most appropriate feed is individualised for patients.

In the absence of an enteral route of administration, parenteral nutrition (PN) should be considered if prolonged fasting is anticipated. The energy reserves in infants are low, lasting as little as 24 hours in premature infants, 4 days in term infants and 7 days in older children. A peripheral route may be used for short-term administration, with line changes every 2–3 days. Both PN and central venous lines have their own complications that must be balanced against the nutritional benefits.

Refeeding syndrome

With a loss of 5–10% of premorbid body mass, careful monitoring of electrolytes, in particular serum phosphate, magnesium and potassium, caused by refeeding should be considered. With chronic weight loss, monitoring urinary electrolytes for Na^+ store depletion as well as trace element depletion should be considered.

Pain management

Pain is common after all surgical procedures. In minor surgery, this may last 2–3 days, whilst in major surgery this may persist during the first postoperative week. The safety and efficacy of analgesic regimes has developed significantly over the last three to four decades. Children dislike suppositories and intramuscular injections. Non-opioid drugs are effective in managing somatic pain, but their efficacy is limited for visceral pain.

Paracetamol

The precise mechanism of action of paracetamol is not clear, but it appears to interact with the more effective oxidised form of cyclo-oxygenase (COX), thereby reducing prostaglandin (PG) synthesis and influencing the endogenous cannabinoid receptors in the synaptic cleft.

Intravenous paracetamol may rapidly achieve peak concentrations within 15 minutes, whilst maintaining an analgesic effect for 4–6 hours and an antipyretic effect for 6 hours.

Non-steroidal anti-inflammatory drugs

Common non-steroidal anti-inflammatory drugs (NSAIDs) in use in children are ibuprofen and diclofenac. They inhibit COX-1 and COX-2 and block PG synthesis. This decreases local inflammation and modulates the PG-related central response to pain. It is important to recognise that it may take 1–2 hours before the maximal analgesic effect is achieved and that pre-emptive treatment does not extend the length of the analgesic effect. The side-effect profile of NSAIDs limits their role in the first 3 months of life and must be a consideration in older children. The use of an NSAID in conjunction with paracetamol is more beneficial than paracetamol or a NSAID alone.

Contraindications to their use are platelet and clotting abnormalities, acute renal or hepatic insufficiency and aspirin sensitivity. Asthma is not a contraindication unless the child is wheezy or has a history of adverse reaction to NSAIDs.

Opiates

The introduction of opiate analgesia enhanced this multimodal role with superior visceral pain control.

Neuronal sensitivity to opiates relates to their binding of receptors on neuronal cells in the brain, spinal cord and nerve plexuses or peripheral nocireceptors. Dependent upon the site of action, opiates can inhibit the release of excitatory and/or inhibitory transmitters. This can produce a wide range of observed physiological responses. Studies have shown that opioid-based analgesia in neonates resulted in clinical benefit, but that there is no simple dose relationship. This is due to developmental changes in infants and children who are involved in the reorganisation of synaptic connectivity (nociceptors), receptor development, enzymatic activity and pharmacokinetic sensitivity opioid analgesia.

The main side effects of opiate analgesia are respiratory or central nervous system depression, vasodilation, reduced gastrointestinal peristalsis, nausea and vomiting and are monitored as part of a pain chart assessment, in the form of a neonatal or infant pain scale or a visual analogue pain scale.

The main delivery systems for opiates in children are the oral route (codeine, morphine) or the intravenous route via patient-controlled analgesia (PCA) or nurse-controlled analgesia (NCA) in the form of infusions, with background or bolus supplementation. The use of fentanyl, instead of morphine, is associated with less nausea and vomiting. The addition of ketamine, (an N-methyl D-aspartate receptor antagonist in the spinal cord and brain) to a morphine PCA or NCA increases analgesic efficacy.

Typical protocols prescribed by the pain team are as follows:
- Loading dose of morphine usually administered in theatre:
  - < 1 month – no loading dose
  - 1–6 months – 50 µg/kg
  - > 6 months – 100 µg/kg
- Infusions:
  - 2 mg/kg morphine in 100 mL 0.9% NaCl solution
  - Bolus = 20 µg/kg in 1 mL
  - Background infusion 4–10 µg/kg/h (maximum 20 µg/kg/h)

Gabapentin

There is evidence that gabapentin reduces opiate requirements when administered postoperatively. It binds to presynaptic voltage-gated calcium channels, inhibiting calcium influx and suppressing the release of excitatory neurotransmitters in the spinal cord, and also modulates glutamate receptors in the spinal cord.

Local or regional anaesthesia

Amide local anaesthetics (LA) are liposoluble and are soluble across nerve cell membranes. Their mechanism of action is to block the propagation of a nerve impulse along the fibre by inactivating the voltage-dependent sodium channels which initiate the action potential. The mechanism of binding and clearance is important as α-acid glycoprotein binds LAs in the serum. Its serum level is reduced in infancy and increases to adult levels by 12 months. The free proportion of LA in the serum relates to toxic complications, which can be neurotoxic and/or myotoxic. A rapid rise in serum concentrations can cause neurological and cardiac toxicity.

LA compounds can be administered locally, regionally, into the caudal or epidural space and by an intrathecal route.

Local	Bupivacaine 0.8 mL/kg (2.5 mg/mL solution)
Regional	Bupivacaine 0.25 mL/kg (2.5 mg/mL solution) (Caudal 0.5 mL/kg for sacral block, 1.25 mL/kg for T10 block) Levobupivacaine 0.25–0.5 mL/kg (2.5 mg/mL solution)

The use of adrenaline (1:200,000) as a vasoconstrictor decreases the absorption rate and therefore has a slower effect but prolonged action, and is usually restricted to the subcutaneous route and contraindicated in digital ring blocks.

Behavioural therapy

There is now a significant body of evidence supporting distraction techniques, with reduced analgesia requirements in the postoperative period, and should be considered as part of a multimodal package.

Further reading

Bingham R, Lloyd-Thomas A, Sury M (eds). Hatch & Sumner's Textbook of paediatric anaesthesia, 3rd edn. London: Hodder Arnold, 2008.

Lee CA. Postoperative analgesia in children: getting it right. South Afr J Anaesth Analg 2011; 17:359–361.

National Patient Safety Agency. Reducing the risk of hyponatraemia when administering intravenous infusions to children. Patient safety alert. London: National Patient Safety Agency, 2007.

Related topics of interest

- Central venous access techniques (p. 38)
- Paediatric anaesthesia (p. 227)
- Perioperative care: surgical safety and human factors (p. 274)

Prenatal diagnosis and counselling

Learning outcomes

- To appreciate the importance of multidisciplinary team working during antenatal care provision
- To understand the principles of effective counselling
- To be aware of the role of palliative care
- To be familiar with the impact of the common trisomies on the outcome of pregnancy

Overview

Many conditions are diagnosed prenatally as a result of routine antenatal screening. This provides the opportunity to plan the type and place of delivery and the postnatal management of the neonate. Antenatal counselling helps parents to adequately prepare for the birth of a baby who may require surgical or other intervention.

Counselling

Counselling is a two-way confidential communication process, which helps parents understand problems detected in their unborn baby and which provides them with the opportunity to be involved in decision making and in making plans for their baby, once born.

Basic skills in counselling include the use of active listening, encouraging parents to talk and ask questions freely and focusing on relevant issues in relation to their baby. The standard set by the National Fetal Anomaly Screening Program is that all pregnant women should undergo a booking scan at 9–11 weeks and a mid-trimester anomaly screening scan at 18–22 weeks. These scans may not be performed initially in a specialist unit.

If abnormalities are detected, the woman is referred to an obstetrician, with some fetal medicine training or a fetal medicine specialist in a designated fetal medicine centre. Following identification of an abnormality, there should be clear definition of the pathology, followed by agreement within the multidisciplinary maternity/neonatal/surgery healthcare team about diagnosis and prognosis.

Where a condition requiring surgery is detected, it is important that the counsellor is fully aware of the details of each individual case. This is so that parents are given the correct individualised information about their baby's condition, using written leaflets to support counselling. These may be available in surgical units and are also available through Fetal Anomaly Screening Program and Bliss (Baby Life Support Systems).

Ideally both parents should be present. They should be counselled in a private and quiet room and given information about postnatal management, the likely requirement for surgery, including the full range of operative options, possible complications and prognosis. They should be given the opportunity to visit the unit where their baby will be delivered, the surgical unit the baby will be transferred to (if the maternity and surgical units are not co-located), and have the opportunity to meet representatives from the surgical, medical and nursing teams (Neonatal Toolkit DH 2009). The method of feeding should be discussed and mothers should be encouraged to breastfeed and/or express breast milk. Mothers should be advised to express breast milk within 6 hours of delivery.

Where conditions are likely to be life-limiting, it is important that parents receive the best possible antenatal information, with involvement of all relevant parties. Parents may choose to terminate the pregnancy and it is important that this important decision is informed, based upon accurate, high-quality information.

While some parents may opt to continue with the pregnancy, others may choose a palliative care pathway for their baby. Perinatal palliative care is the holistic provision of supportive care and end-of-life care. The eligibility of the fetus or neonate for such care should first be established using a multidisciplinary model that is centred on the family.

Approximately 5% of pregnancies are complicated by congenital structural malformations, up to 15% of which are potentially lethal, such as bilateral renal agenesis or hypoplasia, with oligo- or anhydramnios and pulmonary hypoplasia. Late termination of pregnancy is legal at any gestation until birth if the child has a substantial risk of severe mental or physical disability. The Royal College of Obstetricians and Gynaecologists' guideline recommends that after 22 weeks' gestation, termination of pregnancy should involve an offer of feticide. Many parents decide to continue with such a pregnancy, which requires planning for perinatal palliative care. Qualitative evidence suggests that this choice may lessen the potential emotional and psychological effects associated with abortion.

Trisomies
Ultrasound appearances

Prenatal ultrasound is a powerful tool for detecting structural abnormalities in fetuses with the 3 most common trisomies: trisomy 21 (Down syndrome), trisomy 18 (Edward's syndrome) and trisomy 13 (Patau's syndrome). Increased nuchal translucency (>3.5 mm) measured between the 10th and 14th weeks of gestation may be associated with any of the trisomies as well as with Turner's syndrome (karyotype 45,X), triploidies and structural cardiac defects. Antenatal suspicion of trisomies is further increased by the presence of any cardiac,

bowel, brain, renal or limb abnormalities and for this reason, chromosomal testing is offered to confirm or refute such diagnoses.

Down syndrome

Trisomy 21 has an incidence of around 1 in 700–1000 live births and is the most common chromosomal abnormality in humans. If there is associated antenatal hydrops, the fetus is unlikely to survive and if born alive, life is usually limited. Prognosis depends on associated abnormalities at birth, but in general, every attempt should be made to support the medical and surgical needs of a baby with Down syndrome.

Edward's syndrome

Trisomy 18 is the second most common multiple malformation syndrome, with an incidence of approximately 1 in 3000 live births. This is usually a life-limiting condition within the first weeks to months of life, although there are case reports of babies surviving into early childhood. If born alive, palliative care is usually offered and is a valid treatment.

Patau's syndrome

Trisomy 13 has an incidence of approximately 1 in 4000–10,000 live births. Around half of fetuses have holoprosencephaly, with some having exomphalos and/or renal abnormalities. Median survival is 7 days and very few have been reported to survive until the first year. Hence palliation is offered to those born alive.

Given the role of palliation in the management of neonates with Edward's and Patau's syndrome, it is essential that these diagnoses are made at birth before embarking upon complex surgery, so that the full range of management options, including palliation, can be offered to affected families.

Further reading

NHS and Department of Health. Toolkit for high quality neonatal services. London: Department of Health, 2009.

Rennie J. Rennie and Roberton textbook of neonatology, 5th edn. Philadelphia: Churchill Livingstone, 2012.

Jones KL. Smith's recognisable patterns of human malformation, 6th edn. Philadelphia: Elsevier Saunders, 2005.

Related topics of interest

Pyloric atresia

Learning objectives

- To recognise pyloric atresia as the rarest cause of neonatal gastrointestinal obstruction
- To learn the classification of pyloric atresia
- To recognise the importance of the association of pyloric atresia with epidermolysis bullosa
- To review the clinical and biochemical manifestations of gastric outlet obstruction
- To understand the surgical management of patients with pyloric atresia

Overview

Pyloric atresia is a rare cause of neonatal gastrointestinal obstruction but, for the patient with this pathology, it is of extreme importance that this does not lead to delay in its recognition and treatment so that morbidity and mortality are prevented.

The obstruction may manifest itself on antenatal scans or postnatally, with non-bilious vomiting, dehydration and the electrolyte imbalances of gastric outlet obstruction. Surgical correction is mandatory. If pyloric atresia is an isolated defect and is corrected early, the prognosis is excellent. The prognosis is significantly worse in patients with the association of pyloric atresia and epidermolysis bullosa.

Epidemiology and pathology

Pyloric atresia has an incidence of 1 in 1,000,000 live births and it accounts for < 1% of all gastrointestinal atresias. It can be sporadic or familial. There does not seem to be a difference in sex distribution.

Definition and classification

Congenital complete obstruction of the pyloric lumen. It is classified into three types:

- Type I – a mucosal membrane or web is present
- Type II – there is a cord instead of the pyloric channel
- Type III – a gap is present between the antrum of the stomach and the first portion of the duodenum

Associations

Mostly pyloric atresia happens as an isolated lesion. However, rates of 30–40% of associated congenital anomalies have been reported. Associated anomalies include aplasia cutis congenita, malrotation, intestinal duplication, multiple intestinal atresias, oesophageal atresia and agenesis of the gall bladder.

The most common association is with epidermolysis bullosa, which is an heterogeneous group of skin fragility syndromes with the diagnostic hallmark of blistering and erosions of the skin with minor trauma. The cutaneous findings include tissue separation either within the basal cells at the level of the hemidesmosomes or within the lamina lucida of the dermal-epidermal basement membrane.

Aetiology

Pyloric atresia is thought to result from arrested development between the 5th and 7th weeks of fetal life. It has been suggested that this could arise from a vascular accident. Another hypothesis that has been considered is a failure of recanalisation of the pyloric channel.

It is thought that pyloric atresia arises from an autosomal recessive genetic defect. This is supported by studies of affected families, the absence of parent to child transmission, frequent consanguinity in parents, equal sex distribution among affected patients and 1:3 ratio of affected to non-affected children.

Epidermolysis bullosa associated with pyloric atresia has an autosomal recessive inheritance pattern. Defects in the genes *ITGA6*, *ITGB4* and *PLEC1* have been identified in patients with the association of epidermolysis bullosa and pyloric atresia. This association has given rise to new theories regarding the pathogenesis of pyloric atresia. It has been suggested that as a result of poorly functional or absent hemidesmosomal complexes, there might be separation of the intestinal mucosal layer which will lead to inflammatory responses and development of secondary fibrosis.

Clinical features

Pyloric atresia can present antenatally with polyhydramnios. The hallmark of the clinical features is non-bilious vomiting. With time, this will lead to clinical signs of dehydration. The baby can have abdominal distension, but this may not be marked, given that the level of obstruction is high. Some have described visible peristaltic gastric movements. Biochemically, the baby will present with electrolyte disturbances typical of gastric outlet obstruction: hypochloraemic hypokalaemic metabolic alkalosis. This is a direct result of the loss of chloride (Cl^-), potassium (K^+), sodium (Na^+) and hydrogen (H^+) in vomiting and is made worse owing to the following:

- Paradoxical aciduria – extracellular volume contraction activates the renin-angiotensin II – aldosterone system. Angiotensin II increases bicarbonate (HCO_3^-) reabsorption by stimulating Na^+–H^+ exchange and aldosterone increases H^+ excretion in the renal and collecting tubules, particularly when potassium becomes depleted
- Reduced pancreatic HCO_3^- excretion. This is normally stimulated by acid arriving in the duodenum
- Contraction alkalosis – extracellular contraction stimulates isosmotic HCO_3^- reabsorption in the proximal tubule

Differential diagnosis

Other causes of neonatal gastrointestinal obstruction have to be considered in the list of differential diagnosis, predominantly causes of high obstruction like duodenal atresia, gastric volvulus and malrotation with midgut volvulus. Other causes of pyloric obstruction are pyloric duplication, retrograde duodenogastric intussusception and aberrant pancreatic tissue obstructing the pylorus.

Investigations

- X-ray abdomen: will not show any gas beyond the stomach if the obstruction is complete
- USS: may show a long, stretched-out pylorus
- Contrast upper gastrointestinal study: should confirm the diagnosis. Pathognomonic sign of complete obstruction is a long, stretched-out beak

Of note is that prenatal testing in families at risk for epidermolysis bullosa associated with pyloric atresia has been performed from chorionic villus sampling, which can be done as early as the 10th week of gestation.

Management

- Type I: excision with Heineke-Mikulicz pyloroplasty – longitudinal incision through the pylorus from the distal antrum to the proximal duodenum which is closed transversely
- Type II: if the atresia is short – Heineke-Mikulicz pyloroplasty; if the atresia is long – excision of the atretic segment with gastroduodenostomy
- Type III: gastroduodenostomy (Billroth type 1)

Gastrojejunostomy has a failure rate of 60% and mortality of 55% so it is not advocated.

Some authors have suggested that at laparotomy the gall bladder and bowel rotation should be examined and that a skin biopsy specimen should be taken at the time of surgery for electron microscopy, if there is a family history of epidermolysis bullosa. It is now well accepted that the association with epidermolysis bullosa should not preclude surgical treatment.

Complications and prognosis

Delayed diagnosis may lead to aspiration pneumonia, respiratory compromise, difficulties in ventilation, severe metabolic derangement and gastric perforation which can be fatal. If isolated and corrected early, pyloric atresia has an excellent outcome.

After corrective surgery, morbidity and mortality are usually only due to associated anomalies. In epidermolysis bullosa due to the exudative lesions there can be septicaemia, electrolyte imbalance, protein loss, failure to thrive and death. But the long-term outcome can vary from early death to long-term survival. In some cases, the skin fragility may be relatively mild and age-associated amelioration of the skin fragility allows individuals to conduct normal life activities with relatively minor blistering tendency.

Further reading

Chung HJ, Uitto J. Epidermolysis bullosa with pyloric atresia. Dermatol Clin 2010; 28:43–54.

Okoye BO, Parikh DH, Buick RG, et al. Pyloric atresia: five new cases, a new association, and a review of the literature with guidelines. J Pediatr Surg 2000; 35:1242–1245.

Pfendner EG, et al. Prenatal diagnosis for epidermolysis bullosa: a study of 144 consecutive pregnancies at risk. Prenat Diagn 2003; 23:447–456.

Related topics of interest

Pyloric stenosis

Learning outcomes

- To understand the epidemiology, postulated aetiology and pathophysiology of infantile hypertrophic pyloric stenosis (IHPS), including associated biochemical abnormalities
- To develop the ability to diagnose IHPS on the basis of clinical features
- To gain familiarity with non-operative and operative aspects of management and to develop awareness of potential complications

Overview

IHPS is the most common cause of non-bilious vomiting that requires surgery in infants. Autopsy findings were first reported in 1717 by Blair and it was not until 1888 that the clinical features and pathology were accurately described by Hirschsprung.

Epidemiology and aetiology

The reported incidence is 1–4 in 1000 live births, with Caucasians affected more than Afro-Caribbeans, Asians and Hispanics. The male-to-female ratio is 4:1, with 30% of patients being first-born males. More than 90% of cases occur sporadically. There is a familial predisposition in 7% of cases. Male and female infants of an affected mother have a 20% and 7% risk of developing IHPS, respectively. With an affected father, these risks are 5% and 2.5%, respectively. There is an increased incidence in infants with blood groups B and O. Associated anomalies are rare.

The cause is unknown. The circular smooth muscle fibres of the pylorus are hypertrophied and cause gastric outlet obstruction. Abnormalities in smooth muscle innervation, intestinal pacemaker cells (interstitial cells of Cajal), expression of nitric oxide synthase, extracellular matrix proteins as well as a number of growth factors have all been reported. Living in rural areas may play a role.

Clinical features

The typical infant with IHPS is usually 4–6 weeks old and previously well. The predominant presenting symptom is non-bilious vomiting, which is often described as projectile. The vomitus may occasionally be blood-stained as a result of oesophagitis or gastritis. The infant is usually hungry after vomits. Following prolonged vomiting, severe dehydration and weight loss may be present. Inspection of the abdomen may reveal visible peristaltic waves across the upper abdomen. Jaundice occurs in 2–5% of infants, with IHPS associated with a reduced level of glucuronyl transferase.

Differential diagnosis

- Overfeeding
- Gastro-oesophageal reflux
- Sepsis
- Raised intracranial pressure
- Proximal duodenal obstruction
- Inborn errors of metabolism
- Congenital adrenal hyperplasia

Investigations

Serum urea, creatinine, electrolytes and blood gases

In pyloric stenosis, there is continued vomiting of acid gastric fluid, without the loss of alkaline duodenal fluid. The cardinal findings are dehydration, metabolic alkalosis, hypochloraemia, and hypocalcaemia. Loss of gastric fluid leads to volume depletion and loss of Na^+, Cl^-, H^+ and K^+, resulting in a hypokalaemic, hypochloraemic metabolic alkalosis. The kidneys attempt to maintain normal pH by excreting excess bicarbonate. However, renal bicarbonate excretion is affected by hypochloraemia, hypocalcaemia and reduced glomerular filtration, all of which may occur with prolonged vomiting. The kidneys attempt to conserve Na^+ at the expense of H^+, which can lead to paradoxical aciduria. In more severe dehydration cases, renal K⁺ losses are accelerated in an attempt to retain fluid and Na⁺.

Test feed

A test feed enables a definitive diagnosis of pyloric stenosis to be made. The environment should be a warm quiet room. The infant is placed across the carer's lap and the abdomen is exposed. The infant is offered a bottle of milk or Dioralyte, which pacifies the infant and stimulates peristalsis. The upper abdomen is observed for visible peristaltic waves, but their presence does not constitute a positive test feed. The abdomen is approached from the left side and gently and deeply palpated to feel for the hard pyloric tumour or 'olive', which is located lateral to the rectus muscle above the level of the umbilicus. A positive test feed eliminates the need for radiological imaging.

Ultrasound

In some centres, ultrasound scanning (USS) is used as the primary diagnostic modality whereas in others, it is used when a test feed is negative on two occasions in the presence of continuing symptoms. The advantages of USS are non-invasiveness, lack of radiation, reproducibility, sensitivity above 95% and specificity of 100%. The diagnostic criteria are based on the work done by Rohrschneider, with pyloric muscle thickness ≥ 3 mm, pyloric canal length ≥ 15 mm, and muscle diameter ≥ 11 mm. In preterm and low-birth infants, a pyloric ratio (pyloric muscle wall thickness/pyloric diameter) ≥ 0.27 is diagnostic.

Treatment

IHPS is not a surgical emergency. Resuscitation and operative management are the two components to treatment. The aims of resuscitation are to correct fluid, electrolyte and acid–base abnormalities. The infant is kept nil by mouth and on intravenous fluids. The rate of infusion depends on the degree of dehydration. A commonly used regimen is 0.45% saline + 5% Dextrose (with 20 mmol of KCL per litre) at a rate of 150 mL/kg/day. A nasogastric tube (NGT) is inserted and gastric losses are replaced mL for mL, using 0.9% saline and 20 mmol of KCl/L. Serum electrolytes and blood gases are checked regularly until normality is achieved. Only when the electrolyte abnormalities have been corrected can the infant be considered for surgery. Administration of general anaesthesia prior to correction of metabolic alkalosis carries the risk of postoperative apnoea. It is worth pointing out to anxious parents that correction of electrolyte and/or acid–base abnormalities can take a few days and that it is unsafe to proceed with surgery.

Operative management

Open pyloromyotomy

- Ramstedt originally described the operation of pyloroplasty in 1907 and of pyloromyotomy in 1912, following a postoperative complication, when he realised that sutures to the muscle layers could be dispensed with.
- A single dose of antibiotics is given preoperatively
- A circum-umbilical or right upper quadrant incision is made
- The peritoneal cavity is entered
- The pyloric tumour is gently delivered out of the wound
- It is grasped between the index finger and thumb
- An incision is made anteriorly in the pylorus, avoiding blood vessels
- The tumour is carefully split until the mucosa bulges
- Care is taken not to cause mucosal perforation, which is usually at the duodenal end
- An incomplete myotomy may result if the myotomy incision is not extended far enough onto the stomach
- Integrity of the mucosa is tested by injecting approximately 50–60 mL of air via the NGT
- Bleeding from venous engorgement usually settles

Laparoscopic pyloromyotomy

Laparoscopic pyloromyotomy utilises a 3 or 5 mm umbilical port for the camera and two 3 mm working ports or stab incisions for instruments. A myotomy is made and the muscle layers are split using a spreader. The results from randomised controlled trials, comparing the open and laparoscopic techniques, suggest marginal differences in clinical outcomes such as operating time, postoperative vomiting, time to full feeds, postoperative length of stay, and intra- and postoperative complications.

Complications of both approaches include wound infection, mucosal perforation and incomplete myotomy. The rates for all of these are < 2%.

After the operation, the NGT is removed. Feeding regimens vary between institutions, from ad libitum feeding to nil by mouth for 6–12 hours followed by gradually building up of feeds. Most patients are usually discharged after 24–48 hours.

Further reading

Panteli C. New insights into the pathogenesis of infantile pyloric stenosis. Pediatr Surg Int 2009; 25:1043–1052.

Jia WQ, Tian JH, Yang KH, et al. Open versus laparoscopic pyloromyotomy for pyloric stenosis: a meta-analysis of randomized controlled trials. Eur J Pediatr Surg 2011; 21:77–81.

Krogh C, Fischer TK, Skotte L, et al. Familial aggregation and heritability of pyloric stenosis. JAMA 2010; 303:393–2399.

Related topics of interest

- Gastro-oesophageal reflux disease (p. 133)
- Pyloric atresia (p. 290)

Rectal prolapse

Learning outcomes

- To be able to recognise the features of rectal prolapse from the clinical history and physical examination
- To gain an understanding of the aetiological factors in order to aid selection of an appropriate management strategy
- To be familiar with non-operative and operative management options

Overview

Rectal prolapse consists of the protrusion of either the mucosa or the full-thickness rectal wall through the anus. It may be idiopathic or it may have an underlying cause. Rectal prolapse is a relatively common problem in young children and can cause significant distress to both the child and the parents.

Epidemiology and aetiology

The highest incidence is in the first year of life. Boys and girls are equally affected. Rectal prolapse is thought to be secondary to weak pelvic floor musculature. This weakness may be caused by straining at constipated stools and prolonged periods of sitting on the toilet because of protracted diarrhoea or constipation, allowing the pelvic diaphragm to become stretched. In some children, an additional factor may be the fact that the rectal submucosa is only loosely attached to the underlying muscularis, allowing prolapse. Rectal prolapse can also be associated with:

- Cystic fibrosis
- Neuromuscular disorders such as spina bifida
- Rectal polyps
- Cow's milk protein intolerance
- A posterior sagittal anorectoplasty for anorectal malformation
- Rectal parasites
- Solitary rectal ulcer syndrome (SRUS), in which, there is usually a small ulcer on the anterior rectal wall
- Sexual abuse (a rare, but important cause)

Clinical features

The parents usually consult a physician after seeing a dark or bright-red mass, protruding from the child's anus during defaecation, and some parents will provide photographic evidence. The child may also complain of discomfort during defaecation, which may alert the parents to a potential problem. Often, a history of constipation is clear and parents may remark on the length of time the child spends in the bathroom. Equally, a prolonged period of gastroenteritis with protracted diarrhoea may have led to the first episode of prolapse. Bleeding is rarely the primary symptom. A significant proportion of patients will have associated faecal incontinence.

Features of SRUS include tenesmus, blood and mucus per rectum. Rarely, children with undiagnosed cystic fibrosis present with rectal prolapse and this needs to be borne in mind during history taking and examination.

Rectal prolapse in children will often spontaneously reduce when they stand from the toilet and it is uncommon for them to be able to demonstrate the prolapse in the clinic room. Some older children will have learnt to reduce the prolapse themselves. Prolonged exposure of the prolapsed mucosa predisposes to ulceration, haemorrhage and a discharge of mucus. In rare instances, failure to reduce the prolapse may lead to ischaemia and gangrene of the prolapsed bowel.

Investigations

- Examination awake +/– examination under anaesthetic (EUA)
  - It is important to try and differentiate between a 'mucosal' prolapse (most common in infants) (**Figure 53a**) and a 'full-thickness' prolapse (more common in older children) (**Figure 53b**) because their treatments and outcome differ. A distinguishing feature between mucosal and full-thickness prolapse is that the former has radial folds visible on the

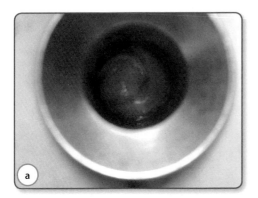

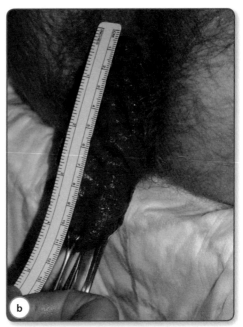

Figure 53 (a) A view of a mucosal rectal prolapse through a proctoscope prior to injection with phenol; (b) an 11 cm full-thickness rectal prolapse in a 15-year-old adolescent.

mucosa whereas the latter has circular folds
- A sweat test to exclude cystic fibrosis

Differential diagnosis

- The most common is a rectal polyp or external haemorrhoids (**Figure 54**)
- Intussusception, on rare occasions; usually obvious on EUA, but if not, either an abdominal ultrasound or a contrast enema may be required
- Older girls may have pelvic floor problems and require a joint surgical/gynaecological review

Treatment

Non-operative management

Appropriately position the child at defaecation avoiding the following:
- Prematurely placing children on 'adult' toilets which causes their pelvis to 'fall' into the toilet

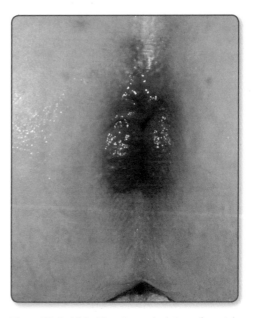

Figure 54 A child with quite marked circumferential external haemorrhoids who had been referred as a patient with a rectal prolapse.

- Children having potty seats which are so low that their bottom is much lower than their knees

Both of these factors make an unnatural angle to defaecate, promoting straining and thus increasing the risk of prolapse.

- Treat constipation with laxatives. Softeners rather than strong stimulants are the treatment of choice
- Prompt manual reduction of prolapse to avoid incarceration and strangulation
- Solitary rectal ulcer syndrome:
  - A trial of short chain fatty acid enemas may 'desensitise' the rectal wall, stop the tenesmus and allow resolution of symptoms and prolapse. This may need to be repeated
  - Biofeedback
- If the sweat test is positive, a referral to a paediatrician with expertise in managing cystic fibrosis is warranted

Operative management

- Injection sclerotherapy:
  - This is the first line of treatment in mucosal prolapse if conservative treatment fails
  - Many compounds have been used namely 5% Phenol in almond oil (beware, 90% phenol which, if used, causes rectal stricturing), isotonic saline, hypertonic saline or ethyl alcohol. The sclerosing agent is injected into the submucosal layer to produce an inflammatory response and subsequent scar tissue formation which prevents the mucosa from prolapsing
  - This treatment may need to be repeated
  - Success rate is reported to be above 90%
- Thiersch suture:
  - It is indicated in persistent mucosal prolapse or in an infant with a full-thickness prolapse but no underlying neurological problem
  - Involves passing a suture around the anus, over a Hegar dilator
  - Treatment tightens the anal outlet and prevents prolapse from recurring

while the musculature of the pelvis regains normal tone. Care must be taken not to make the suture too tight, as this can lead to difficult passage of stool or too loose, as the bowel could prolapse through and subsequently fail to reduce, leading to swelling and ischaemia

  - Success rate is about 90%
- Operative fixation techniques can be described as 'perineal' or 'abdominal':
  - Perineal techniques include:
    - Delorme procedure – plication of muscle with mucosal resection and suturing
    - Altemeier procedure – perineal rectosigmoidectomy
  - Abdominal approaches are
    - Laparoscopic/open rectopexy: the rectum is mobilised and sutured to the sacral promontory in multiple locations with non-absorbable sutures
    - Laparoscopic/open mesh rectopexy: as above but a mesh is placed between the posterior rectal wall and the sacrum
  - Rarely, an open posterior rectopexy: through a natal cleft incision, the coccyx is excised and the rectum is mobilised and suspended from the cut edge of the sacrum

Outcome

- Mucosal prolapse:
  - The vast majority respond to either conservative management or sclerotherapy
- Full-thickness prolapse:
  - The outcome is more guarded due to the more varied aetiology
  - In the younger child, a Thiersch suture alone may suffice but usually, a more invasive procedure is required
  - In older girls, a rectal prolapse may be a sign of 'pelvic floor descent' and merely treating the prolapse does not resolve the underlying problem and leads to recurrence

Further reading

Keighley M, Monson J. Rectal prolapse. In: Keighley MRB, Williams NS (eds). Surgery of the anus, rectum and colon, 3rd edn. Saunders, 2007.

Tou S, et al. Surgery for complete rectal prolapse in adults. Cochrane Database System Rev 2008; (4):CD001758.

Vaizey CJ, van den Bogaerde JB, Emmanuel AV, et al. Solitary rectal ulcer syndrome. Br J Surg 1998; 85:1617–1623.

Related topics of interest

- Anorectal malformation in females (p. 12)
- Anorectal malformation in males (p. 15)
- Child protection (p. 44)
- Faecal incontinence and idiopathic constipation (p. 115)
- Gastrointestinal bleeding (p. 129)
- Intussusception (p. 181)

Renal failure

Learning outcomes

- To recognise acute renal failure (= acute kidney injury, AKI)
- To know the causes of and how to investigate and treat AKI
- To be able to recognise chronic renal failure (chronic kidney disease [CKD])
- To know the causes of CKD
- To be aware of principles of management of CKD
- To be aware of renal replacement therapies (RRTs)

Overview

Acute renal failure (AKI) is a sudden decrease in renal function, with rapid decline in glomerular filtration rate (GFR) and tubular function, resulting in loss of fluid and electrolyte homeostasis. The new terminology for acute renal failure is acute kidney injury (AKI) to reflect different ranges of insults, which lead to a functional or structural change in the kidney. The urine output may be normal, decreased or increased.

Chronic renal failure, now known as chronic kidney disease (CKD), is a state of irreversible kidney damage and/or reduction of kidney function which is usually progressive. There are five stages of CKD (see **Table 15**).

	Table 15 Stages of CKD	
Stages	GFR* (mL/min/1.73 m²)	Description
1	> 90	Kidney damage** with normal or GFR
2	60–89	Usually asymptomatic
3	30–59	Metabolic abnormalities
4	15–29	Growth failure
5	< 15	Renal replacement therapy

*eGFR = (height (cm) × 40)/plasma creatinine (mmol/L)
**Kidney damage is defined as pathologic abnormalities or markers of damage, including abnormalities in blood or urine tests or imaging.

Epidemiology and aetiology

AKI has a yearly incidence of approximately 0.8 per 100,000 population (UK), a fifth of adult AKI. However, AKI is increasing in incidence due to more complex cases with an increasing number of co-morbidities. In neonates, 27% of AKIs are secondary to ischaemia due to congenital heart disease.

In the UK, the prevalence of end-stage renal failure (ESRF) in children younger than 16 years is 65 per million age-related population (pmarp), with an incidence of 7.9 pmarp. ESRF is 1.5 times more prevalent in males than in females and 2.5 times more prevalent in the South Asian population than in the Caucasian population.

The causes of AKI can be classified as:

- Prerenal: results from fall in glomerular perfusion pressure and blood flow
- Renal: vascular, glomerular or tubular/interstitial
- Postrenal: due to obstruction, often precipitated by infection

See **Table 16** for details. Please note that causes are not mutually exclusive and there may be multiple insults leading to AKI. Causes of AKI can also be classified according to age of presentation:

- Neonates: perinatal asphyxia, posterior urethral valves, cardiac surgery
- Young children: haemolytic uraemic syndrome (HUS), cardiac surgery
- Older children: HUS, glomerulonephritides, interstitial nephritis

The causes of CKD in the UK include the following:

- Renal dysplasia ± vesicoureteric reflux (34%)
- Glomerular diseases (16.9%)
- Obstructive uropathy (16.2%)
- Tubulo-interstitial disease (6.3%)
- Congenital nephrosis (8.7%)
- Metabolic diseases (2.5%)
- Renovascular disease (4.3%)
- Polycystic kidney disease (3.3%)
- Malignancy (1.6%)
- Drug nephrotoxicity (0.5%)

Table 16 Causes of acute kidney injurys		
Prerenal	**Volume depletion**	
	• Bleeding (trauma, surgery, gastrointestnal bleed)	
	• Gastrointestnal (vomiting, diarrhoea, ileus)	
	• Urinary (diabetic ketoacidosis, diabetes insipidus, diuretics)	
	• Cutaneous (burns)	
	Decreased effective arterial pressure	
	• Septic shock	
	• Congestive heart failure	
	• Drugs, e.g. angiotensin-converting enzyme inhibitors, cyclosporin A	
	Decreased effective circulating volume	
	• Hypoalbuminaemic state (nephrotic syndrome, cirrhosis)	
	• Drugs, e.g. vasodilators	
Renal	**Vascular**	
	• Thrombosis: arterial and venous	
	• Haemolytic uraemic syndrome	
	• Malignant hypertension	
	• Vasculitis	
	Glomerular	
	• Acute glomerulonephritis	
	Tubular and interstitial	
	• Acute tubular necrosis (secondary to any cause of prerenal failure or nephrotoxins)	
	• Nephrotoxins	
	– Drugs (aminoglycosides, amphotericin, contrast, heavy metals, NSAIDs, cytotoxic agents)	
	– Haem (from myoglobin in rhabdomyolysis or haemoglobinuria in intravascular haemolysis)	
	– Crystal (urate, sulphonamide) nephropathy	
	• Acute interstitial nephritis (usually drugs)	
Postrenal	• Posterior urethral valves	
	• Blocked urinary catheter	
	• Neurogenic bladder	
	• Tumour	
	• Trauma	
	• Stones	
	• Pelvi-ureteric junction obstruction	
	• Vesicoureteric junction obstruction	

Clinical features

AKI

- History
  - Prodromal illness (diarrhoea ± blood, dehydration, pharyngitis and skin infection)
  - Rash
  - Arthropathy
  - Weight loss
  - Convulsions or trauma
  - Urinary symptoms including urinary tract infections (UTIs)
  - Tumour and malignancy
  - Antenatal scans
  - Perinatal history: birth asphyxia, lines,
  - drug history including over the counter medicines
  - travel
  - family history

- Clinical signs
  - Prerenal: intravascular fluid depletion, with or without oedema
  - Renal: fluid overload and oliguria
  - Postrenal: poor urinary stream, palpable bladder or kidney, with or without signs of sepsis

CKD

Depends on severity and underlying disorder

- Symptoms of uraemia: weakness, lethargy, anorexia, vomiting
- Osteodystrophy: faltering growth, rickets, bone fractures
- Symptoms of underlying disease causing CKD, e.g. lupus nephritis or Wegener's granulomatosis: fever, arthralgias and arthritis, rash, pulmonary symptoms
- Glomerular disease: oedema, haematuria, proteinuria, hypertension
- Polyuria (reduced concentrating ability): many congenital anomalies (e.g. obstructive uropathy), inherited disorders (e.g. nephronophthisis), tubulointerstitial diseases
- Incidental finding: abnormality in blood, proteinuria, haematuria
- Detection by imaging: antenatal, post-UTI, incidental
- Poor or faltering growth
- Chronic anaemia
- Hypertension

Investigations

AKI

- Blood
  - Creatinine for eGFR (Schwartz formula: 40x height/creatinine, mL/min/1.73 m^2)
  - Urea, electrolytes, bicarbonate, calcium, phosphate, albumin, liver function tests, glucose
  - Full blood count, blood film and clotting, c-reactive protein
- Urine
  - Urinalysis: blood, protein, glucose, urine microscopy, culture and sensitivity
  - Urine microscopy
    - No casts: likely prerenal or obstruction
    - Red cell cast: glomerular disease
    - White cell cast: tubular and interstitial disease
  - Urine biochemistry: useful to distinguish prerenal and renal AKI (see **Table 17**).
    - Urinary Na excretion, fractional excretion of Na, FENa % = 100x [(urine Na/serum Na)]/[(urine Cr/serum Cr)]
    - Urine osmolality, myoglobin
    - Toxicology
- Imaging
  - Urinary tract ultrasound is very useful
    - Dilated system – postrenal
    - Bright kidneys – renal
    - Small kidneys – CKD
  - Chest X-ray: interstitial infiltrates in vasculitis, pulmonary oedema in fluid overload
- Further investigations:
  - HUS: blood film, stool culture, serology for *E. coli* 0157, LDH, haptoglobins, T antigen
  - Glomerulonephritis: ESR, throat swab, ASOT/anti-DNAseB, C3, C4, immunoglobulins, ANA, dsDNA,

Table 17 Biochemical changes in prerenal and renal AKI		
	Prerenal	Renal
Urine osmolality	>500	<350
Urine sodium (mmol/L)	<10	>20
FENa (%)	<1.0 (<2.5 neonates)	>2.0 (>3.5 neonates)
Urine–plasma osmolality	>1.3	<1.3
Urinalysis	Usually normal	Red blood cells, protein, white blood cells, casts
Fluid challenge ± furosemide	Diuresis	No change
AKI, acute kidney injury		

ANCA, anti-GBM, ENA, anti-cardiolipin antibodies
- Infections: leptospirosis, malaria, meningococcal sepsis
- Rhabdomyolysis: creatine kinase, urine myoglobin
- Tumour lysis: urate

CKD

- Often present with acute-on-chronic exacerbation so investigations as for AKI
- Parathyroid hormone and wrist X-ray for renal osteodystrophy
- Renal biopsy and genetic testing for specific conditions

Differential diagnosis

AKI

- Consider different causes of AKI (prerenal, renal and postrenal) and to remember there may be multiple causes of AKI.

CKD

- CKD can present with acute-on-chronic exacerbation and important to treat reversible causes aggressively.

Treatment

AKI

1. Fluid balance: shock, overload, hypertension
- Meticulous fluid balance: daily weights, hourly input and output, hourly observations, including blood pressure, toe-core temperature gap
- If intravascular fluid depletion, resuscitate with 10–20 mL/kg fluid bolus
- If signs of volume overload
  - Furosemide bolus up to 5 mg/kg IV
  - Restrict fluids to insensible losses (300 mL/m^2/day) and urine output replacement
  - Urinary catheterisation useful to assess fluid balance
- Renal replacement therapy (RRT)
  - Dialysis
    - Haemodialysis
    - Peritoneal dialysis
  - Central veno-venous filtration
- Indications for renal replacement therapy include fluid overload and hypertension, uncontrolled acidosis, refractory hyperkalaemia, severe hypo- or hypernatraemia, symptomatic uraemia, urea > 30, presence of dialysable toxin, multi-organ failure, anticipation of prolonged oliguria and to be able to create space for nutrition

2. Electrolyte disturbances: regular biochemical monitoring for hyperkalaemia, sodium (may be low, convulsions), calcium (low), phosphate (high), acidosis, high urea.
   Management of hyperkalaemia is a medical emergency and electrocardiogram monitoring is mandatory
- Stop any potassium-containing fluids or drugs that cause hypercalcaemia
- 10% calcium gluconate 0.5 mL/kg IV over 5–10 minutes
- Nebulised salbutamol 2.5 mg < 5 years, 5 mg > 5 years
- IV salbutamol 4 µg/kg in 10 mL H$_2$O over 10 minutes IV
- Sodium bicarbonate 1–2 mmol/kg of 8.4% IV
- Calcium resonium 1 g/kg PO or PR
- Glucose 0.5 g/kg/min with 0.1 u/kg/h insulin IV
- RRT

3. Adequate nutritional support
4. Treatment of underlying cause

CKD

- Treat reversible causes: for example hypovolaemia aggressively, avoid nephrotoxic drugs
- Slow the progression of renal disease: Strict blood pressure control, prevent UTIs, relieve obstruction
- Treat the complications of CKD
  - Fluid and electrolyte balance: in many congenital nephropathies, there is a poor renal concentrating capacity and sodium supplementation is required; in certain acquired diseases, e.g. focal segmental glomerulosclerosis there is fluid retention so sodium and fluid restriction is required
  - Acidosis: sodium bicarbonate supplements
  - Infection: UTIs common and hasten progression to ESRF

- – Renal osteodystrophy: replace 1-a-hydroxycalciferol; phosphate restriction and phosphate binders
- – Anaemia: iron supplements and recombinant erythropoietin
- Adequately prepare the child and family in whom renal replacement therapy will be required
  - – Renal Replacement therapy options

- Haemodialysis
- Peritoneal dialysis
- Renal transplantation: live related or deceased donor (may be pre-emptive, i.e. before dialysis is required)
- Nutrition: potassium and phosphate restriction; high in calorific value
- Growth hormone

Further reading

Hui-Stickle S, Brewer ED, Goldstein SL. Pediatric ARF epidemiology at a tertiary care center from 1999 to 2001. Am J Kidney Dis 2005; 45:96–101.

Lewis MA, Shaw J, Sinha MD, et al. UK Renal Registry (December 2009). 12th Annual Report of the Renal Association: Demography of the

UK Paediatric Renal Replacement Therapy population in 2008. Nephron 2010; 115:279–288.

Moghal NE, Brocklebank JT, Meadow SR. A review of acute renal failure in children: incidence, aetiology and outcome. Clin Nephrol 1998; 49(2):91–95.

Related topics of interest

Sacrococcygeal teratoma

Learning outcomes

- To understand the pathology and embryology of sacrococcygeal teratoma
- To be familiar with the methods of clinical presentation
- To be aware of the operative management

Overview

Sacrococcygeal teratoma (SCT) is a germ cell tumour that classically presents with buttock swelling in the neonatal period. It can occasionally be identified on fetal ultrasound scanning and confirmed on fetal magnetic resonance imaging. Primary resection at an appropriate time is the mainstay of management, but neonates with large tumours can present with high output cardiac failure and emergency surgery is required for vascular control or debulking. Because these tumours can become malignant, follow-up with tumour markers is mandatory. Generally, those diagnosed outside of the neonatal period have a higher risk of malignant disease.

Epidemiology and aetiology

SCT is the most common congenital neonatal tumour. The incidence is 1:27,000 to 1:40,000 births, with a male-to-female ratio of 1:4. SCTs are classified morphologically by their relative extent internal and external to the body by the Altman classification (**Figure 55**)

- Type I (46.7%)   Entirely external
- Type II (34.7%)   Mostly external but with significant intrapelvic component
- Type III (8.8%)   Predominantly internal but with visible external component
- Type IV (9.8%)   Entirely internal

Histologically, they are characterised by a wide variety of tissue types derived from all three germ cell layers – endoderm, mesoderm and ectoderm.

Many will contain malignant-looking cells, but if they are completely excised, they do not recur and the diagnosis of malignancy is, therefore, made on the presence of distant metastases.

Age at diagnosis is an important prognostic factor, with children >2 months of age (or 6 months for some authors) often presenting with a metastatic malignant SCT rather than a mature teratoma. Late diagnosis is usually related to Altman type IV SCT because these are difficult to diagnose antenatally and postnatally.

Studies show that 24% of all SCTs are malignant, with 84% occurring in girls. Malignancy rates were 0% with Altman I, 3% with Altman II, 40% with Altman III and 57% with Altman IV tumours.

Aetiology

SCT is defined as an extragonadal germ cell tumour and arises due to abnormal migration of primordial germ cells from the allantois to the genital crest.

SCTs are thought to originate from Hensen's node (an area of the primitive streak), which is an aggregation of totipotential cells that are the primary organisers of embryonic development. As the mesoderm proliferates, the primitive steak moves further caudally where the remnant of Hensen's node descends to the tip of the coccyx or its anterior surface.

The primitive streak diminishes in size and becomes an insignificant structure in the sacrococcygeal region of the embryo, eventually disappearing. If a remnant persists, it may give rise to an SCT because the pleuripotential cells escape from the control of embryonic inducers and organisers and differentiate into tissues not usually found in the sacrococcygeal region.

Clinical features

Antenatal

- Extra- and/or intrapelvic cystic or solid swelling
- Polyhydramnios
- Non-immune fetal hydrops
- High-output cardiac failure manifest by

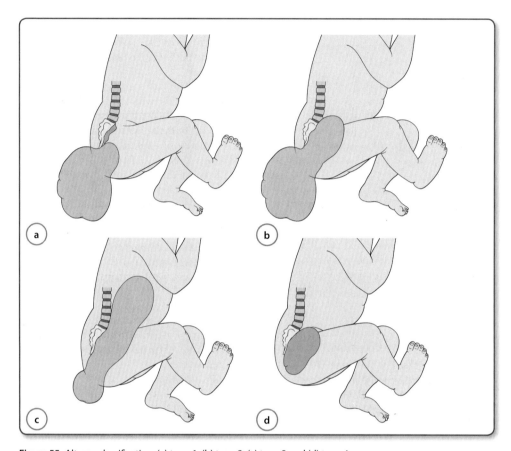

Figure 55 Altman classification: (a) type 1, (b) type 2, (c) type 3 and (d) type 4.

cardiomegaly and a dilated inferior vena cava (IVC) consistent with increased venous return. Reversal of end-diastolic flow indicates a deteriorating condition and mandates urgent management
- Maternal mirror syndrome (maternal hypertension and oedema and fetal hydrops)

Postnatal
- Buttock mass of varying size
- High-output cardiac failure
- Haemorrhage
- Tumour rupture

Infants and young children
- A palpable mass in the sacropelvic region compressing the bladder or rectum.

Investigations
- Preoperative full blood count and alpha-fetoprotein (AFP) (as a baseline level)
- Magnetic resonance imaging to assess the intra-abdominal extent of the tumour
- Sacral and pelvic radiographs to assess for Currarino triad (sacral anomaly, presacral mass, anorectal malformation)

Differential diagnosis
- Myelomeningocele
- Tumours: extraspinal ependymoma, ependymoblastoma, neuroblastoma and rhabdomyosarcoma

Treatment

Antenatal

This can be early delivery and surgery and EXIT (ex utero intrapartum treatment) to resection, maternofetal resection, radiofrequency ablation, major vessel laser ablation or vessel alcohol sclerosis with amniodrainage and cyst decompression to prevent predelivery rupture. Infants requiring antenatal management have a mortality rate of 16–63%, with a large study from Japan showing a mortality rate of 16%, excluding terminations.

If the fetus and mother are well and if the tumour is larger than 5 cm or if there is polyhydramnios, delivery by Caesarean section at 37 weeks is advised in some centres. If unwell, fetal management or termination may be considered.

Postnatal

Surgical excision in the first 24–48 hours of life is the mainstay of management. During resection, it is mandatory that a coccygectomy is performed. Without it, the recurrence rate increased from 0% to 40% in Gross' initial series.

The inverted Y or chevron incision is predominantly utilised during resection for Altman I, II and some Altman IIIs with control of the median sacral artery the primary aim. The secondary aim is resection of the devascularised tumour. Most Altman III and IV tumours require a combined perineal and abdominal approach. The perineal approach is discussed here.

Operative technique for perineal approach is as follows:

- Following urethral catheterisation, the patient is placed prone with the buttocks raised using a roll under the hips and a smaller one under the shoulders to ensure that ventilation is not compromised
- An inverted Y-shaped or chevron incision over the dorsum of the mass is made to preserve as much normal skin as possible and with the apex over the lower sacrum
- This first step is to enter a plane outside the tumour capsule and deep to the very thin levators and gluteus maximus muscles.

The tumour is dissected free from the gluteus maximus muscles

- The coccyx is transected and removed en bloc with the tumour
- The median sacral vessels are ligated and divided
- Blunt dissection is performed in the plane anterior to the median sacral vessels until the superior tumour margin is reached
- The tumour is dissected out from the pelvis and rolled inferiorly, exposing the proximal rectum
- The rectum is identified with a Hegar dilator and the tumour is dissected off the rectum by sharp and blunt methods. It should be rolled inferiorly to expose the dissection plane. This plane should be maintained close to the tumour capsule to preserve all normal structures
- On reaching the inferior tumour surface, just posterior to the anus, the dissection can de discontinued, providing there is enough of a skin flap to allow easy closure and the tumour delivered
- Ensure haemostasis
- Pelvic floor reconstruction begins with identification of the levator ani sling and suturing the central portion to the sacral perichondrium using a monofilament absorbable suture
- A closed suction drain can now be placed in the presacral space
- Any recognisable levator muscles are approximated in the midline and the medial edge of gluteus maximus closed over the sacrum
- The skin flaps are trimmed to length and the skin is closed

Follow-up

Follow-up comprises AFP monitoring and serial rectal examinations every 3 months for the first three years following resection to detect any possible recurrence.

Outcomes

Complications of the tumour mass effect are hip dysplasia, bowel obstruction, urinary obstruction and hydronephrosis. The majority of recurrences occur within 2 years. Recurrence rates of 8.6% have been reported for benign SCT. Five-year event-free survival is reported to be 92% with negative margins, 69% if microscopic margins and 38% if macroscopic residual.

Survival rate is 95% for benign SCT and 80–90% for malignant ones. At a median follow-up of 10 years, faecal incontinence occurs in 7% and urinary incontinence in 31%. An unsatisfactory scar occurred in 40% usually after having a large tumour resected.

Further reading

Derikx JPM, Hoonaard van den TL, Bax NMA, et al. Long-term functional sequelae of sacrococcygeal teratoma: a national study in the Netherlands. J Pediatr Surg 2007; 42:1122–1126.

Rescorla FJ. Paediatric germ cell tumors. Semin Pediatr Surg 2012; 21:51–60.

Usui N, Kitano Y, Sago H, et al. Outcomes of prenatally diagnosed sacrococcygeal teratomas: the results of a Japanese nationwide survey. J Pediatr Surg 2012; 47:441–447.

Related topics of interest

Salivary gland lesions

Learning outcomes

- To be able to recognise salivary gland pathology
- To know the differential diagnosis of a salivary gland mass
- To be aware of the management options including when to recommend surgery and what surgical options are available

Overview

The salivary glands are composed of paired parotid, submandibular and sublingual glands and minor glands throughout the oral and pharyngeal cavities. They produce up to 800 mL of saliva each day, which is antibacterial, lubricates and moisturises the oral cavity, provides digestive enzymes, protects dentition and modulates taste.

Clinical features

History

- Acute or insidious onset
- Single or multiple glands
- Diffuse or focal swelling
- Recurrence
- Painful or worse on eating
- Associated symptoms – dry mouth, dental decay, facial weakness

Inspection

- Swelling
- Skin discolouration
- Flow of saliva or evidence of pus at the salivary duct openings
- Medialisation of the tonsil in the oropharynx as seen in a deep lobe parotid mass

Palpation

- Diffuse or focal swelling
- Systematic assessment for cervical lymphadenopathy
- Bimanual palpation assessing the glands and ducts for palpable calculi

Assessment of facial nerve function using the House–Brackman scoring system and a complete ENT examination should also be performed.

Investigations

The choice of investigations should be based on the history. They include the following:

- Ultrasonography: for distinguishing cystic and solid masses and assessing for vascular anomalies
- Magnetic resonance imaging or computed tomography: for investigation of potential neoplasia especially involvement of the deep lobe of the parotid or the facial nerve
- Sialography: is a less frequently utilised investigation in children because it may not be well tolerated. It involves cannulating the salivary duct and injecting contrast for assessment of duct stenosis, calculi and sialectasis.
- Haematological investigations: in diffuse salivary gland enlargement serology can be sent to investigate for mumps, cytomegalovirus or coxsackie virus and angiotensin-converting enzyme level is useful in sarcoidosis
- SSrho/SSla antibodies, antinuclear factor and rheumatoid factor (RF) may all be positive in Sjögren's syndrome. However, the gold standard is a sublabial biopsy that characteristically demonstrates periductal lymphocytic infiltration
- Fine needle aspiration cytology is difficult to perform in children but can provide useful information when investigating a potential neoplasm

Differential diagnosis

Congenital and developmental abnormalities

- Congenital vascular anomalies: Haemangiomas, vascular and lymphatic malformations may occur in the salivary glands. Haemangiomas are common, affecting 1 in 10 Caucasian babies. They are of endothelial origin and appear after a few weeks of life and grow rapidly with involution commencing at 12–18 months and regression from 3 to 8 years. Lesions may have a cutaneous component giving a red hue. Complications include consumptive coagulopathy, (Kasabach–Merrit syndrome) and high output cardiac failure. Most haemangiomata can be managed conservatively allowing time for spontaneous regression. Steroids can be used to control proliferation. Surgery is occasionally required, but this has been largely superseded by treatment with propranolol.

- Vascular anomalies: These are subdivided into low and high flow and further subdivided by the dominant vessel type. If asymptomatic no treatment is required.
- First branchial cleft anomalies: These rare developmental anomalies can present as a mass in the parotid or submandibular region.

Infective disorders of the salivary glands

- Bacterial infection: Acute suppurative sialadenitis is typically caused by *Staphylococcus aureus* and *Streptococcus pyogenes* and affects patients of any age. Management includes hydration, sialogogues (e.g. citrus juices), antibiotics and, if present, abscess drainage. An immunology assessment is required if attacks are recurrent.
- Viral infection: Mumps usually affects both parotid glands and is accompanied by fever and malaise. Complications include nephritis, orchitis, pancreatitis, encephalitis or sudden sensorineural hearing loss. Management is supportive. Other viral infections causing salivary gland swelling include coxsackie and cytomegalovirus. Parotid cysts are a feature of human immunodeficiency virus infection. Their management is conservative and should be conducted by a paediatrician with a specialist interested in human immunodeficiency virus.
- Atypical mycobacteria infection: This typically affects children < 6 years and presents with a painless parotid or submandibular swelling with no systemic upset. The skin may become discoloured and a discharging sinus may be present.

The natural course of this condition is spontaneous resolution, which can take months. Long-term treatment with macrolide antibiotics has been advocated, however, if skin breakdown is imminent surgical excision with preservation of the facial nerve is recommended to eradicate the disease.

Inflammatory disorders of the salivary glands

- Sjogren's syndrome: This systemic autoimmune condition is rare in children. It manifests with intermittent bilateral parotid swelling, xerostomia, dental caries and dry eyes. Management includes artificial saliva and tears, dental care and consideration of steroids in an acute exacerbation. It is associated with non-Hodgkin's lymphoma in 10%
- Sarcoidosis: This idiopathic multi-system granulomatous condition is rare in younger children and more likely in teenagers. It may present with cervical lymphadenopathy or bilateral parotid swelling. Angiotensin-converting enzyme levels are elevated and chest X-ray may demonstrate mediastinal lymphadenopathy. Non-symptomatic lesions may be managed conservatively and symptomatic exacerbations with corticosteroids
- Obstructive disorders: Salivary duct calculi are unusual in children but are more frequent in the submandibular gland due to the mucoid nature of the saliva it produces. They present with an acute painful swelling of the gland, which is exacerbated by eating. The calculus may be palpable on bimanual palpation. If accessible, it may be removed orally or by sialoendoscopy

Salivary gland neoplasms

Less than 5% occur in children and most in those >10 years of age; 85% occur in the parotid, 12% in the submandibular gland and the remainder in minor salivary glands.

- Benign epithelial salivary neoplasms: Pleomorphic salivary adenoma is the most common paediatric tumour, comprising 30% of paediatric salivary tumours, and is most often found in the parotid gland. Treatment is performed by surgical resection

- Malignant epithelial salivary neoplasm: Clinical presentation is typically with a rapidly enlarging mass, with pain or facial weakness. In children < 10 years, lesions are typically more aggressive and high grade. Mucoepidermoid carcinoma is the most common (60%) and affects 10- to 16-year-olds. Five-year survival of low-grade disease is 85–95% and 30–50% in high-grade disease. Acinic cell carcinoma is the second most common (20%) and is also usually low grade with good prognosis. Other types include adenoid cystic, adenocarcinoma, carcinoma expleomorphic adenoma, undifferentiated carcinoma and sialoblastoma. The differential diagnosis includes lymphoma and rhabdomyosarcoma

Children should be managed by a specialist multidisciplinary team and management is by wide excision with facial nerve preservation; however, if the nerve is involved, it will need to be sacrificed and facial nerve grafting, with a greater auricular or sural interposition graft performed. Radiotherapy is considered in high-grade tumours, nodal involvement, unclear margins and perineural spread. Chemotherapy is not routinely used.

Treatment

The medical management of the common infective and inflammatory conditions are described previously.

Surgery to excise lesions of the parotid region involves identification of the facial nerve. This can be more superficial in children and branches are much finer than those in adults. Facial nerve monitoring should be routinely utilised. Landmarks for the facial nerve include the tragal pointer, the posterior belly of digastric muscle and the temperozygomatic suture. An incisional/trucut biopsy of potential neoplasia is not recommended due to the risk of tumour seeding. Potential complications include facial weakness, greater auricular hyperaesthesia, Frey's syndrome and salivary fistula. Submandibular gland resection warrants attention to preservation of the marginal mandibular nerve and lingual nerve.

Further reading

Bentz BG, et al. Masses of the salivary gland region in children. Arch Otolaryngol Head Neck Surg 2000; 126:1435–1439.

Bradley PJ, Guntinas-Lichius O. Salivary gland disorders and diseases: diagnosis & management. Thieme, 2011.

Bull P. Salivary gland neoplasia in childhood. Int J Paediatr Otorhinolaryngol 1999; 49:235–238.

Related topics of interest

Short bowel syndrome

Learning outcomes

- To be able to define short bowel syndrome and intestinal failure
- To understand the management principles
- To be able to identify patients with short bowel syndrome requiring surgical management
- To be familiar with the indications for surgical procedures and the range of available surgical options

Overview

Short bowel syndrome (SBS) is the most common cause of intestinal failure in the Western world. In 1967, Rickham defined short bowel as small bowel length of < 75 cm or < 30% of the total gut length, respectively, in the newborn. Intestinal failure is defined as a reduction in the functioning intestinal mass below the amount necessary for adequate absorption to allow for growth.

Although the historical definition of SBS was based on the residual length of the small bowel, the current definition is a functional one, because length of the residual bowel is not predictive of function, especially if it is affected by the underlying disease process. The prognosis of children with significant small bowel resection was poor until the recent advances made in the field of parenteral nutrition (PN).

Most children with SBS achieve good bowel adaptation with expert multidisciplinary input and management.

Complications should be identified early and referral should be made to centres with expertise in managing children on long-term PN. A few children need bowel reconstruction or transplantation to achieve freedom from PN.

Epidemiology and aetiology

In the UK, the incidence of SBS is estimated to be 2 patients per million population, based upon patients requiring long-term home PN. Due to the progress in intensive care and better survival of extremely premature neonates who have had massive bowel resection, the prevalence of SBS has increased.

SBS arises most commonly as a result of bowel resection secondary to:

- Necrotising enterocolitis (NEC)
- Gastroschisis
- Jejunal/ileal atresias
- Long segment Hirschsprung's disease
- Volvulus
- Trauma
- Crohn's disease
- Intestinal tuberculosis (in the developing world)

Clinical features

Children with SBS are unable to maintain growth on enteral feeds only and are dependent on PN. They may suffer from malabsorption, diarrhoea, steatorrhoea, high stomal output and failure to thrive. The ability to reabsorb fluid and electrolytes is usually limited in infants with SBS, and this could result in dehydration and electrolyte abnormalities. Trace elements are also poorly absorbed and lost in excess. D-Lactic acidosis may occur on rare occasions as a result of bacterial overgrowth and these children could present with hyperventilation, confusion and sometimes coma. They also suffer from complications of PN and central lines. Many infants with SBS have cholestasis due to intestinal failure-associated liver disease and cholestasis could contribute to ongoing malabsorption of fat and fat-soluble vitamins.

Investigations

The diagnosis of SBS should be obvious in children with extensive bowel resection. However, the possibility of any coexisting medical gastrointestinal problems like congenital diarrhoea or pancreatic insufficiency should be considered, if the response to treatment is not satisfactory.

Blood and urine

Monitoring of serum electrolytes, renal and liver functions, vitamins and micronutrients (copper, manganese, selenium and zinc) levels is essential for the management of these children. D-Lactate assay in the blood or urine would be helpful in infants with suspected D-lactic acidosis. These children will have acidosis with an increased anion gap in the absence of elevated serum lactate as measured by standard techniques, which measure L-lactate.

Stool

Stool microscopy for fat globules or steatocrit estimation would help to identify fat malabsorption and similarly faecal reducing substance testing would identify carbohydrate malabsorption.

Radiology

Contrast study of the gastrointestinal tract would be helpful if there is clinical suspicion of a stricture. Ultrasound study of the hepatobiliary system would be helpful to assess the severity of intestinal failure-associated liver disease (IFALD) and also to look for any other causes of cholestasis, like biliary atresia. Doppler ultrasound or computed tomography or magnetic resonance venography would be helpful in children on long-term PN to assess the patency of major veins for central venous catheter insertion.

Differential diagnosis

Causes of malabsorption such as congenital diarrhoea and pancreatic insufficiency should be considered.

Treatment

Medical management

This needs a multidisciplinary team approach with paediatric gastroenterologists, surgeons, hepatologists, vascular access team, dieticians, pharmacist, nutritional care nurses, social workers and occasionally, transplantation team members.

The principles are to promote bowel adaptation to enable transition to oral and enteral diet and weaning off PN, to avoid long-term complications and to ensure appropriate growth and development.

Soon after bowel resection, the process of adaptation starts. There are two main types of adaptation:

1. Structural adaptation involves both an increase in villous height and mucosal surface area and an increase in bowel luminal circumference and wall thickness
2. Functional adaptation is characterised by an increase in the rate of nutrient absorption

The majority of children who undergo bowel resection are weaned from PN within a few months and only a small proportion require long-term PN.

Different factors influence the pace of adaptation:

- It is difficult to achieve complete intestinal autonomy if residual small bowel length is ≤25 cm
- Children who had bowel resection for NEC tend to adapt less well than those who had resection for atresias
- The presence of the ileocaecal valve and the colon in continuity with the small bowel favour adaptation
- Residual ileum appears to adapt better than residual jejunum
- Premature babies adapt less well than term infants and are more susceptible to long-term complications

Enteral nutrition

The key principle is to promote intestinal hyperplasia, which drives bowel adaptation.

- Enteral feeds need to be started as soon as the child is stable. Most infants will need supplemental nasogastric feeding to ensure adequate fluid and calorie intake
- Most children benefit from specialised formulae, such as extensively hydrolysed or amino acid-based formulae
- It is important to promote non-nutritive sucking in infants to prevent oral aversive behaviour in future life
- Continuous feeds may have some advantages over intermittent bolus feeding, especially in the early stages of bowel adaptation
- Feed volume is advanced on the basis of the number of liquid stools or the amount of stomal output

- Some infants need tailor-made modular feeds with the type of carbohydrate, fat and protein that the infant can tolerate
- Different pharmacological agents have been tried to increase enteral feeding and drive bowel adaptation:
  - Loperamide slows down intestinal transit time to promote fluid and nutrient absorption (caution needs to be exercised in infants who had previous NEC because loperamide-associated NEC has been reported)
  - Cholestyramine is helpful in the setting of bile salt-associated diarrhoea, absence of ileocaecal valve and small bowel anastomosed to the colon
  - Small bowel bacterial overgrowth could impair bowel adaptation and non-absorbable antibiotics like Neomycin and Rifaximin could be helpful
  - Probiotics can be useful in selected patients with small bowel bacterial overgrowth
  - Pectin can be added with the aim that colonic bacteria will produce short chain fatty acids by fermenting it, hence contributing 15–20% of the enteral energy intake
  - Growth hormone, insulin-like growth factor and glutamine-like peptide have been tried in trials but are not used in day-to-day clinical practice

Parenteral nutrition

- Provides the necessary fluid, calories, electrolytes, vitamins and trace elements, which are important to ensure growth and development while all steps are undertaken to promote bowel adaptation
- It is important to provide vitamins and trace elements at the appropriate doses in the PN and to monitor them, because for some children on PN, this may be their only source
- Home PN is considered when it is anticipated that PN may be needed for >6 months. PN is usually infused at home over 12–14 hours and this helps avoid long-term complications and improves psychosocial development

Complications

Intestinal failure-associated liver disease

This is defined by the British Society of Paediatric Gastroenterology Hepatology and Nutrition Working Group as a persistent (>6 weeks) elevation of liver function tests (alkaline phosphatase and γ-glutamyl transpeptidase) 1.5 times above the normal reference range in a patient receiving PN. This entity is more commonly seen in preterm than in term infants. The principles of management are as follows:

- Rule out other causes of neonatal cholestasis in these infants
- Line infections and malnutrition can worsen the liver disease and every effort should be made to increase the enteral feeds to limit liver disease progression
- Ursodeoxycholic acid is used to promote bile flow with the aim of reducing the degree of cholestasis
- Cycling of PN over 12–14 hours a day is helpful to prevent the progression of liver disease. Lack of sufficient enteral feeding tolerance and hypoglycaemia when the infant is off PN usually limit the ability to cycle
- Prevention of central line-associated infections and prompt treatment of catheter infection, with appropriate antibiotics, are important to prevent liver disease. Sometimes removal of an infected line results in significant improvement of the cholestasis
- Soya-based lipid emulsions used in PN are believed to contribute to the development and progression of IFALD. In the last few years, fish oil-based lipids have been used when children have developed IFALD and in most children, cholestasis has been reversed
- A discussion with a paediatric intestinal transplant team is important for children with persistent cholestasis (serum bilirubin >150 µmol/L). Coagulopathy and portal hypertension are usually very advanced features of liver disease in these children

- Care should be taken to supplement fat-soluble vitamins and monitor micronutrient levels especially manganese because of the high risk of manganese toxicity in cholestatic infants

Central line complications

The various types of complications and approaches to prevention are as follows:
- Thrombosis of major veins is a major problem associated with long-term PN
- Episodes of dehydration and frequent central line infections contribute to thrombogenesis
- Insertion by an experienced vascular access team, using ultrasound-guided techniques, is preferable to minimise the risk of complications
- Infection is mostly due to inappropriate care although bacterial translocation from the bowel has a role to play
- Carers should be taught about the need for aseptic handling; administration at home carries a lower infection risk compared to hospital PN
- Early signs of line infection or fever without a clear focus in a child on long-term PN should be treated with antibiotics after obtaining blood cultures from all the lumina
- Choice of the initial antibiotics should be guided by the local microbiology guidelines
- Prompt removal is recommended if no response to treatment is obtained in 24–48 hours or if there is evidence of fungal infection
- Antibiotic-coated catheters, antibiotic line locks and taurine have been tried with limited success in the prevention of central line infection
- Involve the intestinal transplantation team, if the long-term PN patient has two or less major veins which remain patent
- Frequent life-threatening central line infections are an indication for bowel transplantation

Surgical management

The indications for surgery are as follows:
- Structural problems such as bowel dilatation or strictures
- Failure to wean off PN

The aim of surgery in patients with SBS is to increase bowel transit time, hence increasing contact time of nutrients with the mucosa. Various surgical procedures are available to achieve this aim.

An increase in bowel transit time can be achieved by insertion of a reversed bowel segment or colon interposition and the construction of intestinal valves. This procedure should be mainly considered in patients with enough bowel length (> 90 cm) and rapid transit but dependent on PN.

In patients with dilated bowel and severe dysmotility, the objective is to improve intestinal propulsive activity by reducing bowel dilatation. In patients with sufficient bowel length (> 90 cm), tapering or a stricturoplasty is the procedure of choice. PN-dependent patients with dilated short bowel (30–60 cm) may benefit from tapering or a bowel-lengthening procedure. In 1984, Bianchi described the technique of longitudinal intestinal lengthening and tailoring (LILT). In 2003, the serial transverse enteroplasty (STEP) technique was reported.

Both lengthening procedures achieve similar lengthening effects and can almost double the length of the treated bowel segment. The LILT procedure is described by many surgeons as the technically more challenging procedure. Furthermore, a prerequisite is that the bowel segment being lengthened needs to be significantly dilated throughout its length to allow a division of the dilated segment into two halves in order to create two bowel segments.

The main advantage of the STEP procedure is that the bowel is left in continuity and the lumen is not opened during the lengthening procedure. In addition, time to enteral feeding seems to be quicker following the STEP in comparison to the LILT. The mean relative increase in overall intestinal length has been reported to be between 80% and 90% for both procedures. More than 70% of the patients who undergo a lengthening procedure can be successfully weaned off PN and tolerate full enteral feeds. A poor prognostic factor is failure to wean off PN beyond 18 months from the lengthening procedure. The survival of patients following the lengthening procedure has been reported to be as high as 80%.

In patients with < 20 cm of remaining small bowel, bowel with severe dysmotility or lack of absorptive capacity combined with PN-related complications, small bowel transplantation is the surgical procedure of choice.

Given the good outcome following autologous gastrointestinal reconstruction, non-transplant surgery should be considered the procedure of choice in selected patients with SBS who fail to wean off PN. Although substantial progress has been made in transplant surgery, outcome data would suggest that intestinal or combined liver and bowel transplantation in SBS should be considered only in patients with severe liver damage and impaired venous access status.

Further reading

Bianchi A. Intestinal lengthening: an experimental and clinical review. J Roy Soc Med 1984; 3:35–41.

Gupte GL, Beath SV, Kelly DA, et al. Current issues in the management of intestinal failure. Arch Dis Child 2006; 91:259–264.

Kim HB, Fauza D, Garza J, et al. Serial transverse enteroplasty (STEP): a novel bowel lengthening procedure. J Pediatr Surg 2003; 38:425–429.

Reinshagen K, et al. Long-term outcome in patients with short bowel syndrome after longitudinal intestinal lengthening and tailoring. J Paediatr Gastoenterol Nutr 2008; 47:573–578.

Wales PW, Christison-Lagay ER. Short bowel syndrome: epidemiology and etiology. Sem Pediatr Surg 2010; 19:3–9.

Related topics of interest

Skin lesions

Learning outcomes

- To be able to recognise common paediatric skin lesions and be aware of rarer clinical manifestations
- To be aware of the aetiology and natural history of common skin lesions
- To be able to construct a list of differential diagnoses and management plan for the common and important paediatric skin lesions

Overview

Lesions arising from the skin are a common presentation to the paediatric surgeon. The vast majority are benign following an indolent course but may be the cause of significant concern for both child and parent.

Skin lesions presenting during childhood can be either congenital or acquired and may arise from any component of the ectoderm. As such the underlying cause is different for each lesion. Broadly speaking, lesions can be divided into cystic and solid lesions.

Cystic lesions

- **Dermoid cysts**: They are congenital cysts lined by skin and mature sebaceous gland commonly arising in the region of embryonic fusion lines. Their natural history is to progressively enlarge over time due to continued sebum production into the cyst, resulting in its characteristic 'cheese-like' contents. Dermoids present to the paediatric surgeon as a painless, small, soft, round subcutaneous mass that is often tethered to underlying structures. Lesions are predominantly found in the region of the head and neck and most commonly at the external angle of the eye; however, they can be found throughout the body mainly in the midline. Any suspected midline dermoid found in the head region requires careful preoperative investigation and planning because the lesions may have a 'dumb-bell'-like intracranial extension.

- **Epidermoid cysts:** They are also skin-lined but unlike dermoids, they do not contain sebaceous glands but produce their content through continued desquamation of the cells lining it. Epidermoids can be congenital or acquired and commonly arise from hair follicles (alternatively known as sebaceous cysts), although they may also result from the implantation of epidermal cells, following any disruption of the dermis. The lesions are usually round and mobile and rarely grow larger than 4–5 cm and are most commonly found in hair-bearing regions, i.e. head, neck and shoulders. The presence of multiple epidermal cysts should raise the possibility of the rare but important familial colorectal polyposis (Gardner's) syndrome. Small cysts may be left alone; however, recurrent infection, abscess formation or prominent locations may be indications for surgical excision.

Solid lesions

- **Pilomatrixomas:** They are benign calcifying lesions, arising from hair follicles within the epidermis (also termed calcifying epitheliomas of Malherbe). They most commonly present during childhood as small (< 1 cm), single, hard, mobile lesions that may cause a slight yellow or blue discolouration of the overlying skin. Similarly to epidermoid cysts, pilomatrixomas are predominantly found in the hair-bearing regions of the head and neck but may be found elsewhere. They do not involute and treatment is by local excision; recurrence is rare with complete excision

- **Hamartomatous polyps:** They are commonly present as skin tags in children and are comprised of a disorganised overgrowth of components of the dermis and underlying connective tissue. They follow a benign course and excision is performed only for cosmetic concerns or for persistent irritation

- **Pyogenic granulomas:** They are not true granulomas but result from a disordered capillary overgrowth (dermal capillary haemangiomas) following local trauma or irritation. They usually present as bright red raised lesions that may bleed on contact. Occasionally these lesions may regress spontaneously but will often require treatment
- **Neurofibromas:** They are benign tumours derived from Schwann cells surrounding peripheral nerves. In general, they can be divided into two types: dermal neurofibromas and plexiform neurofibromas. Dermal neurofibromas are benign tumours, arising from a single nerve, and may present as either fleshy, non-tender pedunculated lesions or deeper subcutaneous nodules that may be tender. Plexiform neurofibromas arise from multiple nerve bundles and present as poorly defined 'worm-like' thickenings. Neurofibromas may be solitary; however, the diagnosis of either multiple dermal neurofibromas or a single plexiform neurofibroma in a child should prompt investigation for the autosomal dominant disease neurofibromatosis type I (NF1). Patients diagnosed with NF1 have a risk of malignant transformation within existing plexiform lesions, although this usually occurs in adulthood. In patients with multiple neurofibromas or plexiform lesions the role of surgery is limited
- **Histiocytic lesions:** These are rare, but do present in childhood. Juvenile xanthogranulomas are benign lesions, with a yellow or red colouration, usually found either as a single lesion or clusters in the region of the head, neck or trunk. Most present before the age of 2 and are comprised of histiocytes, eosinophils and giant cells. Lesions tend to regress over time and children with cutaneous disease only have a good prognosis. Langerhans cell histiocytosis is the other cutaneous lesion seen in childhood; these are derived from dendritic cells and in contrast to juvenile xanthogranulomas are thought to represent a neoplastic process. Surgical intervention for histiocytic lesions is usually limited to obtaining biopsies for histological diagnosis

Investigations

Not all skin lesions require further investigation because the diagnosis may be made clinically and confirmed with histology following excision. When there is diagnostic doubt, an ultrasound should be performed. Further investigation, if required, is with computed tomography (CT) or magnetic resonance imaging (MRI) and is essential for any midline head lesion to exclude the presence of intracranial extension.

Treatment

Topical treatments

- Careful application of topical silver nitrate or liquid nitrogen for pyogenic granulomas
- Surgical excision
- The use of curettage or diathermy may be possible for persistent pyogenic granulomas, but the majority of other pathologies require formal surgical excision
- Lesions within the dermis require an ellipse excision to remove the involved skin, whereas deeper lesions, e.g. dermoids, can be removed through a simple linear incision
- When planning incisions care should be taken to minimise scarring by locating the incision within or parallel to Langer's lines
- Cysts should not be routinely excised in the presence of active infection, any abscess cavities present should be drained and definitive surgery planned for a later date
- Care should be taken not to rupture cysts because recurrence rates are higher if residual tissue is left behind

Further reading

Cozzi DA, Mele E, d'Ambrosio G, et al. The eyelid crease approach to angular dermoid cysts in pediatric general surgery. J Pediatr Surg 2008; 43:1502–1506.

Elder DE, et al (eds), Lever's histopathology of the skin, 10th edn. Philadelphia: Lippincott Williams and Wilkins, 2008.

Wright TS. Cutaneous manifestations of malignancy. Curr Opin Pediatr 2011; 23:407–411.

Related topics of interest

Small bowel atresia

Learning outcomes

- To know the presentation and relevant investigations to perform
- To be able to describe an appropriate management plan
- To know the operative steps

Overview

Small bowel stenosis or atresia is one of the most common causes of neonatal intestinal obstruction. Less than 1% have other anomalies. They are are thought to arise secondarily to an in utero ischaemic insult, with subsequent necrosis.

Presentation is in the early postnatal period with bilious vomiting and abdominal distension. X-ray and contrast studies are the mainstay of investigation. Management is surgical and although single atresias are most common, 6–12% may have multiple atresias and up to 5% will have a concomitant colonic atresia.

Epidemiology and aetiology

Atresia is 20 times more common than stenosis. Jejuno-ileal atresia has an incidence of 1 in 330 to 1 in 1500 live births, with 33% of infants born premature or small for gestation.

Hereditary forms and familial patterns are rare with a genetic basis established for types IIIb and IV. Associated chromosomal and extra-abdominal anomalies occur in 7% of affected patients.

A localised intrauterine vascular accident leading to ischaemic necrosis, liquefaction and resorption is the commonly accepted hypothesis. This is supported by incarceration of bowel in anterior abdominal wall defects and fetal events, such as mid-gut volvulus leading to small bowel atresias. Meconium ileus and Hirschsprung's disease are also possible aetiological factors in ileal atresia.

Classification (Figure 56)

- Stenosis (7%): localised narrowing, 'windsock' effect
- Type I atresia (16%): transluminal septum/short atretic segment. Bowel is in continuity with no mesenteric defect and is of normal length
- Type II atresia (21%): two blind ending atretic ends connected by a fibrous cord. No mesenteric defect or foreshortening

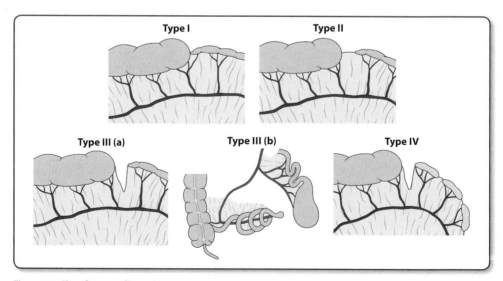

Figure 56 Classification of bowel atresia.

- Type IIIa atresia (24%): similar to type II except there is no fibrous cord. There is a V-shaped mesenteric defect and bowel may be foreshortened. Associated with cystic fibrosis (CF)
- Type IIIb atresia (apple peel) (10%): proximal jejunal atresia often with malrotation. Large mesenteric defect and absence of most of the superior mesenteric artery. The distal bowel is coiled helically around a single artery arising from the right colic arcade. The blood supply to the distal bowel is therefore retrograde from the inferior mesenteric artery via the marginal artery in the watershed region of the splenic flexure of the colon. Further type I and II atresias may be found distally. There is a significant bowel length reduction
- Type IV atresia (22%): described as a string of sausages or a combination of types I, II and III. Bowel length is reduced, but terminal ileum is usually spared. Multiple anastomoses are required

The disparity in lumen diameter varies from a two- to eightfold difference or more between the proximal and distal segments. There is a deficiency in coordinated peristalsis of the bulbous end of the proximal segment that may be due to hyperplasia of ganglion cells in the dilated proximal segment and absent acetylcholinesterase activity at the ends of the blind proximal and distal atretic segments.

Clinical features

- There may be dilated bowel loops on antenatal ultrasound. This may be accompanied by signs of vigorous peristalsis, especially in pregnancies with third-trimester polyhydramnios
- Postnatally there may be vomiting of gastric content, and then bilious vomiting
- Abdominal distension. The more distal the atresia, the greater the distension
- In 20%, symptoms are delayed for 24 hours or more
- Atresia of the proximal jejunum may present with gastric distension, with loops of bowel decompressable by nasogastric aspiration in an otherwise-gasless abdomen

Investigations

- Plain abdominal X-ray:
  - this may show a triple bubble in proximal jejunal atresia or dilated small bowel loops in a more distal obstruction
  - Intraperitoneal calcification may be present, implicating an antenatal perforation, with subsequent meconium spillage and dystrophic calcification
  - It may be gasless due to fluid-filled obstructed bowel loops
- Contrast enema: in complete obstruction this can show the size and position of the colon, exclude colonic atresia and determine if there is a meconium ileus
- Upper gastrointestinal contrast study: to exclude a malrotation and midgut volvulus

Differential diagnosis

- Hirschsprung's disease, meconium ileus, small left colon syndrome, colonic atresia
- Duodenal atresia
- Malrotation and midgut volvulus
- Incarcerated or strangulated internal hernia
- Duplication cyst
- Ileus secondary to sepsis, birth trauma, maternal medications, premature bowel or hypothyroidism

Treatment

Initial treatment is with nil by mouth, intravenous fluids and nasogastric tube decompression.

Once the diagnosis of atresia is established, treatment is surgical. In addition to a laparotomy the neonate may require central venous access for postoperative parenteral nutrition.

Standard surgical approach

- Incision – supraumbilical transverse or paraumbilical from the 8 to the 4 o'clock position
- Dissection through muscle into the abdomen
- Bowel is delivered and inspected for atresias, stenoses, malrotation and

meconium ileus. Volvulus, if present, should be detorted
- The level of proximal dilatation identifies the level of the atresia in the majority of cases. A distal enterotomy allows access for a feeding tube and injection of normal saline to exclude further distal small bowel or colonic atresias
- The bowel length should be accurately measured along the anti-mesenteric border
- Proximal bowel excision is then performed with resection proximally until normal calibre bowel is reached. If this leaves < 80 cm of small bowel with or without the ileocaecal valve, then this resection should be restricted to the bulbous portion or compromised bowel only
- The proximal bowel should be divided at 90° and the distal bowel at an oblique angle to leave both resection margins of similar size
- Anastomosis with an absorbable 5/0 or 6/0 sutures, interrupted or continuous
- Closure of the mesenteric defect if possible
- Closure of the abdomen

Special considerations

- High jejunal atresia
  - Derotate the proximal bowel and resect proximally into the fourth or even third part of the duodenum. Bowel tapering can then be performed.
  - Once complete, the bowel should be left in a non-rotated configuration

- Type IIIb (apple peel)
  - May require division of the mesenteric avascular constricting rings, releasing the blood supply. Replace the bowel in a non-rotated configuration
- Type IV
  - If localised, this facilitates an en bloc resection. However, ensuring that maximal bowel length is preserved may require multiple anastomoses.
- Plication/tapering
  - Used if there is reduced intestinal length or large disparate lumen sizes
- Stoma
  - Primary anastomosis is preferred, but a stoma can be fashioned if there is doubt over the viability of the intestine

Outcome

The majority of neonates with small bowel atresia have a satisfactory outcome although following massive intestinal loss parenteral nutrition and enteral support is required until full adaptation has occurred. Graduated oral feeding should be introduced as soon as it is practical for adaptation to begin. Full enteral feeding may take many months to achieve.

Problems with postoperative bowel dilatation occasionally require further surgery in the form of tapering or further bowel resection because these dilated segments do not drain adequately, leaving the patient at risk of functional closed loop obstruction or bacterial overgrowth.

Further reading

H Rode, Numanoglu A. Jejuno-ileal atresia. In: Puri P, Höllwarth, M (eds), Paediatric surgery. Diagnosis and management. Springer-Verlag, 2009.

Stollman TH, et al. Decreased mortality but increased morbidity in neonates with jejunoileal atresia; a study of 114 cases over a 34-year period. J Pediatr Surg 2009; 44:217–221.

Related topics of interest

Small bowel duplications

Learning outcomes

- To be aware of the types and possible origins of enteric duplications
- To be familiar with the clinical manifestations of small bowel duplications
- To understand the principles of management

Overview

Fraenkel described the first cystic duplication in 1882 and Fitz coined the term 'intestinal duplication' in 1884. These lesions were subsequently classified by Gross in 1953, according to their anatomic location. Enteric duplications can occur anywhere along the alimentary tract. Small bowel duplications are the most common form and account for 50% of all enteric duplications. Although they may be clinically silent, duplication cysts can cause obstruction, bleeding and infection. Large bowel duplications have the highest risk of malignancy, but adenocarcinomas have also been reported in small bowel duplications. Surgical excision is, therefore, recommended where technically possible.

Epidemiology and aetiology

The incidence is 1 in 5000 for all duplications and 1 in 10,000 for small bowel duplications. The majority present within the first 2 years of life. They are more common in boys than in girls, and small bowel duplications are seen most commonly in the ileum, followed by the duodenum. Duplications are cystic in 80% of cases and tubular in 20% (**Figure 57**). Cystic duplications are usually closed, whereas tubular duplications often communicate with the normal bowel. They are situated on the mesenteric border of the bowel and usually share a common blood supply with adjacent bowel. The duplication usually shares a common muscle wall, with the adjoining normal bowel, and

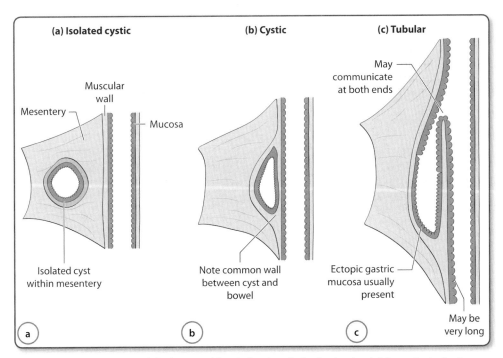

Figure 57 Types of small bowel duplications: (a) an isolated cystic duplication (rare); (b) a cystic duplication sharing a common wall with the small intestine; (c) a tubular duplication.

often communicates with its lumen. Ectopic gastric mucosa is present in 20% of cystic duplications and 80% of tubular duplications.

The aetiology is unknown in most cases and several theories have been postulated, namely:

- 'Split notochord theory' to account for the association of duplications with vertebral defects. The notochord and the endoderm of the primitive gut roof are normally fused until the 4th week of gestation, when the two structures separate. If separation is not complete, differential growth between the two structures results in a cord of endoderm being pulled from the gut roof forming a diverticulum or an enteric cyst and a vertebral defect is present at the dorsal end of the attachment
- Failure of normal regression of embryonic structures, resulting in enteric cysts
- Persistence of digestive tract diverticuli is normally seen between the 6th and 8th weeks of gestation
- Median septum formation, whereby opposing walls of the bowel become adherent, resulting in the formation of a septum and doubling of the lumen
- Failure of proper recanalisation which may account for small duplications, particularly in the duodenum

Clinical features

Small bowel duplications may present in a variety of ways:

- Detected on antenatal ultrasound
- Incidental finding on abdominal ultrasound
- Neonatal abdominal mass
- Abdominal pain secondary to distension of the duplication or compression of adjacent structures
- Intestinal obstruction
- Pancreatitis
- Intussusception, with duplication as pathological lead point
- Volvulus
- Ectopic gastric mucosa may give rise to gastrointestinal bleeding, acute or chronic abdominal pain or intestinal perforation

- Vertebral defects are unusual with small bowel duplications, and are more commonly associated with oesophageal and giant abdominal diverticuli
- Spinal compression and meningitis secondary to neurenteric cysts

Investigations

Duplications are often not diagnosed until surgery.

Blood

- Full blood count
- Urea and electrolytes
- Coagulation screen in patients with gastrointestinal bleeding
- Amylase if pancreatitis is suspected

Radiology

- Plain abdominal radiograph when intestinal obstruction is suspected
- Abdominal ultrasound, which shows a two-layer pattern, provides useful diagnostic information
- Magnetic resonance imaging is indicated in the presence of spinal cord compression or vertebral defects visualised on plain radiography
- Computed tomographic scan may have a role to play
- If a technetium-99m pertechnetate scan (Meckel's scan) shows heterotopic gastric mucosa but does not seem to be typical for a Meckel's diverticulum, a duplication cyst should be suspected

Differential diagnosis

The differential diagnosis depends on the mode of presentation:

- In the antenatal period, this includes ovarian cysts and meconium pseudocysts
- In the postnatal period, other possible cysts are ovarian, Meckel's, choledochal, omental and lymphatic cysts
- In patients with gastrointestinal bleeding, causes of upper or lower gastrointestinal bleeding need to be excluded
- If intussusception is the mode of presentation, other possible causes of intussusception would need to be identified.

Treatment

Because of the potential complications of a small bowel duplication, it should be surgically resected, if at all possible. This could be achieved with a laparotomy, a laparoscopic or laparoscopic-assisted approach.

Small, isolated cystic duplications that do not communicate with the bowel or share a common blood supply may be simply removed by performing a cystectomy but these are unusual. More commonly, it will be necessary to resect the duplication with the adjacent bowel and perform a primary anastomosis.

Long tubular duplications are the hardest to treat, because resection may result in the loss of so much small intestine that a short bowel syndrome would result. In this case, the recommended technique is to multiply incise the duplication and strip the entire mucosa, thereby removing the risk of future bleeding or malignancy. The communication(s) with the bowel itself should then be closed. Care should be taken that it does not compromise the vascularity of the adjacent bowel. Other techniques for giant unresectable duplication cysts include Roux loops to drain the duplications in the absence of heterotopic gastric mucosa and drainage of the duplication into the stomach when gastric mucosa is present.

Further reading

Bentley JFR, Smith JR. Developmental posterior enteric remnants and spinal malformations: the split notochord syndrome. Arch Dis Child 1960; 35:76–86.

Holcomb GW 3rd, et al. Surgical management of alimentary tract duplications. Ann Surg 1989; 209:167–174.

Related topics of interest

Soft tissue tumours

Learning outcomes

- To be able to differentiate between rhabdomyosarcoma and non-rhabdomyosarcoma soft tissue tumours
- To appreciate the patterns of favourable and unfavourable rhabdomyosarcoma
- To understand the importance of the surgical biopsy and how to avoid harm

Overview

Soft tissue sarcomas are generally considered in two groups: rhabdomyosarcomas (RMS) and non-rhabdomyosarcoma soft tissue sarcomas (NRSTS). This separation is justified because RMS is largely a tumour of children, with a reasonably uniform treatment plan and prognosis. This is reflected in the body of research that underpins management of rhabdomyosarcoma in children. The current (2012) relevant European trial is entitled RMS 2005. The current North American equivalent is the Intergroup Rhabdomyosarcoma Study, IRS-V.

In contrast, NRSTS are a heterogeneous tumour group, occurring mainly in adults and differing widely in their biological and clinical characteristics and in their response to therapy. Since these diseases are most common in adults, most of the knowledge of paediatric NRSTS is derived from adult studies.

Epidemiology and aetiology

RMS is the third most common extracranial solid tumour in children. It comprises 4% of childhood malignancies, with an incidence of five per million children under the age of 15 years. There is a bimodal age distribution: 65% at 2–5 years, 35% at 10–18 years and with the overall 'mean' at 5 years. Male:female ratio is 3:2. NRSTS have a similar incidence, but the heterogeneity of the tumour types that comprise this group makes further epidemiological description valueless.

RMS is microscopically a small blue round cell tumour, in common with neuroblastoma,

Ewing's and osteogenic sarcomas, non-Hodgkin's lymphoma and leukaemia. It probably arises from primitive mesenchyme, destined to form striated muscle. It can arise anywhere, including sites where striated muscle is not normally found. The histology is described as embryonal in 80% and alveolar in 15–20%. The pathology of the diverse NRSTS is perhaps best illustrated by listing the more common subtypes: fibrosarcoma, synovial sarcoma, malignant peripheral nerve sheath tumours, malignant fibrous histiocytoma and extraosseous Ewing's sarcoma.

Both RMS and NRSTS occur more commonly in patients with Li-Fraumeni syndrome, a family cancer syndrome characterised by p53 mutations in the germ cell line. Equally, children with neurofibromatosis (NF1) and with congenital anomalies of the CNS and genitourinary systems have a propensity for soft tissue sarcomas. The genetic alterations in RMS, such as reciprocal translocations t (2; 13) t (1; 13) in alveolar and deletion (11p15) in embryonal histology, are well characterised. There are similar genetic alterations in NRSTS, such as t (x; 18) (p11; q11) in 90% of synovial sarcomas.

Clinical features

RMS arises in sites which confer either a favourable (*) or unfavourable (#) prognosis. The clinical picture usually comprises mild pain, discharge if related to mucosal surfaces and features arising secondary to compression of adjacent tissues. Approximately 35% arise in head and neck sites: orbits*, non-parameningeal* and parameningeal#. Genito-urinary tumours comprise 26%, split into 16% which are non-bladder/prostate* and 10% which are bladder/prostate#. RMS of extremity and other sites# constitute 20% and 15% metastatic at presentation.

NRSTS may arise anywhere, usually as painless masses. As with RMS, symptoms generally relate to compression of adjacent structures.

Both RMS and NRSTS are staged using the Intergroup Rhabdomyosarcoma Study (IRS) group pre- and postoperative clinicopathological system, although it has been modified for the current RMS 2005 trial. This more modern risk grouping system, preferred in Europe, depends on six variables. The first of these, the postsurgical (IRS) status, distinguishes those with: (1) localised disease, completely resected; (2) total gross resection, but evidence of regional spread; (3) incomplete resection with gross residual disease; and (4) distant metastatic disease. To this is added the other five variables:

- Favourable or unfavourable site
- Histology (embryonal or alveolar)
- Size (> or ≤ 5 cm tumour)
- Nodes 0/1
- Age (< 10 or ≥ 10 years).

In NRSTS, the histology (which will not be a simple dichotomy between embryonal or alveolar) is adjusted for, but in principle, the end result for both RMS and NRSTS is a risk stratification of low, standard, high or very high risk. To add confusion, it needs to be noted that the North American IRS system retains a three-category stratification of low, intermediate and high.

The intensity of adjuvant therapy will be tailored according to the risk group.

Investigations

Radiological investigation is usually with ultrasound, followed by cross-sectional imaging with computed tomography and magnetic resonance imaging, largely chosen on the basis of surgical and radiological preference. For these choices to be made rationally, it is essential to have a discussion at a multidisciplinary meeting soon after presentation. The purpose of imaging is to ascertain the spread of the disease and to inform the decision on whether a safe biopsy, or unusually, a safe primary resection, should be performed.

Differential diagnosis

- Neuroblastoma
- Ewing's sarcoma
- Osteogenic sarcoma
- Lymphoma
- Leukaemia
- Metastatic carcinoma
- Benign mesenchymal tumours
- Inflammatory masses

Treatment

The treatment of soft tissue tumours is usually multimodal, incorporating adjuvant chemotherapy, surgery and sometimes radiotherapy. The main contribution of the surgeon is to ensure that the prognosis is not jeopardised by irrational biopsies, which may inadvertently (and entirely unnecessarily) upstage the patient's tumour. The other guiding principle is that the patient should be neither endangered nor mutilated. It must be recognised that there is a divergence of opinion between adult and paediatric surgeons as to the role and performance of the incisional biopsy but for the sake of certainty, the following summarises the European position in 2012.

An incisional biopsy is the correct initial surgical procedure, except when primary resection with adequate margins is possible. In reality, with the exception of paratesticular RMS, the opportunities for primary resection are rare. The incisional biopsy must anticipate the later excision of the resultant scar, together with the track of a needle, if a Tru-Cut biopsy could not initially be avoided. The incisional biopsy must avoid opening adjacent musculofascial compartments and both haematomas and drains should be avoided. If the latter must be used, its skin exit site should be in line with the incision, to facilitate excision at the second operation.

If a Tru-Cut needle must be used, it is important to ensure a direct straight track from puncture to sampling area, lying within a single compartment and to consider tattoo of the track. A fresh sample, delivered fast to the laboratory, is mandatory.

The successes of apparent surgical 'resections' are graded histologically: R0 – radical, microscopically complete, either wide or compartmental; R1 – marginal, microscopically incomplete, includes wound contamination; R2 – Intralesional, an inadvertent incisional biopsy.

Subsequent surgery ('Secondary Operation') after an incisional biopsy and adjuvant therapy will aim for a staged R0 resection of any residual mass, together with any necessary reconstruction. Neither secondary operations nor multiple biopsies are indicated in the absence of a residual mass that can be demonstrated clinically, endoscopically or radiologically. When a secondary R0 resection is not possible, an R1 resection may be acceptable, when combined with radiotherapy.

Further reading

Carachi R, Grosfeld JL, Azmy AF. The surgery of childhood tumors, 2nd edn. Berlin: Springer, 2008.

Hayes-Jordan A. Recent advances in non-rhabdomyosarcoma soft-tissue sarcomas. Sem Ped Surg 2012; 21:61–67.

RMS 2005. A protocol for non metastatic rhabdomyosarcoma. European Paediatric Soft Tissue Sarcoma Study Group. CCLG Data Centre, 2005.

Related topics of interest

Spleen disorders

Learning outcomes

- To understand the microscopic morphology, applied anatomy and physiology of the spleen
- To be aware of disorders which affect the spleen in children
- To be familiar with the indications for splenectomy
- To be aware of the vaccination regimen prior to splenectomy
- To understand the operative steps of laparoscopic splenectomy

Overview

The majority of children having splenic surgery are afflicted with chronic diseases and make contact only with the surgical team when a splenectomy is being considered. Paediatric surgeons should have an understanding of the anatomy and physiology of the normal and abnormal spleen and not act as technicians.

An understanding of the microscopic morphology of the splenic parenchyma helps explain the pathophysiology of splenomegaly as well as some clinical features. The splenic parenchyma is composed of two major components, red pulp and white pulp. Red pulp accounts for 75% of the volume of the spleen and contains large vascular spaces, called venous sinusoids, which drain into splenic veins. The red pulp acts as a mechanical filtration device for red blood cells. Macrophages arranged in strips of tissue called splenic cords surround venous sinusoids and phagocytose old or abnormally shaped red blood cells. White pulp comprises lymphoid tissue, which is responsible for mediating humoral and cell-mediated immune responses.

Epidemiology and aetiology

The median age of children undergoing splenectomy is about 12 years.
Disorders of the spleen can be characterised as follows:

Splenomegaly

Aetiology is best understood by correlating structure and function:

- Increased filtration and phagocytosis of red blood cells secondary to abnormal red blood cells (spherocytosis, sickle cell disease and thalassaemia)
- Storage disorders, such as Gaucher's disease, Hurler syndrome and Niemann–Pick disease, arising as a result of inherited deficiencies of enzymes, which would normally break down products of cell metabolism. These conditions are characterised by accumulation of glycolipids in cells and their membranes. Phagocytosis of red cells by macrophages leads to accumulation of these products within the spleen causing splenomegaly, which can be massive
- Mechanical obstruction to venous outflow from sinusoids (portal hypertension, portal vein thrombosis and splenic vein thrombosis)
- Proliferation of the B cells and/or T cells within the white pulp as a result of humoral and/or cell-mediated immune responses secondary to viral infections, such as infectious mononucleosis and human immunodeficiency virus, and bacterial infections such as tuberculosis
- Tumours of lymphoid tissue arise from the white pulp and most are lymphomas or leukaemias
- The spleen can be the site of extramedullary haematopoiesis in certain conditions, such as osteopetrosis, where the space occupied by bone marrow is limited by excess bone formation

Congenital disorders

Asplenia and polysplenia

Congenital asplenia or polysplenia may be a feature of the heterotaxy syndrome, characterised by congenital heart defects, such as Fallot's tetralogy and transposition of the great vessels, midline stomach or liver, intestinal rotational anomalies and vascular anomalies, such as azygos or hemiazygos continuation of the inferior vena cava and preduodenal portal vein.

Splenunculi (accessory spleens)

Splenunculi are present in about 30% of patients and the majority are located near the hilum of the spleen or the tail of the pancreas. Awareness of their presence is important when performing splenectomy as recurrence of certain diseases may be noted if all splenunculi are not removed.

Wandering spleen

Wandering spleen is more common in boys and usually presents before the age of 10 years. There is abnormal attachment of the splenic ligaments and often the only attachment to the spleen are the hilar vessels and the gastrosplenic ligament. The spleen can be found in abnormal positions in the abdomen or pelvis and is prone to torsion.

Splenogonadal fusion

There is either a band connecting the spleen to the testis or ovary (continuous type) or ectopic splenic tissue is attached to the gonad (discontinuous type). It is more common in boys.

Splenic cysts

Cysts of the spleen in children are usually epidermoid cysts and can arise from any part of the spleen. They have the potential to grow, compress and eventually replace the entire normal splenic parenchyma. They need to be differentiated from parasitic cysts.

Splenic abscesses

Abscesses arise secondary to trauma, immunosuppression or splenic infarction. Multiple abscesses are more common than single abscesses. Responsible organisms are staphylococci, anaerobic gram-negative bacteria, salmonella or candida.

Clinical features

The clinical modes of presentation of children in need of splenectomy are as follows:
- Symptoms of anaemia such as tiredness and lethargy

- Transfusion dependency
- Left upper quadrant or shoulder-tip pain
- Acute splenic sequestration crisis (red blood cells are trapped in the spleen and there is a sudden fall in serum haemoglobin; it is associated with sickle cell disease)
- Symptomatic gallstones
- Petechiae secondary to thromboctypaenia (as seen in idiopathic thrombocytopaenic purpura or hypersplenism)
- Recurrent infections
- Splenic trauma

A thorough physical examination should be performed and specific features to elicit are as follows:
- Pallor
- Jaundice
- Palpable spleen and liver
- Murphy's sign secondary to symptomatic gallstones
- Thickening of facial bones as a consequence of extramedullary haematopoiesis

Investigations

Blood

- Full blood count
- Liver function tests including split bilirubin if obstructive jaundice present
- Coagulation profile
- Group and cross match

Radiology

- Abdominal ultrasonography is the only radiological investigation performed in the majority of cases. Its aim is to assess splenic size and establish whether gallstones are present.
- Patients with sickle cell disease often have a preoperative cranial magnetic resonance imaging to establish the presence of abnormalities, such as cerebral infarction, atrophy and haemorrhage, which are present in about 13% of children.
- In children with large splenic cysts, contrast-enhanced computed tomography is helpful to delineate vascular anatomy and help plan the feasibility of partial splenectomy.

Liver biopsy

Liver biopsy is occasionally indicated intraoperatively to assess tissue iron deposition secondary to multiple blood transfusions.

Treatment

Vaccinations

It is recommended by the British Committee for Standards in Haematology that the following vaccines are administered:
- Pneumococcal vaccine at least 2 weeks prior to splenectomy (in children under the age of 2 years, the seven-valent conjugate vaccine is recommended)
- Haemophilus Influenza type B vaccine
- Meningococcal group C conjugate vaccine
- Influenza vaccine

Indications for splenectomy

Common indications are as follows:
- Tiredness and lethargy
- Transfusion dependency
- Thrombocytopaenia
- Acute splenic sequestration crisis

Operative technique for laparoscopic splenectomy

- Laparoscopic splenectomy is the operation of choice for children needing a splenectomy
- A detailed understanding of the ligamentous attachments of the spleen is essential for a safe splenectomy to be performed (**Figure 58**)

- Benzylpenicillin or erythromycin is given at induction of anaesthesia
- Children with sickle cell disease should be kept well-hydrated throughout the perioperative phase
- A large orogastric tube is inserted to decompress the stomach
- The patient is placed supine, in slight reverse Trendelenburg with the left flank raised by a beanbag and the patient secured to the table, which is then rotated to have the patient in right lateral decubitus
- Port sites are infiltrated with local anaesthetic and a four-port technique is used with the primary port at the umbilicus for a 30° laparoscope
- The entire procedure may be performed using an energy device, such as the bipolar Ligasure vessel sealing device
- The gastrosplenic ligament is opened and the lesser sac is entered. The short gastric vessels are divided up to the upper pole of the spleen
- A search is then made for splenunculi, which are removed
- The main splenic artery is dissected free above the tail of the pancreas where it lies just above and anterior to the vein. It is coagulated but not divided. The aim is to stop arterial inflow into the spleen as this manoeuvre significantly decreases bleeding during the rest of the operation and causes the spleen to reduce in size
- The sustentaculum lienis is divided and the splenic flexure retracted inferiorly. The splenocolic ligament is divided and the hilar splenic vessels within the lienorenal

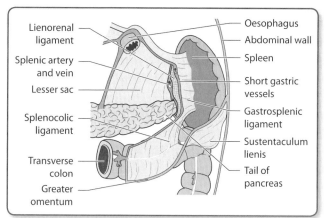

Figure 58 Ligamentous attachments of the spleen.

Lienorenal ligament
Splenic artery and vein
Lesser sac
Splenocolic ligament
Transverse colon
Greater omentum

Oesophagus
Abdominal wall
Spleen
Short gastric vessels
Gastrosplenic ligament
Sustentaculum lienis
Tail of pancreas

ligament are approached from below and divided. An inferior polar artery is present in 39% of cases, a superior polar artery in 31% of cases and both superior and inferior polar arteries in 13% of cases

- Great care is taken to prevent injury to the tail of the pancreas lying in the lienorenal ligament
- The phrenicocolic ligament is divided and the spleen freed of all attachments
- The spleen is bagged and removed piecemeal using a combination of finger fracture and extraction, with sponge-holding forceps
- It is essential to avoid spillage of splenic tissue within the peritoneal cavity or else splenosis may ensue

Gallstones

For many surgeons performing splenectomies, the presence of asymptomatic and symptomatic gallstones constitutes an indication for cholecystectomy. Some surgeons have advocated cholecystostomy and removal of stones only. However, the latter approach carries the risk of recurrence of gallbladder stones. Gallstone surgery during splenectomy occurs in about 22% of cases.

Antibiotic prophylaxis

Lifelong antibiotic prophylaxis, with oral phenoxymethylpenicillin or erythromycin, is recommended to minimise the risk of overwhelming postsplenectomy infection.

Partial splenectomy

The author's preference is to treat large or symptomatic cysts with laparoscopic partial splenectomy. The recurrence rate is lower than with deroofing of the cyst.

Outcomes

- **Conversion to open:** In the author's personal series of 78 laparoscopic splenectomies, the conversion to open rate has been 2% and the quoted figure in the literature is < 5% in larger series
- **Early complications:** Early postoperative complications are pneumonia, intraabdominal bleeding, pancreatitis, wound infections, port-site herniation and sickle cell crises. Such complications arise in < 5% of cases
- **Postsplenectomy sepsis:** A literature review from 1952 to 1987 showed:
  - The incidence of infection postsplenectomy in children under 16 years to be 4.4%, with a mortality rate of 2.2%, compared with figures of 0.9% and 0.8%, respectively, in adults
  - The infection rate is 15.7% in infants and 10.4% in children under 5 years
  - Children are more susceptible to pneumococcal infection than any other infection
  - Children predominantly develop meningitis

Further reading

Davies JM, Barnes R, Miligan D. Update of guidelines for the prevention and treatment of infection in patients with an absent or dysfunctional spleen. Clin Med 2002; 2:440–443.

Hery G, Becmeur F, Mefat L, et al. Laparoscopic partial splenectomy: indications and results of a multicenter retrospective study. Surg Endosc 2008; 22:45–49.

Wood JH, Partrick DA, Hays T, et al. Contemporary pediatric splenectomy: continuing controversies. Ped Surg Int 2011; 27:1165–1171.

Related topics of interest

Thoracic trauma

Learning outcomes

- To appreciate the significant anatomical and physiological differences between children and adults
- To learn when to suspect and how to diagnose thoracic injury
- To appreciate that the immediately life-threatening injuries must be diagnosed and treated during the primary survey
- To develop a structured approach to investigation and treatment of thoracic injuries

Overview

Isolated thoracic trauma in children is associated with a 5% mortality rate, which rises to 40% when other organ systems are also involved.

Children have a compliant ribcage, which allows direct transmission of force to the thoracic and abdominal viscera. There is greater mobility of the mediastinal structures. Thus, visceral injury is more likely than rib fractures. Flail segments and paradoxical respiration are seldom seen and are more likely in adolescents, whose anatomy progressively resembles that of adults.

The diaphragm is relatively flat, and the liver and spleen are comparatively larger than in adults. The trachea is short and narrowest at the cricoid cartilage. Minor changes in calibre, combined with apparently trivial injury or small foreign bodies, can cause rapid respiratory embarrassment. In addition, children have lower functional residual capacity and higher oxygen consumption per unit body mass as a result of which, young children are prone to the rapid evolution of hypoxia.

Aetiology

Toddlers and infants are passive victims of blunt injury due to motor vehicle accidents and non-accidental injury. School-age children are involved in transport-related mechanisms from skateboards, scooters, roller-skates and bicycles. Teenagers are more likely to be involved in high-energy motor vehicle accidents, sports injuries, personal violence and suicide. They are also more likely to sustain penetrating injury.

Clinical features

Tension pneumothorax, massive haemothorax, open chest wound, flail chest and cardiac tamponade are conditions that require prompt intervention and should be identified and dealt with during the primary survey.

Tension pneumothorax manifests as severe hypoxia, shock, hyper-resonant hemithorax, with diminished breath sounds, deviation of the trachea to the contralateral side and displacement of cardiac impulse. A massive haemothorax presents similarly but with dullness to percussion on the affected side.

The presence of an open chest wound is usually obvious. Communication between the pleural cavity and the atmosphere causes respiratory compromise by negating the mechanics of respiration. The contralateral side is also affected by paradoxical movement of the mobile mediastinum.

Accumulation of blood in the pericardial cavity causes haemodynamic compromise by progressively impeding venous return to the heart. Typical clinical features are shock, distension of jugular veins and diminished heart sounds.

In the stable patient, chest injury may manifest itself as abrasions, contusions and/or crepitus, signifying rib fractures or subcutaneous emphysema.

Pulseless electrical activity

Pulseless electrical activity (PEA) in the setting of paediatric blunt trauma warrants immediate bilateral needle thoracocentesis and simultaneous pericardiocentesis to ensure that the treatable causes are dealt with.

In the setting of penetrating injury, if an appropriately trained surgeon is present, a resuscitative thoracotomy should be performed. In cases of penetrating chest injury, this will allow control of the bleeding and internal cardiac massage. Apart from providing the ability to perform internal cardiac massage, this allows the descending aorta to be cross-clamped in case of penetrating injury to the abdomen, stemming bleeding and diverting blood to the heart and brain.

Investigations

A chest radiograph is part of the secondary survey and may pick up fractured ribs, haemothorax, pneumothorax, pulmonary contusion and may raise the suspicion of mediastinal injury. A computed tomography (CT) scan of the chest is usually done in the setting of multiple injuries when there is indication to scan the head and/or the abdomen. It is also done when there is a suspicion of mediastinal injury.

Based on clinical and radiological features, further investigations may become necessary. Cardiac enzymes and electrocardiogram may be required to diagnose and monitor injury to the heart. Transoesophageal and transthoracic echocardiogram may be useful to diagnose heart and great vessel injury.

The gold standard test to diagnose aortic injury is aortography. Suspicion of oesophageal injury warrants a contrast swallow or tube oesophagogram.

Treatment

Initial evaluation and management follows the 'ABC' of trauma resuscitation. Large-bore venous access is vital. Intraosseous infusion of fluid is life-saving if venous access is difficult.

Rib fractures

Rib fractures are uncommon in young children and are more often diagnosed in older children and adolescents. In isolation, rib fractures are rarely clinically significant. However, they provide insight into the force of injury and the likelihood of underlying visceral injury. In the age group 0–3 years, non-accidental injury should

be strongly considered, especially if there is no underlying condition, causing bony fragility or plausible explanation for an injury involving considerable force. Presence of rib fractures must prompt further evaluation of underlying organ injury by CT.

The management of rib fractures is supportive with measures to prevent lung atelectasis and pneumonia. Adequate pain relief to ensure comfortable breathing in conjunction with incentive spirometry and deep-breathing exercises are important measures. In addition, drainage of air and fluid collections helps to improve lung expansion and to promote a return to normal physiology.

Pulmonary contusion and laceration

Pulmonary contusion is the most common intrathoracic injury in children. Contusion may occur by direct compression or by tearing and compression of tissues by rapid deceleration. It is characterised by a non-anatomic pattern of lung injury. While chest radiographs tend to miss minor contusions, CT overestimates the severity of these injuries. The involved lung tissue has alveolar haemorrhage, collapse or oedema. This causes respiratory compromise due to ventilation–perfusion mismatch and decreased compliance. Management is by supportive measures, which include adequate pain relief, breathing exercises and fluid restriction. Appropriately managed, these changes can be expected to revert to normal in a few days. While involvement of a small volume of lung may not be very significant, loss of much larger lung volumes may necessitate mechanical ventilation or even extracorporeal support.

Haemothorax and pneumothorax

Parenchymal lung injury is often associated with presence of air or blood or both in the pleural space. Minor collections are probably not of clinical significance, but in the setting of trauma and in the presence of symptoms, it is impossible to separate the effect of a larger collection from that of underlying lung injury. Placement of a chest drain provides the best method of investigating the volume of air leak or blood loss. It also allows the best chance for the lung to re-expand. Blood in the pleural cavity has a high chance of being infected and resulting in an empyema. Organisation of the blood could result in entrapment of the lung by fibrous tissue and chronic atelectasis. For these reasons, complete drainage is beneficial.

Blood loss resulting in ongoing haemodynamic instability constitutes an indication for thoracotomy to control bleeding. Antibiotic prophylaxis in the setting of lung injury is controversial.

Airway injury

Continued massive air leak from chest drains or presence of mediastinal or subcutaneous air signifies larger airway injury. This may necessitate placement of an endotracheal tube beyond the site of injury or selective intubation to allow the injury to heal or indeed for the patient to survive until surgical repair is possible.

Mediastinal injury

Heart and great vessels

Fortunately, these injuries are rare and nearly always occur in older children or adolescents in the context of road accidents in which they are unrestrained passengers.

Aortic injuries are difficult to diagnose in children. Clues on the chest radiograph may be difficult to interpret in the presence of a thymic shadow. CT may reveal a mediastinal haematoma. Aortic injuries result in high mortality, but 60–70% of those who survive to diagnosis will live to discharge. Definitive management is operative, but this may be delayed by use of beta-blocking agents while other injuries are managed.

Blunt cardiac injury is rare and may result in elevation of cardiac enzymes, rhythm disturbance, valvular incompetence, septal defects and pump failure. Management of these injuries is largely supportive.

Commotio cordis refers to the onset of a rhythm disorder, usually ventricular fibrillation, in response to a relatively trivial but sharp impact to the precordium. The majority of those affected die. As a result of these events, chest protection is now mandatory in many baseball leagues and other sports.

Oesophagus

Due to its location, compliance and ability to empty itself into the mouth or stomach, blunt injury to the oesophagus is very rare. It is more likely to be lacerated by penetrating injury traversing the mediastinum. Primary repair is usually indicated.

Diaphragmatic injury

Blunt diaphragmatic rupture is usually associated with other visceral injury, and in 40–50% of cases, the diagnosis is not made in the acute phase but weeks or months later. An abnormal diaphragmatic contour, a high diaphragm or oddly overlapping gas shadows may be clues. Often, visceral herniation only occurs later and therefore, the injury may be missed even on CT.

The potential complications are lung compression and strangulation of the herniated viscera. Therefore, prompt surgical repair is warranted when the diagnosis is made.

Further reading

Bliss D, Silen M. Pediatric thoracic trauma. Crit Care Med 2002; 30:S409–S415.

Tovar JA. The lung and pediatric trauma. Semin Pediatr Surg 2008; 17:53–59.

Related topics of interest

Thyroglossal cyst

Learning outcomes

- To recognise the diagnosis of thyroglossal cyst
- To understand the embryological origin of the condition
- To understand surgical managements and outcome

Overview

Thyroglossal cyst (TGC) is one of the most common midline neck swellings in childhood. It is a congenital lesion but usually presents in childhood. Three quarters present as cysts and 25% as sinuses with or without infection. Surgical management is by use of the Sistrunk procedure.

Epidemiology and aetiology

TGCs are rare and are equally common in men and women. They rarely present at birth, with 40% presenting in the first decade. Thyroglossal duct remnants account for > 50% of all congenital anomalies in the neck region.

A TGC may not be clearly delineated and may histologically be a pseudocyst, without a true epithelial lining. The thyroglossal duct is lined with cuboidal or columnar epithelium and may undergo squamous metaplasia. The duct may be branching and small, and therefore difficult to distinguish from normal tissues at operation. Thyroid gland tissue may be identified in the cyst.

A thyroglossal fistula between the base of the tongue and neck skin due to persistence of the entire thyroglossal duct is very uncommon. Failure of descent of all or part of the thyroid gland results in aberrant thyroid tissue most commonly in the base of the tongue as a lingual thyroid. About 75% of such patients have the entire gland in the aberrant site, and 25% have some thyroid tissue at the normal location.

The thyroglossal duct is an ectodermal remnant which extends from the foramen caecum (at the junction between anterior two-thirds and posterior one-third of the tongue) to the pyramidal lobe of the thyroid gland, marking the line of descent of the thyroid gland (4th to 7th week of gestation). The duct passes immediately anterior to, or through, the middle of the hyoid bone that develops from the second branchial arch at the same time. The duct is usually obliterated by the 5th week of gestation, but if it is not, a cyst can develop at any point in the tract from the base of the tongue to the suprasternal fossa, most commonly around the hyoid.

Clinical features

- History of anterior midline neck swelling – not usually present at birth, but grows slowly, and 75% are midline with the remainder slightly to one side
- If infected may present with hot, red, tender swelling
- On examination – smooth, soft, non-tender midline neck swelling which may move upwards on swallowing or protrusion of the tongue (due to its close relationship to hyoid bone)

TGCs occur in six different variants:
1. Infrahyoid cysts – about 65% of TGCs – mostly found in the paramedian position
2. Suprahyoid cysts – < 20% of TGCs – found in the midline
3. Juxtahyoid cysts – about 15% of TGCs – found close to the hyoid bone
4. Intralingual cysts – about 2% of TGCs – found within the tongue
5. Suprasternal cysts – < 10% of cases
6. Intralaryngeal cysts – very rare – these must be differentiated from other intralaryngeal lesions

Investigations

Ultrasound scanning of the neck is performed to ensure the presence of normal thyroid tissue outside the cyst, as occasionally ectopic thyroid tissue in the cyst is the only functioning thyroid tissue (1.5%). If normal thyroid tissue is not seen on ultrasound, thyroid function tests and radioisotope scanning may be required.

Differential diagnosis

- Dermoid cyst – epithelial lined inclusion cysts account for 25% of median neck swellings in children
- Lymph node
- Thyroid gland swelling or ectopic thyroid tissue
- Lipoma
- Subhyoid bursa
- Epidermoid, branchial cleft or sebaceous cyst
- Cystic hygroma

Treatment

Complete surgical excision is the recommended treatment to avoid infection of the cyst (which makes excision more difficult) and to prevent the small risk of carcinoma (< 1%). Infected cysts should be treated with antibiotics before excision is attempted because the risk of complications and recurrence is higher. Incision and drainage may be required. A ruptured infected cyst may result in a thyroglossal fistula.

Operative details

The Sistrunk procedure – consisting of excision of the TGC and tract described in 1920 – emphasises the importance of excising the thyroglossal tract as it passes near the middle portion of the hyoid bone to prevent recurrence.

- General considerations – the operation can be performed as a day-case procedure (in healthy children) under general anaesthetic
- Position – the patient is positioned supine, with head extended and shoulders elevated
- Incision – transverse skin crease incision over the cyst

Procedure

- The cyst is carefully dissected ensuring haemostasis, and aiming not to rupture the cyst (increased risk of recurrence). If the cyst appears to be attached caudally to a tract, this is dissected with a cuff of normal tissue
- The thyroglossal tract is identified and followed superiorly between sternohyoid muscles to the hyoid bone. If it cannot be clearly identified, dissection should still include a core of tissue cranially as far as the hyoid to prevent recurrence
- The muscle attachments to the hyoid (sternohyoid, mylohyoid and geniohyoid) are freed from the mid portion of the bone, which is excised using a bone cutter or scissors
- The duct is then followed superiorly as far as possible towards the foramen caecum at the base of the tongue, occasionally requiring a further 'step-ladder' incision in the neck
- Closure – absorbable sutures are used to approximate the muscles and close cervical fascia and platysma in layers. Subcutaneous absorbable sutures or steristrips are used for skin closure
- Complications include bleeding, infection and recurrence (< 5%)

Malignancy has been reported in TGCs, with the papillary type of thyroid tumour the most common.

Further reading

Brewis C et al. Investigation and treatment of thyroglossal cysts in children. J R Soc Med 2000; 93:18–21.

Foley DS, Fallat ME. Thyroglossal duct and other congenital midline cervical anomalies. Semin Pediatr Surg 2006; 15:70–75.

Sistrunk WE. The surgical treatment of cysts of the thyroglossal tract. Ann Surg 1920; 71:121–122.

Related topics of interest

Thyroid and parathyroid glands

Learning outcomes

- To know the differentials of paediatric thyroid disease and how to recognise them
- To know the treatments for thyroid disease in childhood and when surgery is indicated
- To understand the physiology and pathophysiology of parathyroid disease
- To understand key points of peri- and postoperative care

Thyroid gland

Thyroid embryology, anatomy and physiology

The gland descends embryologically from the foramen caecum of the tongue to its neck position. Problems in descent can result in an ectopic or lingual thyroid, thyroglossal cyst or fistula formation.

- The thyroid gland is highly vascular, and synthesises and stores thyroid hormones
- Thyroid hormones are essential to growth, metabolism, cardiovascular function and neurological development
- The thyroid gland also secretes calcitonin, important in calcium homeostasis

In response to hypothalamic thyrotropin-releasing hormone, the anterior pituitary produces thyroid-stimulating hormone (TSH) which in turn stimulates thyroxine – tetra-iodothyronine (T4) and tri-iodothyronine (T3) – production by the thyroid gland. A negative feedback mechanism controls the hormone secretion.

Tyrosine is iodinated and two molecules combine to form T4. T3, the active hormone, is converted from T4 in peripheral tissues (e.g. liver, spleen and kidneys).

Aetiology of thyroid disease

- **Congenital hypothyroidism – anatomical (thyroid dysgenesis, agenesis or maldescent):** This is the most common paediatric endocrine problem (incidence 1 in 3000–4000). It is associated with congenital heart disease, and rarely with sensorineural deafness (Pendred's syndrome)
- **Acquired (Hashimoto's) hypothyroidism autoimmune, diffuse lymphocytic infiltration of the thyroid, antibody-mediated:** This most commonly presents in adolescence, and is increased in females and chromosomal disorders, such as Down and Turner's syndromes. The most common cause of hypothyroidism worldwide is iodine deficiency, although this is rare in the UK
- **Hyperthyroidism:** Graves' disease (caused by TSH receptor antibodies) is the most common cause of hyperthyroidism (90%) in children. Hashimoto's disease can initially be indistinguishable from Graves', but patients eventually become hypothyroid.
- **Thyroid cancer:** This is often secondary to environmental or therapeutic radiation exposure, but can be genetic or sporadic. Mainly papillary or follicular, and very rare in children, it usually presents with asymmetric thyroid swelling.

Clinical features of thyroid disease

1. Goitre
- Diffuse or nodular, may be tender
- Smoothly enlarged with a bruit in hyperthyroidism
- Asymmetrical, with regional lymph nodes may indicate malignancy
2. Hypothyroidism
- In the neonate
  - Poor feeding
  - Prolonged jaundice
  - Hypotonia
  - Protuberant tongue
- In older children
  - Poor appetite
  - Weight gain
  - Poor energy
  - Constipation
  - Cold intolerance
  - Dry skin
  - Hair loss

3. Hyperthyroidism
- Tremor
- Sweating
- Deteriorating school performance
- Rapid growth
- Increased appetite but weight loss
- Diarrhoea
- Heat intolerance
- Tachycardia, rarely atrial fibrillation
- Eye changes – exophthalmos, lid retraction or lag, ophthalmoplegia causing double vision

Investigations

- Neonatal blood spot screening: TSH level identifies congenital primary hypothyroidism
- Serum T4 + T3: reduced in hypothyroidism, raised in hyperthyroidism
- TSH level: raised in hypothyroidism, suppressed in hyperthyroidism
- Thyroid antibodies (thyroid peroxidase): positive in Graves' and Hashimoto's thyroiditis (usually higher in the latter), TSH receptor antibodies in Graves' disease
- Thyroid ultrasound: anatomical assessment of the thyroid gland in congenital hypothyroidism, hyperthyroidism and thyroid swelling
- Thyroid scintigraphy: used in congenital hypothyroidism and thyroid nodules
- Fine needle aspiration: of solitary nodules

Treatment

1. Hypothyroidism: treated with thyroxine replacement. Careful consideration of growth and puberty is required
2. Hyperthyroidism
- Medical: antithyroid drugs (carbimazole, and if not tolerated propylthiouracil), with initial beta-blockade
  - Remission is less common in children than in adults, occurring in 15–30% of patients, becoming less likely if not achieved within the first years of therapy
  - Relapse warrants further treatment
- Surgery remains the definitive therapy

Indications for total thyroidectomy: thyrotoxicosis in the young child, relapsing disease, malignancy or tracheal compression.

Patients need to be biochemically euthyroid prior to surgery.
Specific surgical complications and their management include:
- Hormonal
  - Hypocalcaemia + tetany and carpopedal spasm
    - Calcium monitoring and replacement
  - Hypothyroidism
    - Replacement with levothyroxine
  - Late recurrence of hyperthyroidism
    - Retreatment
  - Thyroid crisis (rare with careful preoperative preparation)
    - Cooling blanket and propanolol, diuretics for heart failure, intensive care
- Anatomical
  - Laryngeal oedema (may be secondary to haematoma compression)
    - May require intubation and usually resolves spontaneously
  - Recurrent laryngeal nerve damage
    - Hoarseness (unilateral)
    - Airways obstruction (bilateral)
    - Hoarseness and vocal weakness
  - Superior laryngeal nerve
    - If neuropraxia usually resolves within 3 months
- Radioactive iodine is an alternative, with no long-term side effects reported. It is not commonly used in children < 10 years in the UK

Parathyroid Glands
Embryology, anatomy and physiology

The four paired parathyroid glands originate from the neural crest mesenchyme and endoderm of the third (inferior) and fourth (superior) branchial pouch endodermes. They usually lie in two pairs, posterior to the lateral lobes of the thyroid gland, although the inferior glands may lie in the neck or the superior mediastinum.

Parathyroid hormone (PTH) elevates calcium levels by osteoclastic bone resorption and increased renal calcium reabsortion, simultaneously increasing renal phosphate excretion. Calcitonin secreted by the thyroid gland opposes these effects.

Hyperparathyroidism

1. Aetiology
- Primary hyperparathyroidism: gland overproduction of PTH due to adenoma, hyperplasia or, rarely, parathyroid carcinoma It can occur as part of a multiple endocrine neoplasia (MEN) syndrome, either type 1 (mutation in the gene *MEN1*) or type 2a (mutation in the gene *RET*). Other mutations in genes *HRPT2* and *CASR* have been linked to parathyroid neoplasia
- Secondary hyperparathyroidism: due to physiological secretion of PTH by the parathyroid glands in response to hypocalcaemia. The most common causes are vitamin D deficiency and chronic renal failure

Vitamin D deficiency leads to reduced calcium absorption by the intestine, leading to hypocalcaemia and increased PTH secretion. This increases bone resorption. In chronic renal failure, the kidney fails to convert vitamin D to its active form, leading to renal osteodystrophy

2. Clinical features
- Primary
  - About 50% of patients are asymptomatic and finding is incidental
  - Many others have non-specific symptoms
  - Symptoms directly due to hypercalcaemia are relatively rare, being more common in patients with malignant hypercalcaemia, but can include:
    - Weakness and fatigue, depression, bone pain, myalgia
    - Decreased appetite, feelings of nausea and vomiting, constipation, polyuria, polydipsia, cognitive impairment, kidney stones and osteoporosis
- Secondary: clinical problems are due to bone resorption and manifest as bone syndromes such as rickets, osteomalacia and renal osteodystrophy
3. Investigations
- Primary: PTH and serum calcium are high, and serum phosphate is low due to decreased renal reabsorption
- Secondary: PTH is high and serum calcium is low or normal
4. Treatment
- Primary: in those with a parathyroid adenoma management is surgical. A preoperative technetium99m-sestamibi scan can identify hyperfunctioning normally sited or ectopic (commonly anterior mediastinum) parathyroid tissue, guiding the surgical approach and leading to a minimal parathyroidectomy, with less risk of postoperative hypoparathyroidism
- Secondary: treatment is directed at the aetiology of the hypocalcaemia

Hypoparathyroidism

1. Aetiology
- Inadvertent damage or removal of the parathyroid glands during surgery can cause transient or permanent hypocalcaemia
- Autoimmune
- Haemochromatosis
- Hypomagnesaemia
- DiGeorge syndrome (chromosome 22q11 microdeletion syndrome) – congenital absence of the parathyroid glands
- Familial hypoparathyroidism with other endocrine diseases, such as adrenal insufficiency, in autoimmune polyglandular failure syndrome type 1
- Defect in calcium receptor
- Idiopathic
2. Clinical features and investigation: monitoring calcium levels following thyroid surgery is essential. Severe hypocalcaemia (~1.5 mmol/L) causes
- Carpopedal spasm
- Tetany
- Stridor
- Seizures
- Paraesthesia and weakness are more common if hypocalcaemia is mild
3. Treatment
- Severe hypocalcaemia: slow intravenous infusion of 10% calcium gluconate, followed by oral calcium supplementation for up to 3 months
- Vitamin D supplementation (as alfacalcidol)
- Parathyroid recovery in transient hypoparathyroidism can take up to 2 years

Further reading

Butler G, Kirk J. Paediatric endocrinology and diabetes. Oxford University Press, 2011.

Raine JE, et al. Practical endocrinology and diabetes in children, 3rd edn. London: Wiley-Blackwell, 2011.

Rivkees SKA. Pediatric Graves disease: controversies in management. Horm Res Pediatr 2010; 74:305–311.

Related topics of interest

- Thyroglossal cyst (p. 336)

Tracheal anomalies

Learning outcomes

- To be aware of various types of tracheal anomalies
- To know the various presenting signs and symptoms
- To learn the appropriate investigations and management options, including the indications for surgery
- To be aware of the different surgical options and likely outcomes

Overview

Tracheal anomalies involve structural abnormalities of the trachea itself or extrinsic mediastinal anomalies that compress the lower airway.

Intrinsic tracheal anomalies include the following:

- Primary diffuse tracheomalacia – compression of >50% in sagittal diameter of tracheal lumen during coughing or expiration; can be due to inherent weakness or absence of tracheal cartilage, often associated with trachea-oesophageal fistula
- Long segment tracheal stenosis (LSTS) (with complete cartilaginous tracheal rings, exceeding two-thirds the length of the trachea) or short segment stenosis, which may be acquired
- Abnormal branching of trachea – variant branching like tracheal bronchus (bronchus suis or 'pig bronchus') which originates from the right lateral wall of the trachea above the level of the main carina. Not significant unless associated with other problems
- Tracheal web – isolated fibrous constriction with no associated tracheal cartilage abnormality
- Tracheal agenesis and atresia – continuity between the larynx and lungs is absent or underdeveloped
- Tracheo-oesophageal fistula (TOF) with oesophageal atresia (OA)

Extrinsic mediastinal anomalies include the following:

- Vascular – compression from complete rings (double aortic arch, right aortic arch) or incomplete rings [aberrant innominate artery, aberrant right subclavian artery, left pulmonary artery (LPA) sling]
- Cardiac – compression from enlarged left atrium, enlarged pulmonary arteries
- Mediastinal masses – compression from enlarged thymus, bronchogenic cyst, lymphatic malformation, neoplasm
- Musculoskeletal – compression from severe pectus excavatum, scoliosis

Epidemiology and aetiology

The incidence of congenital tracheal stenosis is fortunately low, estimated to be 1 in 64,500 live births in Canada. Primary tracheobronchomalacia is estimated to be 1 in 2100 children. Tracheal anomalies are often associated with mediastinal malformations. At Great Ormond Street Hospital, London, 70% of patients with LSTS have congenital heart disease and 66% of them have a LPA sling. Isolated LSTS occurs only in 10–25% of cases.

During the 4th week of gestation, the trachea develops as a respiratory diverticulum from the foregut. Posteriorly, the common membranous wall of the trachea and the oesophagus is formed. In the 8th week, splanchnic mesoderm differentiates into primitive cartilage and muscles. In the 10th week, the primitive cartilage migrates and forms the C-shaped rings. Due to the complex and inter-related embryologic development of the trachea, oesophagus and cardiovascular system, tracheal anomalies often involve these foregut structures such as OA with TOF.

The cause of intrinsic tracheal anomalies remains unknown. Alterations in expressions of collagen and aggrecans were associated with primary tracheomalacia. Recent studies on cellular differentiation and organ development suggest some possible molecules, for example cell-adhesion protein β-catenin, which converge with transcription factor SOX-9 to play a major role in tracheal ring formation.

Other causes of secondary tracheomalacia are:

- Prolonged intubation

- Post- tracheitis
- Post-tracheal surgery
- Post-fetoscopic tracheal occlusion for congenital diaphragmatic hernia

Classification of tracheomalacia

Several classification systems have been proposed for tracheobronchomalacia, but the one from Mairs and Parsons is the most practical, with type 1 equating to primary malacia and types 2 and 3 relating to secondary malacia:
- Type 1: congenital or intrinsic tracheal abnormalities (i.e. TOF)
- Type 2: extrinsic compression (i.e. vascular or tumour)
- Type 3: acquired malacia (i.e. chronic intubation and infection)

Clinical features

The child could present with one or more of the following symptoms, all of which should make you ask if there is an airway problem:
- Respiratory distress soon after birth
- Barking cough ('brassy, seal-like')
- Chronic wet cough
- Severe stridor (biphasic)
- Recurrent wheeze
- Recurrent respiratory tract infections, pneumonia
- Dyspnoea and shortness of breath
- Chest retractions
- Reduced exercise tolerance
- Dysphagia and regurgitation
- Difficulty in weaning from mechanical ventilation
- Apparent life-threatening events (ALTEs)
- Sudden death

Investigations

Investigations for tracheal anomalies involve both static and dynamic imaging; 3D reconstruction is helpful. It is always best to have these children seen by experts, either local paediatric ENT surgeons or referral to a specialist service (see below).
- Chest X-ray
- Bronchoscopy
- Bronchography
- Echocardiography

- Spiral CT (pulmonary angiography) or MRI
- Optical coherence tomography – measures the thickness of tracheal cartilage
- Swallowing assessment (videofluoroscopy if extubated)

Differential diagnosis

- Croup
- Gastro-oesophageal reflux disorder
- Bronchomalacia
- Laryngomalacia
- Hyperactive airways

Treatment

Management depends on establishment of definitive diagnosis and severity of symptoms. A multidisciplinary team approach provides optimal surgical outcome, thus discussion with a specialist centre is indicated.

Primary tracheomalacia

- Watchful waiting with regular follow-up for mild symptoms
- Continuous positive airway pressure
- Aortopexy – the trachea-aorta complex is pulled anteriorly via lateral thoracotomy, median sternotomy or thoracoscopic routes, with sutures attached to the sternum, to decompress the collapsed trachea. For primary malacia, >90% patients are asymptomatic at follow-up. For malacia associated with the other complex disease, there is both a high mortality and worse late results
- Internal stenting – tracheal stents can be made of silicone, metal or biodegradable material (polydioxanone)
- External stenting or Hagl procedure – external stabilisation of the severely malacic segment by suspending within an oversized and longitudinally opened ring-reinforced PTFE prosthesis. Simultaneous bronchoscopy is performed together with gentle traction of the sutures to ascertain re-expansion of a collapsed segment
- Tracheostomy

Long segment tracheal stenosis

- Non-surgical treatment is an option for those with mild symptoms (10%)

- Slide tracheoplasty – the treatment of choice for LSTS due to favourable outcomes (87% 17-year survival at Great Ormond Street Hospital). The stenotic trachea is transected at its midpoint, and vertical incisions are made on the posterior aspect of the upper segment and the anterior aspect of the lower segment. The two halves are then slid together and anastomosed, doubling the luminal circumference and increasing the cross-sectional area fourfold. The procedure is done under cardiopulmonary bypass.
- Resection with end-to-end anastomosis
- Enlargement patch tracheoplasty
- Tracheal autograft technique
- Tracheoplasty with cadaveric tracheal graft
- Tissue-engineered tracheal transplant – successful case reports

Short segment stenosis

- This is usually managed by the very effective resection and end-to-end repair

- More rarely, laser and balloon dilatation

Tracheal web

- Web rupturing using rigid dilatation, cutting balloon dilatation or laser surgery

Extrinsic mediastinal anomalies

- Vascular repair: division of vascular sling, repair of LPA sling, Kommerell's diverticulum repair
- Musculoskeletal: Nuss bar insertion to address severe pectus excavatum with aortopexy if needed

In all cases, expert follow-up is mandatory because scarring and recurrence may occur. Regular bronchoscopy and bronchography with intermittent balloon dilatation have been most effective in our practice. Longer term detailed regular clinical and pulmonary function exercise tests are necessary for objective outcome analysis.

Further reading

Boogaard R, Huijsmans SH, Pijnenburg MW, et al. Tracheomalacia and bronchomalacia in children: incidence and patient characteristics. Chest 2005; 128:3391–3397.S

Calkoen EE, Gabra HO, Roebuck DJ, et al. Aortopexy as treatment for tracheo-bronchomalacia in children: an 18-year single-center experience. Pediatr Crit Care Med 2011; 12:545–551.

Speggiorin S, Torre M, Roebuck DJ, et al. A new morphologic classification of congenital tracheobronchial stenosis. Ann Thorac Surg 2012; 93:958–961.

Related topics of interest

Ulcerative colitis

Learning outcomes

- To be able to recognise the clinical features of ulcerative colitis
- To be familiar with relevant investigations
- To be aware of surgical management options

Overview

Ulcerative colitis (UC) is part of the spectrum of inflammatory bowel diseases with unknown aetiology. The disease affects the mucosa of the rectum and extends proximally into the colon to a varying extent. Surgery is curative.

Epidemiology and aetiology

The worldwide incidence of UC varies greatly from 0.5 to 24.5 per 100,000 population. Incidence and prevalence are related to the economic situation of the country, with the lowest rates in the developing countries and the highest in Western and Central European countries. At present, the incidence of UC seems to be increasing in Central and Eastern Europe. A family history is the most consistent predisposing risk factor in children. Children with UC are most commonly diagnosed at the age of 5–16 years, especially around puberty. However, a trend towards earlier appearance of symptoms has been noted. In addition, children seem to develop more widespread disease, with pancolitis, than adults. UC and Crohn's disease are the two most common types of inflammatory bowel disease.

Between 40 and 70% of affected children eventually undergo surgery, mainly because of the significant side-effects of high-dose medical treatment on the growing and developing body. About 10–40% of patients in general with UC eventually need a proctocolectomy.

Although UC was described in 1859 by Sir Samuel Wilks, the aetiology of this disease is still unknown. It seems to occur more frequently in susceptible patients in response to environmental triggers. UC is probably an autoimmune disease, initiated by an inappropriate inflammatory response to colonic bacteria. An association between UC and diet has been suggested but remains unproven to date.

Clinical features

The most common symptom in UC is lower abdominal pain, with crampy pain most intense during defaecation. Nearly 95% of patients notice bloody diarrhoea, with mucus and tenesmus, a constant desire to empty their bowels.

Extraintestinal symptoms of UC are tiredness, fatigue, weight loss, delayed growth and anaemia. UC can also cause joint pain, eye irritation, liver disease and osteoporosis due to long-term steroid use.

Investigations

- Full blood count
- Urea and electrolytes
- Liver function tests
- Serum albumin

Common laboratory findings in patients with UC are anaemia, thrombocytosis and hypoalbuminaemia. However, in up to one-third of paediatric patients, blood tests can be normal.

- **Colonoscopy and biopsies:** Endoscopy is used to diagnose and stage the disease. UC presents with a continuous inflammation from the rectum to various levels of the proximal colon. Anal lesions are infrequent. At endoscopy, the mucosa is inflamed and appears red, granular and friable. The serosa is usually not affected and serositis occurs only in fulminant cases. The small bowel is only rarely affected. Pathological findings are erosive, and superficial ulcerations are limited to the mucosa and submucosa. All crypts are involved with cryptitis and crypt abscesses, in combination with generalised goblet cell mucin depletion. A biopsy is essential to diagnose inflammatory bowel disease and to distinguish between Crohn's disease and UC

- **Abdominal radiograph:** In fulminant cases, a plain abdominal radiograph can be obtained to exclude toxic megacolon or perforation

Differential diagnosis

- Crohn's disease
- Coeliac disease
- Acute appendicitis
- Carcinoid tumour
- Gastroenteritis

Treatment

UC is managed medically with corticosteroids in the acute phase and as maintenance therapy to prevent recurrence. However, because of their side effects, steroids are not recommended for long-term use.

Immunomodulators, such as azathioprine, 6-mercaptopurine and cyclosporin, are used in patients with refractory disease, requiring high-dose steroid therapy to control symptoms. Cyclosporin is only used with severe UC because of its toxicity.

Infliximab, a monoclonal antibody against tumour necrosis factor-alpha, has been used more recently in the management of inflammatory bowel disease. It is also important to maintain good nutrition and eliminate growth failure.

More common indications for surgery are:
- Disease refractory to medical management
- Growth failure, unresponsive to medical treatment
- Toxic megacolon
- Haemorrhage and rarely perforation.

Surgery for UC is curative. The aim of surgical therapy is to resect the affected bowel. There are three operative strategies available for patients with UC: proctocolectomy with ileostomy, colectomy with ileorectal anastomosis and restorative colectomy with ileal reservoir (J-pouch). The gold standard had been proctocolectomy and permanent ileostomy, and the long-term outcome was excellent. However, because of significant social restrictions, it has not been well accepted and tolerated in children and adolescents. Colectomy with ileorectal anastomosis was widely performed in children because it was a less challenging operation than J-pouch formation. However long-term outcomes showed a higher failure rate due to poor function from persisting inflammation and increased carcinoma incidence in the rectal stump. Acceptable long-term results have been achieved by restoration of bowel continuity in combination with formation of a J-pouch reservoir as a single-stage operation. This procedure can be performed laparoscopically in children. Depending on the systemic status secondary to immunosuppression and the nutritional status at the time of surgery, a protective ileostomy may be considered. In severe cases, a demucosectomy of the rectum down to the dentate line needs to be performed. Nowadays, a colectomy with ileostomy is initially performed, followed by reconstructive surgery at a later stage in:
- Children younger than 12 years
- Very rarely in emergency situations with extensive bleeding or toxic megacolon

Restorative proctocolectomy with ileoanal pouch anastomosis has a significant risk of early and late complications. Most of them are well known in adults. The incidence in children is less well reported.

Typical early complications are sepsis and pouch leaks (41–56% of children). Risk factors predisposing to these complications are malnutrition, prolonged steroid use, hypoalbuminaemia and anaemia. Patients present with symptoms such as fever, perineal pain, purulent discharge and leucocytosis between the third and sixth postoperative days.

Typical late complications are recurrent pouchitis, fistulae and anastomotic strictures (38% of children). Pouchitis is an acute or chronic inflammation in the ileal reservoir. It causes increased stool frequency, cramps, abdominal pain, bright red bleeding, diarrhoea and fever. The prevalence in children has been reported to be 30–47%. The treatment for pouchitis comprises antibiotics (metronidazole and ciprofloxacin) and bowel rest. Fistulae and anastomotic strictures are observed in patients with intra- and postoperative complications, such as pelvic contamination and anastomotic leakage.

Further reading

Gorgun E, Remzi FH. Complications of Ileoanal pouches. In: Beck DE (ed.), Clinics in colon and rectal surgery, vol 17, number 1. Thieme, 2004:43–55.

Patton D, Gupta N, Wojcicki JM, et al. Postoperative outcome of colectomy for pediatric patients with ulcerative colitis. J Pediatr Gastroenterol Nutr 2010; 51:151–154.

Rintala R, Pakarinen M. Inflammatory bowel disease. In: Puri P, Hollwarth M (eds), Pediatric surgery: diagnosis and management. Heidelberg: Springer-Verlag, 2009.

Related topics of interest

- Crohn's disease (p. 74)
- Gastrointestinal bleeding (p. 129)

Umbilical disease

Learning outcomes

- To be familiar with common umbilical problems
- To be aware of the pitfalls of misdiagnosis
- To be aware of the risk of malignancy

Overview

In the neonate, the cord dessicates and separates within 21 days, leaving a dry, central abdominal scar that forms the umbilicus. Umbilical hernia is the most common abnormality and results from failure of closure of the umbilical ring.

Umbilical discharge or the presence of abnormal tissue commonly indicates an umbilical granuloma, but can be secondary to failure of complete involution of the urachus or vitellointestinal duct. Any discharge, mass or sinus tract is pathological and should be appropriately evaluated and treated.

Vitellointestinal duct remnants

Aetiology

The vitellointestinal duct is an embryonic communication between the primitive yolk sac and the developing midgut. During midgut elongation in week 6, the lumen of the duct begins to obliterate. When the midgut returns to the abdominal cavity in week 10, the duct becomes a thin fibrous band, which undergoes resorption. Persistence leads to a spectrum of anomalies that can present any time in childhood, including Meckel's diverticulum, persistent fibrous cord, umbilical fistula, vitellointestinal cyst or umbilical polyp.

Clinical features

A persistent fibrous cord or cyst may be asymptomatic until the child presents with intestinal obstruction due to volvulus around the cord. Polyps present as a bright red nodule of sequestered ectopic gastrointestinal tissue and reside in the umbilical dimple.

A persistent fistula usually presents in the neonate with discharge of intestinal content from the umbilicus and periumbilical excoriation. Prolapse of a large patent tract presents as a characteristic 'double-horn' deformity, with intestinal lumen evident. In some cases, omphalitis may be the only presenting feature.

Investigations

In those with unresolving polyps or a grossly abnormal appearance, an underlying duct abnormality should be sought with appropriate imaging or at exploration. Contrast fistulogram can confirm aberrant anatomy (**Figure 59**).

Differential diagnosis

- Umbilical granuloma
- Dermoid
- Rhabdomyosarcoma
- Teratoma

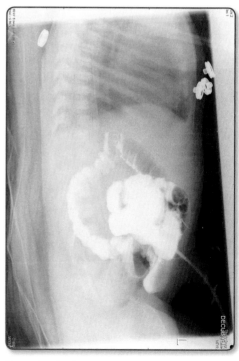

Figure 59 Fistulogram of patent vitello intestinal duct.

Treatment

Management of intestinal obstruction should be by laparotomy, excision of the obstructing band, and resection and anastomosis if needed, via a transverse incision. A cosmetic circumumbilical incision is useful in the case of a patent duct. Polyps can be treated with excision.

Patent urachus

Aetiology

The urachus develops embryologically from the allantois, forming the duct connecting the dome of the urinary bladder to the umbilical ring. It normally obliterates prior to birth and forms the median umbilical ligament.

Entire tract non-closure leads to a patent urachus, whilst closure on the bladder side creates a sinus. Closure of both ends but patency in between occurs in a urachal cyst – the most common urachal anomaly. The rarest urachal anomaly is a bladder diverticulum, which forms when the distal tract involutes.

Clinical features

Patent urachus and sinus may present with clear drainage from the umbilicus, and careful examination demonstrates a sinus at the umbilical base. Because a patent urachus drains urine, presentation may include cystitis or recurrent UTI.

Urachal cysts most commonly present once infected, and the child may present with infraumbilical swelling, abdominal pain and erythema. Patients with delayed separation of the umbilical cord may have a urachal anomaly.

Investigations

Ultrasonography shows a cystic hypoechogenic lesion in the preperitoneal space in the case of urachal cyst, and a longitudinal double line from the bladder dome to the umbilicus indicates a urachal remnant.

Sinogram can be performed in patients with a suspected patent urachus or urachal sinus.

A voiding cystourethrogram is prudent to exclude the presence of posterior urethral valves in the patient with a patent urachus.

Differential diagnosis

Treatment

- Any part of the tract that has failed to obliterate should be completely excised
- Urachal excision should include a cuff of bladder to prevent the risk of developing a urachal adenocarcinoma in later life

Umbilical hernia

Epidemiology

There is an equal sex ratio occurrence, but the incidence in Caucasian newborns is 5–10% while in African infants it is 26.6%.

Aetiology

The umbilical ring is open throughout gestation and becomes relatively smaller. At birth it is surrounded by a dense fascial ring due the linea alba defect. It is reinforced by remnants of umbilical vessels and urachus and a fascial layer, overlying the peritoneum. If the support is weak or absent, a hernia develops.

Clinical features

Most are noticed in the first few weeks of life and almost all by 6 months as an obvious umbilical swelling. Reducible umbilical herniae are rarely painful. Incarceration is rare with a reported incidence of 7.4%. Strangulation of contents, intestine or omentum, is extremely rare with a reported incidence of 0.26%.

Investigations

None unless the child appears syndromic or unwell. Umbilical herniae have been associated with trisomies 13, 18 and 21, mucopolysaccharidoses, congenital hypothyroidism and Beckwith–Wiedemann syndrome.

Treatment

Most close spontaneously during the first 3 years of life, with reports of closure between 5 and 11 years of age.

The majority of paediatric surgeons would avoid operating on an asymptomatic hernia unless it was large (> 1.5 cm) and the child is older than 4 years.

Incarceration is an absolute indication and if reducible then surgery is preferable the following day; if not then emergency surgery is required.

- Elective day case surgery
- Infra- or supra-umbilical incision
- The sac is dissected free and opened with any content being reduced
- The defect is closed transversely with an absorbable suture
- The umbilicus should be inverted with a suture between its underside and the middle of the fascial closure

In African children with giant herniae, the redundant skin and the potential for keloid formation can affect postoperative cosmesis. Removal of redundant skin may be required at a later stage. Complications such as infection (0.8%) and haematoma (1.3%) are uncommon.

Further reading

Lassaletta L, Fonkalsrud EW, Tovar JA, et al. The management of umbilicial hernias in infancy and childhood. J Pediatr Surg 1975; 10:405–409.

Skinner MA, Grosfeld JL. Inguinal and umbilical hernia repair in infants and children. Surg Clin North Am 1993; 73:439–449.

Snyder CL. Current management of umbilical abnormalities and related anomalies. Semin Pediatr Surg 2007; 16:41–49.

Related topics of interest

- Meckel's diverticulum (p. 202)

Undescended testis

Learning outcomes

- To understand the theories of descent
- To identify when surgery is required
- To be aware of the consequences of undescended testis and complications of surgery

Overview

Undescended testis (UDT) occurs due to the failure of normal descent from the abdominal cavity into the scrotum. It is the most common congenital problem seen in children, and its aetiology and ideal management remain controversial. Treatment is aimed at minimising the risks of neoplasia, infertility, testicular torsion and inguinal hernia.

Epidemiology and aetiology

UDT occurs in 3–5% of full term and in 30% of premature boys. Without intervention, in 80% of cases, the testis becomes normally sited within the first 12 months, with most occurring in the first 3 months. The incidence in the > 12 months age group is 1%. It is bilateral in 10%, with a right-to-left ratio of 2:1.

The causes are multifactorial with risk factors including

- Low birth weight, twin pregnancy, prematurity, small for gestational age and maternal oestrogen exposure in the first trimester
- Siblings and parents of affected boys have a higher incidence of this condition, indicating possible genetic susceptibility

It is associated with epididymal cysts (90%), hypospadias and genital ambiguity.

The presence of penile abnormalities (hypospadias and/or small phallus) and undescended testes warrants investigations for disorders of sexual differentiation. Early gonadal differentiation occurs in the urogenital ridge and is regulated by at least two genes, *ZFY* and *SRY*, located on the short arm of the Y chromosome. The *SRY* (sex-determining region of the Y chromosome) gene encodes for a testis-specific DNA-binding protein that stimulates development of the embryonic gonad towards a testis.

Testicular descent is a complex, two-stage process, involving anatomical and hormonal regulators. Stage 1 (transabdominal) occurs at 8–15 weeks' gestation. The testes begin high up in the abdomen and are held by the cranial suspensory ligament (CSL) and gubernaculum caudally. The gubernaculum swells and helps to anchor each testis close to the site of the internal inguinal ring. The CSL regresses to allow relative movement to the external ring by the end of stage 1.

Müllerian-inhibiting substance (MIS) has previously been implicated as the main hormone of the Y chromosome in stage 1. Abnormalities in the *MIS* gene or receptor lead to anomalies, including persistent uterus and tubes, elongated gubernaculum and intra-abdominal testes. Recent data in mice with *MIS* gene mutation show normal testicular descent, and insulin-like growth factor 3 (INSL-3) released by testicular Leydig cells is now thought to be the key stage 1 hormone. MIS and INSL-3 interaction needs further clarification.

Stage 2 (inguinoscrotal) occurs at 25–35 weeks' gestation and is mainly controlled by androgens and the genitofemoral nerve (GFN). Innervation of the gubernaculum contributes to descent because androgens produced by the fetal testis act to irreversibly virilise the sensory dorsal root nucleus of the GFN. The gubernaculum everts and elongates, and the blind pouch forming inside is the processus vaginalis (PV). The PV undergoes active growth within the gubernaculum and the neurotransmitter, calcitonin gene-related peptide (CGRP), released through the sensory fibres of the GFN, acts on the CGRP receptor-rich gubernaculum, inducing strong rhythmic contractions and drawing the testis into the scrotum via the PV.

Recent studies implicate cremaster muscle playing an important role in stage 2 descent in rodents, and new theories question the role of the sympathetic nervous system and striated and smooth muscles within the gubernaculum.

Clinical features

- Group1: impalpable testis – intra-abdominal testis or in utero torsion/infarction of an intra-abdominal or inguinoscrotal testis with testicular demise
- Group 2: testis palpable within the inguinal canal and unable to be brought down to the scrotum
- Group 3: testis palpable within the inguinal canal, able to be brought down. It does not remain once tension released
- Group 4: testis palpable within the inguinal canal, able to be brought down. It remains within the scrotum once tension released (retractile testis)
- Group 5: ectopic testis (lateral abdominal wall, femoral, base of penis, perineal, crossed ectopia)

Investigations

- Imaging for an impalpable UDT is of no value
- A karyotype in patients with a UDT and penile abnormalities
- Endocrine referral and/or investigations may be warranted in patients with bilateral UDT, particularly if impalpable

Elevated gonadotrophins, especially follicle-stimulating hormone, likely represent bilateral anorchia. If gonadotrophins are normal, a human chorionic gonadotropin (HCG) stimulation test has clinical use, although surgical exploration remains indicated whatever the result. HCG (100 IU/kg) is injected looking for a testosterone response at 72 hours.

Differential diagnosis

- Inguinal hernia
- Disorder of sexual differentiation

Treatment

Groups 1–3 and 5 require surgery. Group 4 patients should have yearly follow-up because the chance of permanent ascension is 3%.

Patients in groups 1–3 should be examined once anaesthetised to ascertain whether the testis is palpable or retractile because this may alter both anaesthetic and surgical strategies.

All those in group 1 require a laparoscopy. Findings and intraoperative plans would be as follows:

- If no testis is in the line of descent (they can have blind ending vessels and vas deferens (vas) at or near the internal ring), offer a peripubertal insertion of a prosthesis
- If vas and vessels are passing through the internal ring, undertake a groin exploration
- Intra-abdominal testis
  - If the testis cannot reach the contralateral internal ring laparoscopically, stage 1 Fowler-Stephens (FS) procedure with the second stage 3–6 months later
  - If it does reach the contralateral ring, single-stage laparoscopic procedure
- Stage 1 FS: laparoscopic division of testicular vascular pedicle
  - Dissect the testicular vessels from retroperitoneal position on lateral abdominal wall
  - Clip and divide the vessels well above the testis
- Stage 2 FS: laparoscopic assisted orchidopexy
  - Confirm testicular viability
  - Divide gubernaculum distally
  - Dissect a tongue of peritoneum that includes the vas (and vessels if present) with laparoscopic monopolar electrocautery. Be aware of the position of the vas, iliac vessels and ureter at all times
  - Check cord length – if the testis reaches contralateral external ring, there is enough length for it to reach the scrotum
  - Scrotal incision
  - Insert a 5–12 mm Versastep or similar port via the scrotum into the abdominal cavity. The entry point should be medial to the internal ring and lateral to the bladder
  - Place a Johannes grasper through the port and grasp the testis
  - Pull testis down as the port is removed and suture into the scrotum, ensuring minimal or no tension

Groups 2 and 3 require an inguinal orchidopexy.

Inguinal orchidopexy is performed as follows:

- Cosmetic groin crease incision, dissection down through layers
- Open external oblique from the external ring before and after locating the testis
- Divide gubernaculum watching for low looping vas
- Separate and ligate patent processus vaginalis
- Divide adhesions and lateral bands
- Ensure enough length on the cord to bring the testis down to a reasonable position

- Scrotal incision and dissection up to the external ring in the line of the canal, with mosquito forceps
- Attach the testis to forceps and bring down to scrotum and suture or place in subdartos pouch
- Ensure the cord is not twisted by checking position via the groin wound
- In all cases epididymal cysts should be excised

Specific complications are

- Ascending testis
- Testicular atrophy
- Damage to vas and vessels
- Bladder injury

Further reading

Lie G, Hutson JM. The role of cremaster muscle in testicular descent in humans and animal models. Pediatr Surg Int 2011; 27:1255–1265

Tanyel FC. The descent of testis and reason for failed descent. Turk J Pediatr 2004; 46:7–17.

Related topics of interest

Urethral anomalies

Learning outcome

- To understand anomalies of the urethra and the principles involved in their treatment

Overview

Posterior urethral valves are the most common and important developmental anomaly of the posterior urethra and are considered separately. Other anomalies include

- Urethral duplication
- Urethral hypoplasia and atresia
- Urethral polyps
- Anterior urethral valves and anterior urethral diverticula
- Cowper duct cysts and syringocele
- Megalourethra
- Urethral prolapse
- Lacuna magna

Urethral duplication and fistula

Urethral duplication

Urethral duplication is an extremely rare anomaly, and although it occurs almost exclusively in men, isolated reports in women associated with bladder duplication also exist. The aetiology is unknown, but the association with pubic symphysis diastasis suggests a relationship with the exstrophy–epispadias complex.

Complete or incomplete forms occur and are best described by the plane of duplication (sagittal or coronal), the dominant urethra and the position of the meatus. The most common form is the Y duplication, with a single urethra proximally. The ventral urethra is usually dominant and passes through a normal bladder neck, and the orthotopic or epispadiac urethra is incomplete or does not pass to the bladder neck, so does not tend to give rise to incontinence. The ventral meatus may lie in any hypospadiac position from shaft to perineum, with a few approaching or fusing with the rectum.

Effmann's classification is as follows:
- Type I: blind partial duplication of the urethra
- Type II
  - Type IIA1: both urethras arise from separate bladder necks
  - Type IIA2: if one channel arises from the other
  - Type IIA2: Y duplication occurs when one urethra arising from the bladder neck or posterior urethra opens to the perineum
- Type III: a component of complete or partial caudal duplication

Congenital urethroperineal fistula

Congenital urethroperineal fistula resembles Y-type urethral duplication, except that the dorsal urethra is the functional urethra and the ventral urethra (fistula) is hypoplastic.

Investigation and management

Patients may present with urinary tract infection, discharge or double stream. Ultrasound scan identifies associated anomalies, whilst antegrade voiding cystography via a suprapubic catheter and cystoscopy are diagnostic. Asymptomatic patients may not need anatomical correction.

If the two meatuses are close and orthotopic, intervention may not be required or one may be marsupialised into the other. Identification of the dominant urethra is essential to the management because the dominant urethra must be preserved. Surgeons disagree as to the basic technique of mobilisation of the dominant urethra or progressive gradual dilatation of the dominant orthotopic urethra, with anastomosis of the duplication urethra to it. The technique will be based on individual anatomy, including the presence of chordee or dorsal angulation.

Urethral hypoplasia and atresia

Urethral hypoplasia and atresia are associated with severe infra-vesical obstruction antenatally and follow a pathway similar to that of severe posterior urethral valves. The exception, however, is the association with prune belly, urethral duplication and patent urachus, with urethral hypoplasia. Fetuses without a method of spontaneous decompression have a high incidence of perinatal death associated with oligohydramnios and renal failure. The treatment involves vesicostomy, followed by urethral substitution, or where possible the PADUA technique of progressive urethral dilatation, popularised by Passerini–Glazel, which may result in a functionally normal urethra with minimal morbidity.

Müllerian duct remnants: utricles and prostatic cysts

The prostatic utricle is a functionless gland-lined midline cyst in the dorsal aspect of the prostatic urethra. It is derived from Müllerian duct remnants, which normally regress in the male under the influence of Müllerian-inhibiting substance. Abnormality of Müllerian regression is common in intersex conditions and proximal hypospadias, but may occur in isolation. If the Müllerian remnant opens into the urethra, a prostatic utricle is formed; if it is isolated, a prostatic cyst is formed.

The majority of utricles are asymptomatic, but if they extend above the bladder neck, post-void dribbling, infection, epididymitis and stone formation can occur. Müllerian duct cysts may enlarge into adulthood and result in obstructive azoospermia, and there is a small malignant potential.

Congenital urethral polyps: urethral polyps

These fibroepithelial polyps are almost entirely found arising from the posterior prostatic urethra in males, but scattered examples in females have occurred. They are associated with bladder outlet obstruction, infection, haematuria and prolapse. They are smooth and epithelium covered, usually measuring between 1 cm and 2 cm and are distinct from postpubertal polyps that contain prostatic tissue. Treatment is by transurethral resection.

Anterior urethral diverticula and anterior urethral valves

These rare conditions may occur anywhere in the anterior urethra (40% bulbar urethra, 30% penoscrotal junction and 30% penile urethra). Anterior urethral valves are associated with urethral dilatation proximal to the obstruction, whereas the anterior urethral diverticula have a saccular or globular dilatation, arising from a ventral defect within the urethral wall and with the lip, which is associated with valve-like obstruction. Whether these represent the same or separate conditions, in both there is a defect in the corpus spongiosum and bladder outlet obstruction occurs during the antenatal period. Although the incidence is only 10% of that of posterior urethral valves, the effects are similar – usually less severe with proximal urethral dilatation, bladder outlet obstruction and hypertrophy and occasionally with secondary upper tract changes. Antenatal ultrasound may pick up the penile or penoscrotal cyst and be diagnostic.

Most cases present in infancy with infravesical obstruction, leading to poor urinary stream with dribbling, difficulty in voiding, incontinence, hesitancy or urinary retention, poor urinary stream and recurrent urinary tract infections. Later presenting children may have enuresis, post-void dribbling or a palpable cyst, with a history of relief by manual expression of the cyst.

Investigation and management

Ultrasound scan may suggest infravesical obstruction, but an antegrade micturating cystogram, and occasionally a retrograde urethrogram, is required for definitive diagnosis. Like posterior urethral valves, the management is transurethral resection of the valve or marsupialisation of the cyst into the urethra. A cold parrot beak blade is used with no or minimal irrigation flow to stop the compression of the filmy walls of the cyst or valves. Following resection the edges of the cyst or valve may give the impression of persisting obstruction on micturating cystourethrography, but the dilation usually gradually resolves and pressure is relieved.

However, low-pressure dilatation may persist where the spongiosum is widely defective, giving a megaurethra effect, and a more definitive open treatment may then be necessary.

Cowper duct cysts and syringocele

Cowper's glands are exocrine structures in between the layers of urogenital diaphragm; they secrete, pre-ejaculate into the genitourinary tract and occasionally become obstructed and dilated. Presentation is usually in childhood, but adult cases are increasingly recognised. Melquist's review suggests that the presentation depends on whether the cyst has ruptured. The ruptured cyst presents with infection, dribbling and haematuria, whilst the closed cyst, recurrently refilled via the patulous Cowper's duct, presents with urinary obstruction and perineal pain.

Treatment, as with anterior urethral valves, is largely by transurethral resection. However, if the spongiosum defect is large or a large deep cyst is present, the approach to the bulbous urethra may be difficult, and some authors have suggested a laparoscopic approach to large cysts.

Megalourethra

Megalourethra differs from the last two categories of urethral dilatation in that it is primarily non-obstructive urethral dilation. In scaphoid megalourethra the ventral spongiosum is deficient, whilst in fusiform the corpus spongiosum is circumferentially deficient. In both varieties, the urethra lacks structural support so that it dilates. Chordee or torque occurs where the corpora cavernosa are also abnormal. Megalourethra is strongly associated with prune-belly syndrome, and a common pathology of abnormal mesodermal development has been suggested. Vesicoureteric reflux and bladder diverticulum are common, and megacystis–microcolon–hypoperistalsis syndrome and VACTERL are recognised associations. Concomitant obstructive urethral anomalies have been described. In only 15% of cases is the megalourethra an isolated anomaly, and thus for the majority the approach to treatment is dictated by the associated conditions.

Urethral prolapse

In the contrast to postpubertal urethral prolapse, which is associated with significant lower urinary tract symptoms, the majority of girls with urethral prolapse are asymptomatic. The urethral prolapse is a circumferential prominence and congestion of the distal urethra at the meatus. The mucosa may be ulcerated and may bleed on contact, and the swelling may be tender to palpation and in some cases spontaneously painful. It is differentiated from a polyp by the presence of the central urethral opening. It is rare and may be confused with genital trauma, with the associated worry of non-accidental injury.

There is no associated upper tract abnormality, but the diagnosis of ectopic ureterocele or rhabdomyosarcoma should be considered. Authors vary in their treatment protocols and outcomes; both antibiotics and oestrogen creams have been suggested whilst others recommend conservative management. The condition may be persistent or recurrent, but is benign, with no serious sequelae.

Lacuna magna (sinus of Guérin)

The lacuna magna is a small dorsal diverticulum in the roof of the fossa navicularis, which may be present in as many as 30% of boys. It occasionally causes voiding symptoms or haematuria. It can be treated by dividing the common wall endoscopically.

Further reading

Effmann EL, Lebowitz RL, Colodny AH. Duplication of the urethra. Radiology 1976; 119:179–185.

Levin TL, Han B, Little BP. Congenital anomalies of the male urethra. Pediatr Radiol 2007; 37:851–862.

Melquist J, Sharma V, Sciullo D, et al. Current diagnosis and management of syringocele: a review. Int Braz J Urol 2010; 36:1.

Related topics of interest

Urinary tract infection

Learning outcomes

- To understand the definition of a urinary tract infection (UTI)
- To understand the natural history of UTI
- To understand how to investigate and manage a UTI

Overview

UTI is one of the most common bacterial infections and method of presentation of underlying urinary tract abnormality. It is defined as a combination of clinical features and the presence of bacteria in the urine.

In young children, the presentation is non-specific with similar symptoms and signs to many acute self-limiting viral illnesses, and obtaining an uncontaminated urine specimen is difficult. The National Institute for Health and Clinical Excellence (NICE) guidelines should be the standard of care for children with UTIs, excluding those who have underlying abnormalities. UTIs can have long-term sequelae, including renal scarring and permanent renal damage, which become more likely with recurrent infections.
UTIs can be classified by the following method:

- Upper – kidney
- Lower – bladder, urethra
- Complicated – infant and neonate, fever, foreign body or stone, underlying abnormality
- Uncomplicated – simple lower UTI and apyrexial
- First infection – complicated or uncomplicated
- Recurrent
  - Unresolved: urine culture contains the same pathogen
  - Bacterial persistence: sterile cultures after first infection, but the same organism implicated
  - Reinfection: infection with a different bacterium with the original eradicated

Epidemiology and aetiology

In the first year of life, the incidence is 2.7% in boys and 0.7% in girls, but overall during childhood approximately 5% of girls and 1.5% of boys develop symptoms. Between 30–50% of children investigated for UTI have an underlying abnormality.

Mechanical factors preventing urine flow and dysfunctional voiding, constipation and periurethral bacterial colonisation increase the incidence of UTI. Foreskin and preputial colonisation have been implicated as factors causing the higher incidence of UTIs in the first year of life in boys.

Escherichia coli accounts for 77–93% of cases, with *Klebsiella* (0–11%) and *Enterococcus* (2–9%) the next common. *E. coli* has a significant predilection for UTIs due to its fimbriae. Type 1 fimbriae bind uroplakin, a protein cap receptor on the urothelial cell.

Individuals with a blood group P phenotype have increased susceptibility for UTIs due to the blood group antigen, acting as a receptor for bacterial P fimbriae. Those *E. coli* strains with P fimbriae are highly associated with causation of pyelonephritis.

Risk factors include female gender (beyond the first year of life), previous infection and non-circumcision (although psychosocial aspects of circumcision outweigh the medical benefits). It is postulated that native immunity, urinary immunoglobulin A and breastfeeding may have protective effects.

Clinical features

In infants younger than 3 months, fever, vomiting, lethargy and irritability are the most common features. Others include failure to thrive (FTT), poor feeding, abdominal pain, jaundice, haematuria and offensive urine.

In non-verbal children older than 3 months, fever is the predominant feature. Abdominal pain, loin tenderness, vomiting, poor feeding, lethargy, irritability, haematuria, offensive urine and FTT also occur.

In verbalising children, older than 3 months, the most common features are frequency and dysuria. They also exhibit dysfunctional voiding, continence issues, abdominal pain, loin tenderness, fever, lethargy, vomiting, haematuria, offensive and cloudy urine.

There is not normally a great deal to find on examination, but care should be made to examine the abdomen, spine and lower limb neurology for neurological abnormalities, indicating possible neuropathic bladder.

Investigations

A clean catch urine sample is the gold standard. If this is not possible, then collection pads or urine bags are alternatives. Catheter sampling or suprapubic aspiration, preferably ultrasound scan (USS) guided, can also be undertaken. If upper tract sampling is required, then a ureteric or nephrostomy sample should be obtained. Treatment should not be delayed if a urine sample is unobtainable.

Send a urine culture for urgent microscopy and culture in infants younger than 3 years. In children older than 3 years, dipstick testing is as useful as microscopy and culture.

- Further investigations are aimed at identifying the underlying abnormalities and assessing the extent of upper tract pathology.
- Ultrasound during acute infection – for an atypical UTI in a child of any age or in a child younger than 6 months, with recurrent UTIs
- Ultrasound within 6 weeks – for recurrent UTIs, in those older than 3 years, the USS should include pre- and post-void bladder volumes
- Dimercaptosuccinic acid (DMSA) scan 4–6 months after infection when the UTI is atypical or recurrent

Micturating cystourethrograms are used to investigate children younger than 6 months, with recurrent or atypical UTIs.

Differential diagnosis

- Any cause of acute or chronic abdominal pain

Treatment

NICE defines an atypical UTI to include
- Children who are seriously ill, with poor urine flow, abdominal or bladder mass, raised creatinine, septicaemia, failure to respond to treatment with suitable antibiotics within 48 hours or infection with non-*E. coli* organisms

And a recurrent UTI as
- Two or more episodes of UTI with acute pyelonephritis or upper tract infection, or
- One episode of UTI with acute pyelonephritis or upper tract infection as well as one or more episodes of UTI with cystitis or lower tract infection, or
- Three or more episodes of UTI with cystitis or lower tract infection

Parenteral antibiotics should be given to infants younger than 1 month, all infants aged 1–3 months who appear unwell and infants aged 1–3 months, with white blood cells < 5 or > 15 × 10^9/L.

Any child between 3 months and 3 years who has urinary tract-specific symptoms or non-specific symptoms, but is high risk, should receive intravenous antibiotics. If indeterminate or low risk, then antibiotics should be delayed until the microscopy result is known. If urgent microscopy is unavailable, then the presence of nitrites suggests infection and antibiotics should be commenced.

In children older than 3 years, dipstick testing with leucocyte and nitrite positivity is sufficient to diagnose a UTI. If it is a recurrent UTI, the sample should be sent for microscopy and culture. If only either nitrites or leucocyte esterase are positive, then the sample should be sent for microscopy and culture.

Antibiotic treatment can be given as follows:
- In all children older than 3 months with upper tract infection, 7–10 days of oral cephalosporin or co-amoxiclav

- If oral antibiotics cannot be used, intravenous cefotaxime and ceftriaxone for 2–4 days then oral antibiotics for a total of 10 days
- In those with lower tract infection, 3 days of oral antibiotics using local guidelines
- Antibiotic prophylaxis can be considered in children with recurrent UTIs

Management of other factors is also important:
- Reduce residual volume – regular, frequent, complete or double voiding
- Treat constipation
- Drink at regular intervals, avoid irritants
- Prevent local irritation

If vesicoureteral reflux is identified, this has its own management strategy.

Further reading

National Institute for Health and Clinical Excellence. Urinary tract infection in children. Diagnosis, treatment and long term management. London: NICE, 2007.

Soccorso G, et al. Infantile urinary tract infection and timing of micturating cystourethrogram. J Ped Urol 2010; 6:582–584.

Related topics of interest

- Vesicoureteral reflux (p. 371)

Urolithiasis

Learning outcomes

- To be able to recognise the symptoms and signs of urinary tract calculi
- To understand the underlying aetiology
- To be aware of the management options and the rationale
- To be aware of the indications of each option

Overview

Urinary tract calculi in the paediatric age group are infrequent compared with the adult population in the UK. It is estimated that there are approximately 150 new cases a year, although the reporting of the data precludes accurate assessment of the true incidence. However, paediatric urolithiasis is endemic in the 'stone belt' across Eastern Europe and the Asian subcontinent (e.g. Turkey, Middle Eastern countries, Pakistan and India)

Epidemiology and aetiology

The pathophysiology of stones is multifactorial and is determined by a combination of urine flow and volume, crystal saturation and the urinary pH. Any factors affecting these components may give rise to urinary tract stones. Supersaturation is a prerequisite to stone formation. This may occur due to reduction in urinary volume (e.g. dehydration), urinary stasis (e.g. anatomical abnormalities causing urinary tract obstruction) or metabolic factors that may produce higher concentration of solutes (e.g. primary hyperoxaluria, cystinuria, hypercalciuria and dietary causes). Once supersaturation occurs, this acts as a nidus for further crystallisation, thereby forming a stone.

Substances in the urine known as inhibitors reduce the propensity to form calculi, whereas promoters are substances that favour formation of calculi. An imbalance of promoters and inhibitors will make the individual more susceptible to calculi formation. Promoters are mainly calcium, oxalate, phosphate and urate.

Inhibitors include citrate, pyrophosphate, glycosaminoglycans and glycoproteins.

Urinary infection, particularly with urease-producing organisms, causes alkalinisation of the urine and crystallisation or supersaturation of several compounds such as struvite or carbapatite and ammonium urate.

Clinical features

Stones may be discovered incidentally or due to symptoms. A high index of suspicion is required.

Symptoms may be:

- Those of urinary tract infection (UTI) – dysuria, frequency, pyrexia, haematuria
- Pain typical of UTI, although younger children may be unable to localise or describe the typical pain of renal and ureteric calculi
- Renal and/or ureteric colic
- Obstructive renal failure, particularly in patients with a single functioning kidney
- Passage of grit and small stones or matrix
- In babies, nonspecific symptoms of irritability, poor feeding, lethargy and poor weight gain

Investigations

Diagnosis

The diagnosis is based on a high index of suspicion. The various diagnostic modalities can be used:

- **Plain X-ray kidneys–ureters–bladder (KUB):** A plain KUB film is a useful adjunct to detect stones (**Figure 60**). However, faecal loading and bowel gas may obscure the view, and hence a plain X-ray is not as sensitive as an ultrasound
- **Renal ultrasound – sensitive and specific for renal calculi:** In the kidney, it can demonstrate the location of the stones in the collecting system (**Figure 61**). However, it is operator dependent and may miss stones in the mid-ureter or distal ureter, especially if obscured by bowel gas and if the bladder is empty

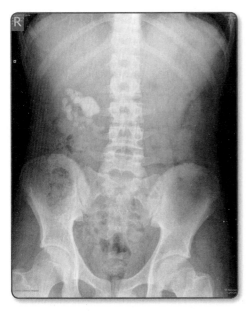

Figure 60 X-ray showing multiple calculi in the right kidney.

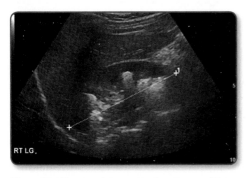

Figure 61 Ultrasound demonstrating stones with posterior acoustic shadowing in the kidney.

- **Computed tomography (CT) scan:** Unenhanced spiral CT is the diagnostic modality of choice in adults. However in children, it involves radiation and should only be used when ultrasound and plain X-ray fail to detect a stone and there is a high index of suspicion, or for accurate anatomical localisation at surgical treatment planning

Further investigations

- **DMSA scan (Dimercaptosuccinic acid tagged with technetium 99m):** For renal tract calculi, a DMSA scan should be performed with or without a combined intravenous urogram to ascertain the function of the kidney and the presence of structural anomalies
- **Other imaging such as voiding cystourethrogram or Mag3 scan (mercaptoacyl triglycine tagged with technetium 99m):** Renogram will depend on the findings on the original diagnostic imaging
- **Urinalysis:** 24-hour urine collection is recommended but difficult to perform in children. A spot urine can also be analysed for a metabolic stone screen. However, the best biochemical investigation is the chemical analysis of a stone fragment.

Treatment

Treatment of the stones is aimed at:
- Removal of the stones by techniques that will reduce morbidity for the child
- Complete clearance of the stones
- Prevention of recurrence

Surgical options

- Open surgery
- Minimally invasive techniques – percutaneous nephrolithotomy (PCNL), extracorporeal shock-wave lithotripsy (ESWL), ureterorenoscopy (URS), laparoscopy

Open surgery

- Indications for open surgery are limited
- This may be an option if there is a large stone burden or with associated anatomical abnormality that needs correction at the same time, such as ureteropelvic junction obstruction

PCNL

- Multiple renal stones
- Staghorn calculus
- Part of multimodality therapy
- Involves percutaneous access to the collecting system of the kidney and use of fragmentation techniques such as ultrasound lithotripsy, laser or lithoclast for stone retrieval
- May be complicated by bleeding, urine leak, residual stones

URS

- Ideal for ureteric stones
- Flexible URS with laser can also manage upper urinary stones

ESWL

- Single stone < 2 cm
- Can be used in several sessions for larger stone burden such as a staghorn calculus
- Can be used as multimodal therapy with PCNL

Laparoscopy

- Solitary stones in renal pelvis
- Bladder calculi or calculi in augmented bladders
- Requires expertise in laparoscopy

Stones once retrieved are sent for chemical analysis.

The management of urinary tract stone disease is multidisciplinary and should involve the paediatric nephrologist and dietician.

Further reading

Dogan HS, Onal B, Satar N, et al. Factors affecting complication rates of ureteroscopic lithotripsy in children: results of multi-institutional retrospective analysis by Pediatric Stone Disease Study Group of Turkish Pediatric Urology Society. J Urol 2011; 186:1035–1040.

Lottman H, Gagnadoux MF, Daudon M. Urolithiasis in children. In: Gearhart J, Mouriquand P, Rink R (eds), Pediatric urology, 2nd edn. Philadelphia: Saunders, 2010:631–663.

Raju GA, Norris RD, Ost MC. Endoscopic stone management in children. Curr Opin Urol 2010; 20:309–312.

Related topics of interest

- Pelvi-ureteric junction obstruction (p. 270)
- Urinary tract infection (p. 358)
- Vesicoureteric junction obstruction (p. 374)
- Vesicoureteral reflux (p. 371)

Varicocele

Learning outcomes

- To be able to define and classify varicocele
- To know the investigations to perform and why
- To know the management options

Overview

Varicoceles are defined as an abnormal dilatation of the pampiniform plexus of veins draining the testis. They usually occur in adolescence and are usually left sided. They can be asymptomatic and are commonly referred as a scrotal mass, or with asymmetry in testicular size. They are implicated in infertility and have been found in 35% of males with primary infertility. It is important to document testicular size on ultrasound prior to management, which can include interventional radiology or surgical options.

Epidemiology and aetiology

Varicoceles are extremely rare in boys under the age of 9, and their prevalence is reported as 15% in the 10–19 years age group. This is roughly equal to the prevalence in adult males. The incidence may be higher due to their mainly asymptomatic nature. Bilateral varicoceles occur in 2–20% and isolated right-sided varicoceles in 1–7%.

The ipsilateral testis is abnormally small compared with the contralateral testis, and histologic studies have revealed seminiferous tubule sclerosis, small vessel degenerative changes, and abnormalities of Leydig, Sertoli and germ cells. These have been documented in patients of 12 years, and effects on semen parameters have been extensively studied in adults. Consistent findings include decreased sperm motility, lower total sperm counts and an increased number of abnormal sperm forms. A limited number of studies in adolescents have also shown altered seminal parameters.

Reasons for changes in sperm, testicular size and morphology are not clearly understood and proposed mechanisms include

- Dilated veins with pooling of venous blood, resulting in increased scrotal and testicular temperature, may alter DNA synthesis within the testicle, leading to morphologic changes in sperm and testicular tissue
- Renal and adrenal metabolites, refluxing into dilated spermatic veins affect testicular tissue damage through undefined mechanisms. Testicular hormone function may be compromised, leading to impaired spermatogenesis
- Low oxygen content in the dilated veins, resulting in local tissue hypoxia, affects testicular architecture and sperm production
- Paracrine imbalances in the testicle, due to any of the above conditions, lead to impaired testicular function

These findings may be reversed with corrective surgery, and testicular catch-up growth is observed following varicocele ligation.

Aetiology is multifactorial, and various theories attempt to explain varicocele formation in view of the fact that 90% are left-sided. These include

- Congenital absence of valves in the left testicular vein that normally prevent retrograde flow of blood in the upright position. Anomalous branches may also bypass the valves
- A predisposition to slower drainage in the left testicular vein because the right testicular vein drains directly into the inferior vena cava and the left inserts at a right angle into the left renal vein
- The 'nutcracker' phenomenon – the left renal vein can be compressed between the superior mesenteric artery and the aorta, thus creating a higher pressure in the left testicular vein
- Increased length of the left testicular vein that is 8–10 cm longer than the right
- An isolated right varicocele is very rare. Investigations for inferior vena cava thrombosis and occlusion or retroperitoneal mass, including Wilms'

tumour and neuroblastoma, must be undertaken in all patients who present with a solitary right-sided varicocele or any varicocele in children younger than 9 years

Clinical features

Most adolescent varicoceles are asymptomatic. Some patients describe a dragging sensation within the testis, especially following physical activity and occasionally present with acute scrotal pain. Other presentations include traumatic haematoma, subfertility or testicular asymmetry.

The patient should be examined standing, and the scrotum should be inspected and palpated for distended veins, usually on the lateral side. These should increase in size when a Valsalva manoeuvre is performed. Then, the patient should be examined in a supine position; if the varicocele does not diminish, a venous obstruction should be sought. Testicular size can be documented with an orchidometer. A large varicocele is reported to feel like a 'bag of worms', but a small one may feel like a thickened spermatic cord.

Grading (on physical examination) is as follows:

- Grade 0 – subclinical, generally identified on ultrasound scanning (USS)
- Grade 1 – palpated with difficulty (< 1 cm), size increases with Valsalva
- Grade 2 – easily detected without Valsalva (1–2 cm)
- Grade 3 – obvious on inspection (> 2 cm)

Investigations

- Scrotal USS is performed in some centres to confirm the diagnosis and document testicular size
- In adolescents a testis that is smaller by > 10% compared to the contralateral side is considered hypoplastic
- Abdominal USS is mandatory in right-sided varicoceles and in varicoceles occurring in patients younger than 9 years or those who are prepubertal

Differential diagnosis

- Hernia
- Hydrocele
- Tumour

Treatment

If the patient has no size discrepancy and is asymptomatic, then yearly follow-up with a USS is justifiable. Surgical treatment is based on ligation or occlusion of the internal spermatic veins, while minimising complications such as recurrence, hydrocele or atrophy. Surgery is recommended in patients who have symptoms or hypotrophy.

There is no gold standard approach with the subinguinal microscopic approach, giving superior results in adults, but is difficult in children due to the arterial diameter. Interventional radiology can be used to embolise the vein, but the failure rate varies from 5 to 20% and the hydrocele rate is high at about 14%.

The most recent meta-analysis in children shows that

- Results after laparoscopic technique are similar to those after open with a recurrence rate of 8.6% and 4.7%, and the postoperative hydrocele rate of 6.7% and 7.1%, respectively
- Laparoscopic lymphatic sparing has a lower incidence of the postoperative hydrocele, 4.3% versus 17.6%, but a higher incidence of recurrence, 3.5% versus 2.2%, than the Palomo procedure
- There is no risk of testicular atrophy following division of the artery due to sufficient collaterals

Palomo procedure

- Using the open or laparoscopic technique, the spermatic vessels are isolated within the retroperitoneal space, where they course along the posterolateral abdominal wall
- They are then clipped and divided
- The lymphatics can be spared by delineation, following preincision intrascrotal methylene blue injection, but this can cause local tissue ischaemia and fat necrosis

Ivanissevich procedure

- The vessels are approached via an inguinal incision, with preservation of the vas, and if possible, the artery. The veins are then divided

Further reading

Borruto F, Impellizzeri P, Antonuccio P, et al. Laparoscopic vs open varicocelectomy in children and adolescents: review of the recent literature and meta-analysis. J Pediatr Surg 2010; 45:2464–24649.

Diamond DA, Zurakowski D, Bauer SB, et al. Relationship of varicocele grade and testicular hypotrophy to semen parameters in adolescents. J Urol 2007; 178:1584.

Tekgul S, Riedmiller H, Gerharz E, et al. European Association of Paediatric Urology Guidelines on Paediatric Urology. Arnhem: European Association of Urology, 2012.

Related topics of interest

- Inguinal hernia (p. 176)
- Hydrocele (p. 165)
- Wilms' tumour (p. 377)

Vascular anomalies in paediatrics

Learning outcomes

- To know the types of vascular anomalies presenting in children
- To understand the natural history
- To know the treatment strategies and when to offer surgery

Overview

Vascular anomalies are divided into vascular tumours and vascular malformations although some manifest in both categories. As the skin is the largest organ, vascular lesions are relatively common, with haemangioma the most frequent. Management options include observation, medical treatment, interventional radiology and surgical resection.

Vascular tumours

Epidemiology and aetiology

Haemangiomas are the most common type and occur in 1–2.6% of children perinatally. They may affect 4–12% of caucasian children. Preterm infants < 1 kg have an incidence of 30%. There is a 3:1 to 5:1 male:female ratio.

Their pathogenesis is unclear, but evidence indicates their development from a clonal expansion of endothelial cells that have been subjected to either abnormal local cellular signals or a somatic initial mutation, favouring rapid expansion.

Theories include a population of angioblasts arrested in early development, giving rise to these endothelial cells, or their derivation from a distant population, with haematogenous spread from the bone marrow or placenta. A placental origin would account for the increased risk of haemangiomata in infants whose mothers have had chorionic villous sampling. In addition, some haemangioma markers are expressed in the placenta.

There is no clear genetic tendency although there is a family history in approximately 10%. A small subset of them have a missense mutation in the genes encoding vascular endothelial growth factor receptor 2 or tumour endothelial marker 8.

Clinical features

- Haemangiomas appear in the first 2 weeks of life
- Approximately 33% present at birth as a pink macular spot, pale spot, telangiectasia or ecchymosis
- Approximately 60% occur in the head and neck; 25% on the trunk and 15% on the extremities; 80% are isolated and 20% proliferate in multiple sites. With multiple skin lesions, there may be visceral organ involvement
- Cutaneous (strawberry or capillary) haemangioma: This invades the dermis and the overlying skin becomes raised, red and bosselated
- Deeper (cavernous) haemangioma: This is located in the lower dermis, subcutaneous tissue or muscle. It presents as raised blue-coloured lesions, with indistinct borders at 2–3 months of life or later
- Congenital haemangiomas: These are tumours that evolve in utero and are fully grown at birth. Their appearance varies, but they are commonly raised purple masses, often with a pale halo, and occasionally, a central area of necrosis. There are two forms:
  1. Rapidly involuting congenital haemangioma – regresses during early infancy and is fully involuted by 12–14 months
  2. Non-involuting congenital haemangioma: grows in proportion to the child and never regresses
- Gastrointestinal (GI) haemangiomas may present with anaemia or rectal bleeding
- Hepatic haemangiomas are generally asymptomatic, but a small percentage can manifest as cardiac failure due to shunting, hypothyroidism (overproduction of type 3 iodothyronine deiodinase), fulminant

liver failure and abdominal compartment syndrome

Associations include

- PHACES syndrome
  - P: posterior fossa and other structural brain abnormalities (Dandy–Walker cystic malformation)
  - H: haemangioma(s) of the cervical facial region
  - A: arterial cerebrovascular anomalies (absent ipsilateral carotid or vertebral vessels)
  - C: cardiac defects, aortic coarctation and other aortic abnormalities
  - E: eye anomalies (e.g. micropthalmia, optic nerve hypoplasia and cataracts)
- Lumbosacral haemangiomata (an ectodermal lesion) may signal underlying occult spinal dysraphism

Investigations

- In lumbosacral haemangioma, ultrasound or magnetic resonance imaging (MRI), depending on age, to exclude spinal dysraphism

Differential diagnosis

- Kasabach-Merritt phenomenon occurs only with the invasive vascular tumours such as kaposiform haemangioendothelioma (KHE) or tufted angioma (TA). It is never associated with the common haemangioma of infancy. Both KHE and TA are present at birth; they have no gender predilection and are unifocal. They generally involve trunk, shoulder, thigh or retroperitoneum. The skin overlying them is red-purple, tense and shiny. Peritumoural bruising occurs along with petechiae. Severe transfusion-resistant thrombocytopenia occurs although coagulation is usually normal. These children are at risk of intracranial, pleural or pulmonary, intraperitoneal or GI bleeding, and mortality is of the order of 20–30%. MRI can show the extent of the tumour along with feeding or draining vessels. Histologically KHE shows an aggressive cellular pattern of infiltrating sheets and nodules of slender epithelial cells, slit-like vascular spaces that are filled with haemosiderin and red blood cell

fragments and dilated lymphatic spaces. TA consists of small tufts of capillaries in the middle to lower dermis. Lymphatics are present in the periphery

- Naevus flammeus neonatorum (stork bite or salmon patch) is a non-evolving macular stain, which typically disappears by the end of the first year of life
- Vascular malformation
- Pyogenic granuloma

Treatment

The majority grow quickly in the first 6–12 months of life (proliferative phase), and then they grow in proportion to the child, and finally they enter a slow regression (involution phase). Involution can last 1–7 years during which the haemangioma endothelial matrix is replaced by loose fibrous or fibrous fatty tissue.

Regression is complete in 50% by the age of 5, 70% by 7 and in the rest by 10–12 years. Tertiary referral should be undertaken if there is diagnostic doubt, if the location is dangerous (e.g. obstructing vision and subglottic position) of if there is rapid growth or potential for complications.

Medical management includes

- Propranolol (for haemangiomas of infancy) – appears to inhibit the vascular proliferation during the growth phase. Theoretically it causes vasoconstriction and possibly decreased expression of proangiogenic factors in the growth phase, causing apoptosis of capillary endothelial cells. Careful monitoring is required in the initial phase of treatment owing to the risk of adverse cardiovascular events and hypoglycaemia, bronchospasm, diarrhoea and hyperkalaemia
- Intralesional steroid injection – in small, well-localised mucosal haemangiomas in critical locations
- Oral corticosteroid (or intravenous in an acute setting) – in large, problematic, life-threatening haemangiomas
- Vincristine and interferon-α have also been used

Surgical management includes

- Pulsed dye laser – indications include reduction of a unilateral subglottic haemangioma. Complications include

ulceration, partial-thickness skin loss and scarring
- Surgical excision may be indicated for haemangiomas of the upper eyelid or haemangiomas, with demonstrable GI bleeding, which are resistant to medical therapy. Excision can be considered in school-age children if the haemangioma compromises body image. Staged resection may be required due to the residual expanded skin and fibrofatty remnants

Vascular malformations

Vascular malformations are errors of embryonal development, which may be localised or diffuse. They can affect the arterial, venous, capillary and lymphatic vessels and are present in 1.2–1.5% of the population, with the majority being sporadic. Two major categories exist
1. Slow-flow anomalies
   - Simple: capillary, lymphatic and venous malformations (VMs)
   - Complex: capillary–lymphatic, capillary–lymphaticovenous, lymphaticovenous
2. Fast-flow anomalies
   - Simple: arterial, arteriovenous (AVM) and arteriovenous fistulae (AVF)
   - Complex: capillary–lymphatic AVM, capillary–lymphatic AVF

Capillary malformations (port-wine or claret stains)

Capillary malformations are dermal vascular anomalies and occur in 0.3% of neonates, with no gender predilection. They are normally sporadic, but a familial autosomal dominant pattern, with incomplete penetrance, has been reported. They can be localised or extensive and occur anywhere, but are usually single. A mutation in *RA5AI* has been linked with the hereditary form.

They are composed of dilated, ectatic capillary to venule size vessels in the superficial dermis, and immunohistochemistry shows normal endothelium and smooth muscle, but a paucity of normal surrounding nerve fibres. The vessels dilate with age. They can be associated with underlying soft tissue

and skeletal hypertrophy or may indicate an underlying structural abnormality, such as an encephalocele, spinal dysraphism or Sturge–Weber syndrome.
Other syndromes include
- Klippel–Trenaunay – a slow-flow capillary-lymphatic–VM which manifests with axial elongation and overgrowth in one or more extremities. Lymphatic hypoplasia is present in > 50%, with associated lymphoedema, and thrombophlebitis occurs in 20–45% of patients, which can lead to pulmonary embolus. Management includes shoe lifts and compression stockings. Sclerotherapy, embolisation or debulking procedures may be effective, and amputation can also be considered
- Parkes Weber – a fast-flow anomaly of a capillary stain with AVM or AVF. These are obvious at birth, and the asymmetric, enlarged limb is covered by a pink, warm, macular stain, with a bruit or thrill. The patient may have associated lymphatic malformations. Large abnormalities can be associated with high-output cardiac failure
Management includes
- Pulsed dye laser
- Surgery, for soft tissue and skeletal hypertrophy
- Neurosurgical resection, if intractable seizures in Sturge–Weber syndrome

Telangiectasia

Telangiectasias are tiny acquired capillary vascular marks which can spontaneously resolve, but may need pulsed dye laser. Hereditary haemorrhagic telangiectasia (Osler–Weber–Rendu) is an autosomal dominant disease with high penetrance. It occurs in 1–2 per 100,000 Caucasians. Patients exhibit mucocutaneous defects along with cerebral and pulmonary AVMs and some liver vascular anomalies. *HHT1* and *ACLVRL1* genes have been implicated, and both are linked to the loss of tumour growth factor-β function.

Venous malformations

Venous malformations are the most common of all vascular anomalies, and whilst present at birth, they are not always evident. They are composed of thin-walled, dilated spongy abnormal channels, with distorted vascular smooth muscle architecture.

They are a blue, soft, compressible mass and can vary greatly in size, shape and associated deformities. They grow in proportion with the child, and phlebothrombosis is common. The majority are single, but multiple lesions can occur. Blue rubber bleb naevus syndrome is a rare disorder of cutaneous and GI VMs, which can lead to chronic GI bleeding or form the lead point for volvulus or intussusception.

- Imaging: MRI
- Management: elastic support stockings and low-dose aspirin minimises the risk of phlebothrombosis
- Interventions: sclerotherapy, embolisation or surgical resection

AVMs

Most of the AVMs are latent in infancy and childhood, with expansion during adolescence, with the hormonal changes seeming to trigger expansion. They appear as a warm, pink patch and may have a bruit or thrill. Ischaemic changes with ulceration, pain and intermittent bleeding can occur. The Schobinger's staging system documents their natural history:

1. Stage I (quiescence) – pink-bluish stain with warmth and AVM shunting evident on Doppler scanning
2. Stage II (expansion) – stage 1 as well as enlargement, pulsation, bruit and tortuous and tense veins
3. Stage III (destruction) – stage II as well as one of dystrophic changes, ulceration, bleeding, persistent pain or tissue necrosis
4. Stage IV (decompensation) – stage III as well as cardiac failure

- Imaging: MRI or MR angiogram
- Management: embolisation if symptomatic in the neonatal period. If there are symptoms or the lesion is enlarging, then embolisation alone or in combination with surgical resection after 24–72 hours, is often the best option.

Further reading

Hogeling M, Adams S, Wargon O. A randomised controlled trial of propranolol for infantile hemangiomas. Paediatrics 2001; 128:e258–e266.

Léauté-Labrèze C, Dumas de la Roque E et al. Propranolol for severe hemangiomas of infancy. N Engl J Med 2008;358(24):2649 –2651

Sans V, de la Roque ED, Berge J, Hubiche T, et al. Propranolol for severe infantile hemangiomas: follow-up report. Pediatrics 2009; 124(3):e423–431.

Related topics of interest

Vesicoureteral reflux

Learning outcomes

- To understand causes of vesicoureteral reflux (VUR)
- To raise awareness of the complications of VUR
- To discuss the treatment options for managing VUR

Overview

VUR is a retrograde flow of urine from the bladder into the ureter.

Epidemiology and aetiology

VUR occurs in 1–3% of children. It is associated with 7–17% of children diagnosed with end-stage renal failure. It is more common in Caucasians and males (29% males and 14% females). Males are more likely to have high-grade reflux, but their VUR is more likely to resolve.

VUR occurs in 25–33% of siblings of patients with VUR, whilst offspring of parents with VUR have an incidence of up to 66%. Notably, these patients may have high-grade reflux and renal scarring, despite being asymptomatic.

The potential morbidity of VUR includes

- Decreased renal growth
- Reflux nephropathy – does not tend to occur in the absence of urinary tract infection (UTI)
- Hypertension
- Renal failure

VUR may be classified as primary or secondary:

- **Primary VUR:** This is attributed to a short submucosal intravesical tunnel of the ureter. The ureteric orifice (UO) is located in the base of the bladder, rather than the trigone. The ratio of tunnel length to ureteral diameter should be at least 5:1 to prevent reflux. As the child grows, the length of the tunnel increases, which explains the spontaneous resolution of VUR
- **Secondary VUR:** This occurs when the reflux is induced by an abnormality, which increases bladder pressure, e.g. urethral obstruction or neurogenic bladder dysfunction

Clinical features

VUR may be symptomatic or asymptomatic. UTIs remain the most common mode of presentation. Traditionally, the incidence of VUR in patients investigated for UTI was 30%. In reality, the true incidence is unknown and lower because now there is greater awareness and diagnosis of UTIs in milder forms, resulting in a much greater incidence of UTI. On top of this, the indications for a micturating cystourethrogram are much more selective, meaning it would be impossible to accurately define the true incidence.

Occasionally, VUR comes to light during investigation of renal insufficiency and/or hypertension. Asymptomatic VUR tends to be diagnosed on investigation of antenatally detected urinary tract abnormalities or with screening of siblings.

Investigations

The aims of investigations are to

- Make diagnosis and assess severity of VUR
- Assess renal function

Imaging modalities used are as follows:

- **Ultrasonography:** This is good for assessment of upper tract dilatation, size of kidneys and evidence of renal damage. It also enables assessment of the bladder for causes of secondary VUR
- **Micturating cystourethrogram (MCUG):** This is the gold standard test for diagnosing VUR and provides most precise anatomical detail and allows grading of reflux. It is an invasive test and it is now used more selectively. It should not be performed when the patient has a UTI, and all patients should receive prophylactic antibiotic cover
- **MAG3 indirect cystogram (Mercaptoacetyltriglycine tagged with technetium 99m):** Indirect cystography gives poor anatomical detail and may

miss low-grade VUR. However, it uses substantially less radiation (10%) than a MCUG, and does not require the child to be catheterised. The MAG3 also provides information regarding differential renal function, but is less reliable for assessing obstruction because a diuretic is not given
- **DMSA scan (Dimercaptosuccinic acid tagged with technetium 99m):** This is used for the assessment of renal scarring and differential renal function

Based on the findings of MCUG, the International Classification System for VUR allows grading of VUR from grade I to V (**Figure 62**)
- Grade I – reflux into a non-dilated ureter
- Grade II – reflux into the renal pelvis and calyces without dilatation
- Grade III – reflux with mild-to-moderate dilatation and minimal blunting of fornices
- Grade IV – reflux with a moderately dilated tortuous ureter and dilatation of the pelvis and calyces
- Grade V – reflux with gross dilatation of the ureter, pelvis and calyces, loss of papillary impressions and a tortuous ureter

In general, low-grade reflux resolves spontaneously, whereas high grades of reflux do not resolve. The estimated spontaneous resolution rates of VUR by grade are
- Grade I – 83%
- Grade II – 60%
- Grade III – 46%
- Grade IV – 9%
- Grade V – 0%

Occasionally videourodynamic studies are required to define lower urinary tract dysfunction. This is important because antireflux surgery is less effective in patients with secondary reflux.

Differential diagnosis

- Vesicoureteric junction obstruction
- UTI
- Pelvi-ureteric junction obstruction
- Posterior urethral valves
- Voiding dysfunction

Treatment

The aims of treatment are to prevent the sequelae of pyelonephritis, renal

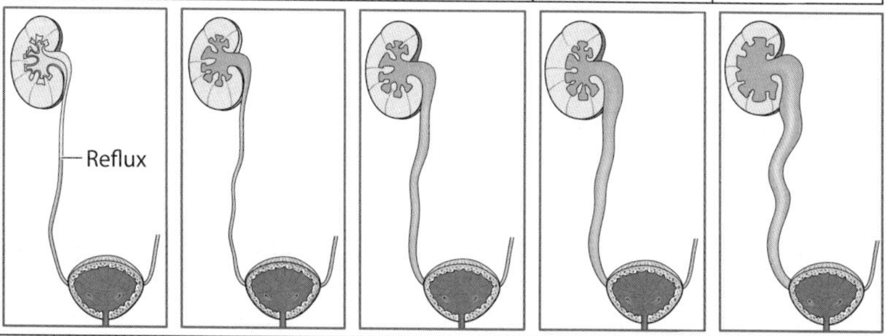

Grade:	I	II	III	IV	V
Reflux into:	Ureter	Ureter, renal pelvis and calyces	Ureter, renal pelvis and calyces	Ureter, renal pelvis and calyces	Ureter, renal pelvis and calyces
Dilatation of ureter, renal pelvis, calyces:	None	None	Present: mild-to-moderate with minimal blunting of calyceal fornices	Present, with ureteral tortuosity	Gross, with ureteral tortuosity and loss of papillary impressions

Figure 62 International Classification System for Vesicoureteral reflux.

scarring, hypertension and chronic renal insufficiency.

Treatment may be conservative or surgical. Conservative management consists of

- Prophylactic antibiotics (e.g. Trimethoprim 2 mg/kg PO nocte)
- Urine surveillance with urine dipsticks
- Management of underlying bladder dysfunction
- Management of constipation

Indications for surgical intervention are relative, rather than absolute. They include

- Failure of conservative management
- Anatomical – high-grade VUR that occurs in the presence of an anatomical abnormality (e.g. a paraureteric diverticulum)
- Parental preference

Options for surgical management include endoscopic correction by subureteric injection of an implant material. Common materials used include Teflon, dextranomer-hyaluronic acid copolymer (Deflux) and Macroplastique (PDMS)

Operative details

- **Endoscopic treatment:** Under general anaesthetic, rigid cystoscopy using a scope with a working channel (9–14 Fr) is performed. A needle is introduced under direct vision and advanced through mucosa under the UO. If the UO is open enough, an intraureteric injection is performed. The implant is then injected to create a 'volcanic' bulge, which makes the UO look like a nipple.
- This technique is most effective in patients with lower grades of reflux. Repeated injections may be required. Some authors report success in up to 93% of cases.
- **Circumcision:** This reduces risk of developing UTI in males younger than 1 year
- **Ureteric reimplantation:** A number of variations of this technique exist. Cross-trigonal (Cohen) technique remains most commonly used. Other options are Leadbetter–Politano with or without a psoas hitch and the Lich–Gregoir extravesical procedure
- **Cohen reimplantation:** Under general anaesthetic, the bladder is opened via a Pfannenstiel approach. The UO is identified and the intravesical ureter is mobilised. It may be necessary to plicate the ureter prior to reimplantation. A cross-trigonal submucosal tunnel is created. The tunnel should be at least three times the diameter of the ureter. The ureter is passed through the tunnel and reimplanted. The bladder is closed in layers and drained postoperatively. A ureteric stent may be used.
  - Nephroureterectomy (if function poor)
  - Transureteroureterostomy

Secondary VUR tends to resolve following management of the underlying bladder pathology.

Further reading

Coleman R. Early management and long-term outcomes in primary vesico-ureteric reflux. BJU Int 2011; 108:3–8.

Diamond DA, Mattoo TK. Endoscopic treatment of primary vesicoureteral reflux (review). N Engl J Med 2012; 366:1218–1226.

Puri P. Vesicoureteral reflux. In: Puri P, Hollwarth M (eds), Pediatric surgery: diagnosis and management. Springer, 2009:855–862.

Related topics of interest

Vesicoureteric junction obstruction

Learning outcomes

- To understand the development of the vesicoureteric junction (VUJ)
- To formulate a rational approach to investigation of the VUJ
- To be aware of the natural history of abnormalities of the VUJ
- To be able to discuss treatment options

Overview

Vesicoureteric junction obstruction (VUJO) is an unusual cause of hydroureteronephrosis. Investigation of VUJO is difficult due to the absence of a good specific test for obstruction at this level. There is a wide range of clinical significance of lesions of the VUJ, and a significant rate of spontaneous resolution of VUJO. The difficulty with this topic is deciphering the nomenclature that is used.

Epidemiology and aetiology

A megaureter is defined as a ureter that measures > 8 mm in diameter. Various classification systems exist. A megaureter can be described as primary or secondary. Another system defines megaureters as refluxing, obstructed, refluxing and obstructed, or non-refluxing and non-obstructed, with this latter category being the equivalent of a primary megaureter. Vesicoureteric reflux (VUR) is covered elsewhere.

Whilst symptomatic megaureters were historically a rarity, they account for up to a fifth of antenatally diagnosed renal tract dilatation. Ureters obstructed at the level of the bladder are frequently associated with an ureterocele. Other pathologies identified include stricture, adynamic segments, abnormal collagen deposition and abnormal neuromodulation.

Discussion of the embryology of the ureteric bud and the VUJ is covered elsewhere. In addition to VUR, VUJO at least in some cases is presumably a result of abnormal integration of the ureter into the trigone. Some instances of VUJ obstruction come to light in later childhood. There appears to be less spontaneous resolution in these cases, and this may result in an inherent abnormality in the wall of the ureter as we see with some non-resolving PUJ obstructions. The presence of a ureterocele can imply VUJO; however, it is possible to have a ureterocele without clinically relevant obstruction. Ureteroceles can exist in single and duplicated systems. Historically single-system orthotopic ureteroceles have been referred to as 'adult-type'; however, this is not a useful or reliable classification.

Clinical features

Due to the widespread use of antenatal scans, many dilated ureters are identified as asymptomatic findings. Others can be identified during childhood when ultrasound scanning (USS) is performed for investigation of abdominal pain, after urinary tract infection or any other reason. Pain solely due to VUJO is uncommon because it is usually a subtle pathology and the dilatation tends to be compensatory; however, it could be complicated by a calculus, or infection. Whilst there is no evidence that VUJO predisposes to infection, reports of greater morbidity associated with urinary tract infection in obstructed systems merit consideration of prophylaxis.

Investigations

The investigations used to establish other renal tract pathologies are also useful for VUJO, but must be interpreted with caution. Both VUR and VUJO can cause distal ureteric dilatation on USS. Investigations that look at drainage, such as nuclear renography and intravenous urography, will both show poor drainage through the VUJ when there is a full bladder; furthermore, when the bladder is full of contrast or isotope, it is difficult to visualise the VUJ. Therefore, it is important to consider a bladder catheter when performing these investigations with a differential diagnosis of VUJO. Nuclear renography is typically used to assess obstruction at the PUJ; it is also important to inform your nuclear physician of the differential diagnosis, so area of interest curves can be obtained for the ureter in addition to the renal pelvis and collecting system.

Differential diagnosis

As discussed previously, the differential diagnosis of a dilated ureter is between pathologies that cause VUR, obstruction or that of non-obstructed or non-refluxing primary megaureter.

As a general rule, in the renal tract, obstruction is the most important pathology to identify and treat. Obstruction can lead to progressive renal damage, and if complicated by infection this is more likely and the poor drainage can lead to a clinically serious course.

Treatment

The majority of megaureters do not require treatment. Spontaneous resolution and non-progression are common. Size > 10 mm and poor drainage on excretion renography are associated with eventual symptoms or loss of function, both of which would mandate repair.

When VUJO is associated with a ureterocele, the first step in treatment is endoscopic incision of the ureterocele. This can be achieved by a variety of techniques. A resectoscope can be employed with either a 'hot' or 'cold' knife (diathermy current through the cutting element), with the author preferring a cold-knife incision. If a resectoscope is unavailable or too large for the patient's urethra, a Bugbee electrode can be used to puncture the ureterocele. These are insulated flexible electrodes which can be obtained down to 3 French size, enabling use down the smallest of cystoscopes. The limitation is that they only create small punctures in the ureterocele,

and after the first puncture it can collapse, making it difficult to add additional drainage. The resectoscope with a curved blade by contrast allows the surgeon to create a generous incision along the ureterocele. Complications of this procedure include any general risks, with anaesthesia and cystoscopy. Specific to the incision itself, the risks are bleeding, creation of VUR, and if diathermy employed risks of damage to other structures. Surprisingly, even with the most generous incisions into a ureterocele, VUR is not inevitable. If its presence is suspected, a micturating cystourethrogram can be performed postoperatively, and if present can be managed as per the surgeon's usual practice.

When there is no ureterocele but other bladder pathology, contributing to dysfunction of the VUJ, this pathology should be treated.

There is growing interest around the use of medium-term double J stents for the management of VUJO. The rationale behind this treatment is that 3–6 months of stenting across the VUJ can act to dilate it so that there is long-term resolution. Whether this occurs or simply relieves the dilatation, while spontaneous resolution occurs through remodelling of the trigone, is a question that could only be addressed by a prospective randomised study.

If a stent is not considered appropriate or is unsuccessful, ureteric reimplantation is the definitive treatment. With the decreasing use of reimplantation in the management of VUR, VUJO has become the main indication for reimplantation at the author's institution. The surgeon should utilise the reimplantation method they are most familiar with, be that Cohen, Politano–Leadbetter or other. There are a few considerations; the first is that this pathology is usually unilateral. The second is that the ureter can be grossly dilated and may have to be tapered to effect a suitable reimplantation. Finally, because obstruction is an important complication of reimplantation, tunnel length and angle should be carefully assessed to ensure this does not occur; a technique like the Paquin can be utilised for this.

Further reading

Liu HY et al. Clinical outcome and management of prenatally diagnosed primary megaureters. J Urol 1994;152:614–617.

Carroll D, et al. Endoscopic placement of double-J ureteric stents in children as a treatment for primary obstructive megaureter. Urol Ann 2010; 2:114–118.

Dewan P. Ureteric reimplantation: a history of the development of surgical techniques. BJU Int 2000; 85:1000–1006.

Related topics of interest

Wilms' tumour

Learning outcomes

- To be able to diagnose Wilms' tumour
- To understand its epidemiology, aetiology and pathology
- To be familiar with the diagnostic modalities and chemotherapy protocols
- To be aware of the operative management options

Overview

Wilms' tumour (WT) or nephroblastoma is the most common renal tumour and the second most common abdominal malignancy in childhood. It frequently presents as an asymptomatic abdominal mass in children between 2 and 4 years of age. The overall survival rate is 85%, with low-stage tumours doing considerably better as a result of multidisciplinary treatment.

Three study groups have been instrumental in establishing the basis for current therapy:

1. The National Wilms' Tumour Study Group (NWTSG), now the Children's Oncology Group Renal Tumor Committee (COG RTC) in North America
2. The International Society of Paediatric Oncology (SIOP) in Europe
3. The United Kingdom Children's Cancer Study Group, now the Children's Cancer and Leukaemia Group

Immediate nephrectomy is the preferred approach of the NWTSG, whereas in continental Europe (SIOP), nephrectomy follows a short course of chemotherapy. The SIOP approach has the advantages of reducing operative tumour rupture and spillage and tends to downstage tumours. The NWTS group believes that the chemotherapy alters staging information and modifies tumour histology and biological information. In the UK, prior to 1991, an immediate nephrectomy approach was followed. The UKW3 trial, which randomised patients to either preoperative chemotherapy or immediate nephrectomy, demonstrated a significant downstaging of tumours, a reduction in the need for radiotherapy and fewer surgical complications in the preoperative chemotherapy group. As a result of this, the UK adopted the SIOP approach.

Epidemiology and aetiology

WT has an incidence of approximately 8 cases per million children, resulting in 80 new cases per year in the UK. There is no gender predilection, but there are racial variations. In the USA, there is a higher incidence in African-American children compared with Caucasian and Asian children. Bilateral tumours account for 4–5% of tumours, and there is a familial association in 2% in cases.

In 10% of cases, WT is associated with a congenital disorder, including syndromes such as Denys–Drash, Beckwith–Wiedemann, Simpson–Golabi–Behmel and WAGR (Wilms' tumour, aniridia, genitourinary anomalies, retardation). Children with these disorders are screened by regular examination and ultrasound (US) for the first 5–7 years of life. These congenital disorders are linked to specific genetic loci implicated in WT genesis. The Wilms' tumour-suppressor gene (*WT1*) is found on the short arm of chromosome 13 (13p), and a deletion of this area is found in WAGR and isolated aniridia. In Denys–Drash, there are point mutations of this area. No familial Wilms' patients have abnormalities of *WT1*, and therefore a second gene, *WT2*, was proposed. Beckwith–Wiedemann syndrome is associated with loss of heterozygosity (LOH) at chromosome 11p, and the *WT2* gene may be situated at this locus. Other genes implicated and associated with familial WT are the *WTX* gene on the X chromosome and the *FWT1* and *FWT2* genes on chromosomes 17q and 19q, respectively. These genetic abnormalities do not seem to have any prognostic significance, but LOH at 1p and 16q is currently being used by COG to upstage a group of favourable histology tumours to more intensive treatment.

WT is also associated with clusters of persistent metanephric blastemal cells, called nephrogenic rests or nephroblastomatosis. Nephroblastomatosis is found in 1% of kidneys at post mortem, but in 20–50% of WT specimens, suggesting it may be a precursor of WT and some other renal tumours.

WT is characteristically a triphasic embryonal neoplasm, with blastemal, stromal and epithelial components. Variations in these components define histologic subgroups associated with prognosis. Anaplasia and blastemal predominance are associated with a worse prognosis.

Clinical features

Presenting features are:
- Abdominal mass
- Haematuria
- Hypertension
- Abdominal pain
- Malaise
- Pulmonary metastases (~15% of cases)
- Involvement of renal vein, inferior vena cava (IVC involved in 8% of cases) or atrium

Investigations

The main purpose of investigations is confirmation of diagnosis and staging of tumours. In SIOP studies, the stage of a tumour is determined after preoperative chemotherapy and surgical excision, whereas a pretreatment surgical stage is used in North America. SIOP staging is as follows:
- Stage I: tumour limited to kidney; complete excision
- Stage II: tumour extends beyond kidney; complete excision
- Stage III: invasion beyond capsule; incomplete excision; tumour rupture
- Stage IV: distant metastases
- Stage V: bilateral renal involvement

Blood tests

- Full blood count
- Coagulation profile and von Willebrand factor assay (acquired von Willebrand disease is associated with WT)
- Urea and electrolytes
- Liver function tests

Urine tests

- Spot urinary catecholamine metabolites – vanillylmandelic acid and homovanillic acid to exclude Neuroblastoma

Abdominal ultrasonography

- To assess renal and venous involvement

Chest radiograph

- To look for pulmonary metastases

Cross-sectional imaging

- Contrast-enhanced CT scan to assess both abdominal (**Figure 63**) and pulmonary diseases
- MRI of the abdomen is replacing CT in some centres and is especially useful in assessing bilateral disease, vascular involvement and nephroblastomatosis

Biopsy

- Ultrasound-guided core biopsy to obtain histological diagnosis (UK only)

Differential diagnosis

- Neuroblastoma
- Other renal tumours such as mesoblastic nephroma, clear cell sarcoma, malignant rhabdoid tumour and renal cell carcinoma
- Benign renal cystic disease

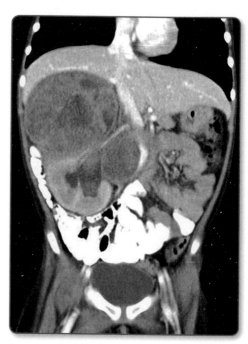

Figure 63 CT scan of the abdomen. Wilms' tumour arising from upper pole of right kidney. Large lymph node mass displacing IVC and aorta.

Treatment

All children older than 6 months with non-metastatic WT receive:

- 4 weeks of chemotherapy with vincristine and actinomycin D
- Radical nephroureterectomy:
  - Long transverse incision, with initial control of the vascular pedicle, outside Gerota's fascia
  - Lymph node sampling essential for staging information
  - If vascular extension or thrombus is present, it is important to remove the tumour thrombus, although this is not always possible
  - Complications of this procedure are tumour rupture, bleeding and late bowel obstruction

Postoperative chemotherapy and radiotherapy is then determined by histological stage.

- Children with metastatic disease (stage IV):
  - 6 weeks of vincristine, actinomycin D and doxorubicin
  - Radical nephroureterectomy
  - Pulmonary metastectomy approximately 2 weeks later, if feasible
- Children with bilateral disease (stage V):
  - 4 weekly cycles of vincristine and actinomycin D until there is maximal shrinkage of the tumour
  - Nephron sparing surgery (NSS), if possible

NSS for unilateral tumours is gaining in popularity in an attempt to reduce the long-term sequelae of nephrectomy, hypertension and renal failure. NSS has previously only been used for those congenital conditions that may predispose to metachronous tumours.

Laparoscopic nephroureterectomy is acceptable in WT, providing the tumour is small and central and oncological principles, including lymph node sampling, are maintained.

Further reading

Ahmed HU, Arya M, Tsiouris A, et al. An update on the management of Wilms' tumour. Eur J Surg Oncol 2007; 33: 824–831.

Ahmed HU, Arya M, Levitt G, et al. Part I: Primary malignant non-Wilms' renal tumours in children. Lancet Oncol 2007; 8:730–737.

Ehrlich PF. Wilms' tumor: Progress and considerations for the surgeon. Surg Oncol 2007; 16:157–171.

Ahmed HU, Arya M, Levitt G, et al. Part II: Treatment of primary malignant non-Wilms' renal tumours in children. Lancet Oncol 2007; 8:842–848.

Related topics of interest

Index

Note: Page numbers in **bold** or *italic* refer to tables or figures, respectively.